全国中医药行业高等教育“十三五”创新教材
National Innovative Textbook Of 13th Five~Year Plan For High Education Of Chinese Medicine Students

生理学（双语）
Physiology (bilingual)

（中医学、针灸推拿学、中西医临床医学、护理学等专业用）

主　编　高剑峰
Editor~in~Chief Jianfeng Gao

中国中医药出版社
National Press For Traditional Chinese Medicine
·北　京·
· beijing ·

图书在版编目（CIP）数据

生理学：双语：英、汉 / 高剑峰主编 . —北京：中国中医药出版社，2018.8
全国中医药行业高等教育“十三五”创新教材
ISBN 978 – 7 – 5132 – 4785 – 6

Ⅰ . ①生…　Ⅱ . ①高…　Ⅲ . ①人体生理学—高等学校—教材—英、汉　Ⅳ . ① R33

中国版本图书馆 CIP 数据核字（2018）第 034243 号

中国中医药出版社出版
北京市朝阳区北三环东路 28 号易亨大厦 16 层
邮政编码　100013
传真　010–64405750
河北省武强县画业有限责任公司印刷
各地新华书店经销

开本 787 × 1092　1/16　印张 22.5　字数 624 千字
2018 年 8 月第 1 版　2018 年 8 月第 1 次印刷
书号　ISBN 978 – 7 – 5132 – 4785 – 6

定价　128.00 元
网址　www.cptcm.com

社 长 热 线　010–64405720
购 书 热 线　010–89535836
维 权 打 假　010–64405753

微信服务号　zgzyycbs
微商城网址　https://kdt.im/LIdUGr
官 方 微 博　http://e.weibo.com/cptcm
天猫旗舰店网址　https://zgzyycbs.tmall.com

全国中医药行业高等教育“十三五”创新教材

《生理学》（双语）编委会

主　审　赵铁建（广西中医药大学）

主　编　高剑峰（河南中医药大学）

副主编　尤行宏（湖北中医药大学）
单德红（辽宁中医药大学）
张松江（河南中医药大学）
徐　颖（上海中医药大学）
谢海源（广西中医药大学）
韩　曼（陕西中医药大学）

编　委　（以姓氏笔画为序）
M.Azizul Haq（广西中医药大学）
王冰梅（长春中医药大学）
甘贤兵（安徽中医药大学）
刘海梅（广州中医药大学）
许　敬（南京中医药大学）
孙世晓（黑龙江中医药大学）
杜　联（成都中医药大学）
闵建新（江西中医药大学）
明海霞（甘肃中医药大学）
郭　健（北京中医药大学）
海青山（云南中医药大学）
谢佐福（福建中医药大学）
谭俊珍（天津中医药大学）

学术秘书　刘　永（河南中医药大学）

编写说明

随着近年教学改革及国际交流的不断深入开展，生理学双语教学越来越受到重视。为了适应新的形势和教学要求，我们有针对性地编写《生理学》（双语）教材作为“十三五”期间的创新教材。

《生理学》（双语）教材以器官系统为单位对人体生理学进行了系统的阐述。本教材共分十二章，第一章主要介绍生理学的基本概念与基本知识，第二章介绍细胞的基本功能，第三章介绍血液，其余章节分别介绍心血管系统、呼吸系统、消化系统、能量代谢与体温、泌尿系统、内分泌系统、生殖、神经系统和感觉器官。为方便教学和学习使用，本教材在每章均对一些重点和难点内容配以表格总结和图示。

本教材的特点是：①编排新颖，本书以全英正文为基础、配合以脚注的形式对重点和难点内容进行中文翻译。希望通过这种创新的教材编排形式，在不影响专业知识掌握的基础上，更好地培养学生专业英语的阅读和理解能力。②语言简洁，重点突出。为了克服学生有限的英语阅读能力对专业知识理解的限制，我们力求英文表达简洁明朗，专业内容介绍重点突出。规避了很多全英文教材甚至双语教材语言晦涩、内容繁杂的特点，确保学生不会因此失去进一步学习的兴趣和信心。本教材适合中医学、针灸推拿学、中西医临床医学、护理学及其他医药相关专业学生使用，也可为广大医学工作者参考利用。

本教材的编写得到了全国18所中医药院校的资深教师的大力支持和帮助，参加编写人员共21人，都是目前正在生理学教学第一线工作的教授、副教授和讲师。在编写过程中，编者对各自负责编写的章节内容都做了认真考虑，参考了国内外著名生理学教材的最新版本。为了确保语言表达的准确性，特邀请广西中医药大学基础医学院生理学教研室的外籍教师M.Azizul

Haq进行语言上的把关，在此一并表示衷心的感谢！由于编写时间仓促及编者水平有限，书中不免存在一些不当之处，敬请各位读者不吝指出，以备再版时更正。

《生理学》（双语）编委会

2018年5月

Catalog

Chapter 1 INTRODUCTION

Section 1 Content of physiology

The goal of physiology is to elucidate the physical, chemical and environmental factors that are involved in the origin, development, maintenance and progression of normal life. Each type of life, from the simple virus to the largest tree or the complicated human being, has its own sets of physical traits and functional characteristics. Therefore, the vast field of physiology can be divided into viral physiology, bacterial physiology, cellular physiology, plant physiology, human physiology, and many more subdivisions[1].

1 Research object and task of physiology

Human physiology is the branch of science that deals with the specific characteristics or phenomena and mechanisms of normal human life's functions as a single entity[2]. It concerns with complex processes that depend on the interplay of many widely separate organs in the body. The tasks of human physiology include revealing the functional mechanisms, functional relationships, functional regulation, functional origin and functional evolution of various organ tissues to their more complex adult forms, their adaptive change to the external environment, and their mutual coordination and reunification at the the integral level[3]. Thus, the intention of physiology is how each part of the body works together at various levels of organization as an integral organism.

Physiology is a very important basic medical course. Without the knowledge of physiology, doctors cannot determine the occurrence and development of disease. Similarly, clinical practices constantly propose new research directions and issues for the study of physiology. Physiology and clinical medicine are mutual promotion and common development. In recent years, with the development of modern science and technology, especially molecular biology

[1] 广义的生理学可以分为病毒生理学、细菌生理学、细胞生理学、植物生理学、人体生理学等。

[2] 生理学是研究正常人体生命活动特征和活动规律的科学。

[3] 生理学的任务就是探讨各种生理活动的发生原理、功能联系、调节机制、功能起源、功能演进，环境因素改变对机体功能的影响，以及整体状态下生理功能的相互协调与统一等。

techniques[1] are widely used in medical research, physiological research has been greatly improved and developed to sophisticated level. Many theories, such as cell cycle regulation, cell apoptosis, receptor physiology, ion channels, and transcription factors theories are proposed. Thus, Our understanding of physiological activities is gradually deepening.

2 Research methods

Experiments are the main research methods of physiology. Modern physiology is a subject which uses a large number of new methods to comprehensively and thoroughly reveal the laws and nature of life activities. Physiological experiments are the studies of the body, organs, tissues or cells. In human studies, the experiment must not endanger human health, so it is mainly observational studies, also known as non–invasive tests[2], such as temperature, blood pressure, electrocardiogram (ECG)[3] measurements or blood, urine test and so on. Intervention studies are mostly animal experiments; animal experiments can be divided into two types of acute and chronic experiments[4]. Acute experiment permits to observe some functions of organism (for instance, heart contraction) and register it during a short time. The acute experiment facilitates study of many functions of organism, though it suffers from grave shortcomings exerting the negative influence on the experimental animals' vital functions. The chronic experiments permit to study the functions of experimental animals during a long period of time, even for many months or years.

2.1 Acute experiment

Acute experiment is divided into two kinds of in vivo experiments[5] and in vitro experiments[6]. In vivo, experiment is to observe how the organ works when the organ is still in the natural state of the body, and how various factors will affect the organ. The advantage of the experiments in vivo is that the experimental conditions are easy to control, and the observation is more objective, such as the cardiac contraction and compensatory intermittent experiments[7].

In vitro, experiments are those experiments that remove the organs (such as heart, kid-

[1] 分子生物学技术。

[2] 无创性检测。

[3] 心电图。

[4] 急性实验和慢性实验。

[5] 在体实验。

[6] 离体实验。

[7] 期前收缩与代偿间歇。

ney), tissues or cells (such as myocardium,[1] smooth muscles, nerve stem cells[2]) by surgery, and place them in a suitable artificial environment for observation, then analyze the principle of their activities. The advantage of the experiments in vitro is that the effects of many unrelated factors are excluded, the experimental factors are simple and the results are easy to analyze.

2.2 Chronic experiments

Chronic experiments are usually carried out under sterile conditions, and exposure, destruction, removal or transplantation of certain organs by surgery, and. then observe the functional activity of the organ after surgery. For example, if the nerve is cut, it is the method of denervation[3] and the physiologist has an opportunity to study the changes in organs' activity when it is not controlled by the nervous system. An advantage of such an approach is the preservation of the natural relationship between the organs, thus experimental conditions are close to the normal state, and the experiment can be repeated many times.

3 Three levels of physiological studies

Physiology is an experimental science, the contents of which are based on observation and analysis of the human or animal. The human body consists of a variety of cells, tissues, organs and functional systems, which constitute a unified whole. In order to investigate the processes of life activities, regularities and principles, physiology research is divided into three levels: the integral level, organ and system level, cell and molecular level[4].

3.1 The integral level

In this level it studies people or animals as a whole object. It studies the function of the whole body, the interaction of our bodies with the external world, and the influence of the environmental and social factors on human body. For example, the temperature regulation. Those body's various physiological parameters are determined by a large number of human investigations and measurements.

3.2 The organ and system level

In this level it tries to understand the rules and principles of activity of an organ or a functional system, as well as their status and role in the overall activities. The main subject is the mechanics of activities of organs and systems. Such as food is digested and absorbed in the

[1] 心肌细胞。

[2] 神经干细胞。

[3] 去神经支配。

[4] 整体水平、器官系统水平、细胞分子水平。

gastrointestinal tract[1], as well as their neuro–regulation and humoral–regulation.

3.3 The cell and molecular level

The individual cell is the basic unit of the structure and function of the human body. The individual human body consists of great numbers of these cells working together as a total organism. The basic functional medium of the human body is the chemical molecules. The various functional activities of the body are ultimately embodied in the physical changes and chemical reactions in the cell. Such as the secretion of glandular cells[2], the biological activity of nerve cells and muscle cell contraction. The research results in the cell and molecular level are important to reveal the nature of life. The structure and interaction of the molecules of the body are one of the most exciting areas in biology today. With the development of molecular biology, the nature of human activities has entered the molecular level. Physiology research area also reaches out to a variety of molecules that makes up cells, especially the physical and chemical properties and functions of biological macromolecules (nucleic acids and proteins), such as the contraction of muscle cells is formed by changing the arrangement of special protein molecules, physiological characteristics and cardiac cycle activity of cardiac myocytes are determined by their electrophysiological characteristics[3].

Three levels of research are artificially differentiated from the research content, which is an integral part of human understanding of life phenomena. The integral functional activity is the result of harmonization under the overall conditions. Activities of cells and organs are not independently carried out, but interrelated and harmonized. Each experiment result must be comprehensive and objectively evaluated to arrive in line with the objective and practical conclusions.

Section 2 The shared basic characteristics of all life's activities

An object that consists of biological macromolecules such as proteins is called an organism. It includes simple organisms (single cell organisms), higher organisms and the human body. Each organism can carry out a variety of life activities with different characteristics, but the most basic life activities are metabolism, excitability, adaptability and reproduction.[4]

[1] 胃肠道。

[2] 腺细胞。

[3] 电生理特性。

[4] 每个生物体都可以进行各自具有不同特点的多种生命活动，但最基本的生命活动特征是新陈代谢、兴奋性、适应性与生殖。

1 Metabolism

The metabolism of the body means simply all the chemical reactions in all the cells of the body, which make it possible for the cells to continue living. Metabolism is the life phenomenon of material metabolism and energy metabolism with the external environment. It includes all the material and energy changes that occur in the body. All the changes fall into two categories: catabolic and anabolic reactions[1]. Catabolic reactions involve the breakdown of the components of the body, the larger molecules into smaller molecules, during which energy is released from the activity of the body. Anabolic reactions are processes that simple molecules in the body to synthesize macromolecular substances. Anabolism and catabolism are two mutually opposing and unified processes of material metabolism. All kinds of life activities are completed in the material exchange and energy conversion with the external environment constantly. Once the metabolism stops, life will end.

2 Excitability

The environment in which the body is located is constantly changing. Changes in the external or internal environment can induce changes in the activity of a living organism, in other words, environmental stimuli can elicit response of the tissues of the body. A change in the living environment that can be felt is called stimulation[2]. Such as electricity, temperature, pressure, chemical stimulation and so on. The change of internal metabolic process or external activity caused by stimulation is called response[3]. The response can be classified into two types: excitatory response or excitation[4], and inhibitory response or inhibition[5]. Excitation signifies an increase in activity, such as secretion of gland, nerve impulses of neurons. Since these different changes are all preceded by bioelectric changes, that is, action potential[6] (AP), action potential appears simultaneously with the conduction of excitation along the nerve fiber, and always precedes the contraction of a muscle, thereby the action potential is usually considered to be an objective indicator of excitement[7]. Nerve, muscle and glandular cells are excitable cells[8].Inhibition, on the contrary, is a decrease in activity, such as the decrease in blood

[1] 分解代谢和合成代谢。

[2] 刺激。

[3] 反应。

[4] 兴奋。

[5] 抑制。

[6] 动作电位。

[7] 动作电位通常被认为是发生兴奋的客观指标。

[8] 可兴奋细胞。

pressure. The property of living organisms that permits them to react to stimuli is defined as excitability. This is a fundamental property common to all tissues and cells.

Metabolism is the basis of excitability. Once the metabolism stops, excitement will disappear, the body will not make any response to the stimulus. Therefore, excitability is the basis of the interdependence between stimuli and reactions, and is a necessary condition for the survival of the body. The excitability of different tissues was different, such as nerve cell excitability is higher than muscle cell's. Even the same kind of cells, in different conditions, its excitability will also change accordingly.

3 Adaptability

The term adaptation denotes a characteristic that favors survival in specific environments. The precise anatomical and physiological changes that bring about increased capacity to withstand change during adaptation are highly varied. They involve the changes in the number, size, or sensitivity of one or more of the cell types that mediate the basic response. Adaptability is the gradual development and improvement of the process of biological evolution to be fitter with better survival power. Human beings are not only able to adapt themselves to the environment they live in, but also take the initiative to use the achievements of science and technology to transform the natural environment in order to achieve the purpose of active adaptation to the environment.

4 Reproduction

Reproduction means generating new beings to take the place of those that are dying. It helps maintain the automaticity and continuity of life. This perhaps sounds like a permissive usage of the term homeostasis, but it does illustrate that, in the final analysis, essentially all body structures are organized such that they help maintain the automaticity and continuity of life. If the reproductive function is lost, the germline cannot be extended, the species will be eliminated, so the reproduction is also one of the characteristics of life activities.

Section 3 Internal environment and homeostasis

1 Body fluid and internal environment

Body fluid[1] is the fluid in the body which composed of water as the universal solvent for ions and other biological substances essential to living organisms, for instance, CSF(Cerebrospinal fluid) (Figure1-1).Approximately 60 percent of the adult human body is fluid. Water is

[1] 体液。

present within and around the cells of the body, and within all the blood vessels. Two–thirds of this fluid are inside the cells and is called intracellular fluid [1]. The remaining one–third of the fluid present in blood and in the spaces surrounding cells is called extracellular fluid [2]. Three quarters of this extracellular fluid is interstitial fluid [3], and the other is plasma. This extracellular fluid is in constant motion throughout the body. It is transported rapidly in the circulating blood and then mixed between the blood and the tissue fluids by diffusion through the capillary walls.

The extracellular fluids are the ions and nutrients needed by the cells for maintenance of cellular life. Therefore, all cells live in essentially the same environment––the extracellular fluid. For this reason the extracellular fluid is called the internal environment [4] of the body. Cells are capable of living, growing, and performing their special functions because several conditions in the internal environment must be maintained within narrow limits. Thus stability of the internal environment is the primary condition for a free and independent existence.

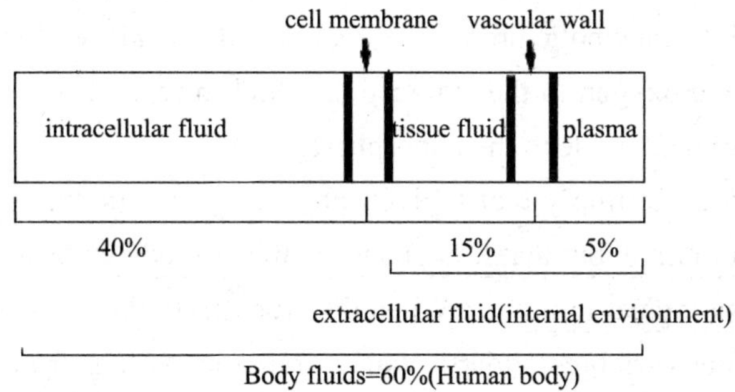

Figure 1–1 Figure of body fluid distribution

Compartmentalization is achieved by barriers between the compartments. The properties of the barriers determine which substances can move between contiguous compartments. These movements, in turn, account for the differences in composition of the different compartments. In the case of the body fluid compartments, the intracellular fluid is separated from the extracellular fluid by membranes that surround the cells. In contrast, the two components of extracellular fluid are separated by the cellular wall of the smallest blood vessels, the capillaries.

As the blood flows through blood vessels in all parts of the body, the plasma exchanges nutrients, oxygen, and metabolic products with the interstitial fluid. Because of these exchanges, concentrations of dissolved substances are identical in the plasma and interstitial fluid,

[1] 细胞内液。

[2] 细胞外液。

[3] 组织液。

[4] 内环境。

except for protein concentration. In contrast, the composition of the extracellular fluid is very different from that of the intracellular fluid. The extracellular fluid contains large amounts of sodium, chloride, and bicarbonate ions and nutrients for the cells, such as glucose, fatty acids, amino acids, proteins and oxygen. It also contains carbon dioxide and other cellular waste products to be excreted. The intracellular fluid contains large amounts of potassium, magnesium, and phosphate ions instead of the sodium and chloride ions found in the extracellular fluid.

2 Homeostasis

The key to maintaining stability of the internal environment is the presence of regulatory mechanisms in the body. Homeostasis[1] was introduced as a concept describing this capacity for self-regulation. It is used to mean the maintenance of nearly steady states in the internal environment by coordinating physiological mechanisms. Essentially all organs and tissues of the body perform functions that help maintain these relatively steady states. For instance, the kidney can discharge the metabolic products to maintain the stability of various ion concentrations, the lungs provide oxygen to the extracellular fluid to replenish the oxygen used by the cells and carry the carbon dioxide to the atmosphere.

Homeostasis does not imply that a given physiological function or variable is rigidly constant with respect to time, but that it fluctuates within a predictable and often narrow range within a normal physiological limits[2]. When disturbed from the normal range, it is restored toward baseline. Some variables undergo fairly dramatic swings around an average value during the course of a day, yet may still be considered in balance. That is because homeostasis is a dynamic, not a static process. For example, if blood glucose concentration is too low, the hormone glucagon[3], from the alpha cells of the pancreas, and epinephrine[4], from the adrenal medulla, will increase it. If blood glucose concentration is too high, insulin[5] from the beta cells of the pancreas will lower it by enhancing the cellular uptake, storage, and metabolism of glucose. Behavioral responses also contribute to the maintenance of homeostasis. For example, a low blood glucose concentration will make people feel hungry and drive him to seek food.

The concept of homeostasis is helpful in understanding and analyzing conditions in the body. In general, if all the major organ systems are operating in a homeostatic manner, a person

---

[1] 稳态。

[2] 稳态并不是一成不变的，而是指各种生理功能相对的、动态的稳定，各项生理指标维持在一个正常的生理范围内波动。

[3] 胰高血糖素。

[4] 肾上腺素。

[5] 胰岛素。

is in good health. Certain kinds of disease, in fact, can be defined as the loss of homeostasis in one or more systems in the body. Homeostatic regulation of a physiological variable often involves several cooperating mechanisms activated at the same time or in succession. The more important a variable, the more numerous and complicated are the mechanisms that keep it at the desired value.

Section 4 The regulation mechanism of body's physiological function

The environment where we lived is ever–changing, and the functional state of the body is varied too. However, a normal body is a rounded system that all of organs constitute a complete, coordinated and unified entirety. The integrity of the body can be expressed as the harmonization of the composition of the body and the unity of body and environment. However, the function of the human body and living conditions of the environment are constantly changing. Therefore, the coordination of the human body and the environment are destroyed at any time. In order to enable life activities to proceed normally, the human body must constantly adjust the function of the various parts of the body, So that they cooperate with each other and maintain stability of the body. The human body detects the internal and external environment changes, adjusts various functional activities accordingly, maintains a steady state by coordinating all organs with each other, and acclimates itself to the changes in the environment, so this functional activity is called regulation. There are three main ways of regulation: neuroregulation, humoral regulation and autoregulation [1].

1 Neuroregulation

Many of the body's homeostatic control systems belong to the general category of stimulus–response sequences known as reflexes. Neuroregulation is the fastest controller to act and adapt to changes between external and internal environment. It is achieved by the reflex activity. A reflex [2] is a specific involuntary, unpremeditated response to a particular stimulus. The knee jerk [3] is an example of the simplest type of reflex. When the knee is tapped, the nerve that receives this stimulus sends an impulse to the spinal cord, where it is relayed to a motor nerve. This causes the quadriceps muscle [4] at the front of the thigh to contract and jerk the leg up. The leg begins to jerk up while the brain is just becoming aware of the tap.

---

[1] 调节方式主要有神经调节、体液调节及自身调节三种。

[2] 反射。

[3] 膝跳反射。

[4] 股四头肌。

Reflection is different from the simple response of an ordinary cell, tissue, or organ to the stimulus; it is an advanced, adaptive response. The reflex activity must be completed by the reflex arc[1]. The reflex arc is the route followed by nerve impulses in the production of a reflex act, from the peripheral receptor organ through the afferent nerve to the central nervous system synapse and then through the efferent nerve to the effector organ. Thus the reflex arc includes five components: receptors, the afferent nerve, an integrating center, the efferent nerve, and effectors[2](Figure 1–2). The integrity of the reflex arc is a necessary condition for the reflection activity, if any of these parts be damaged or defective, the reflex activities will disappear.

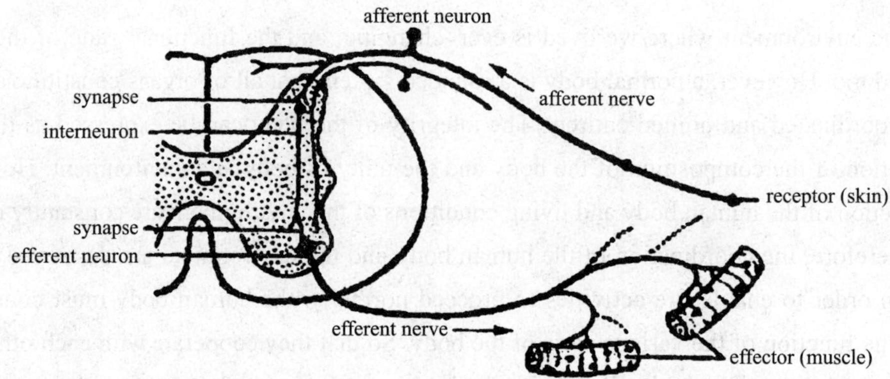

Figure 1–2 Reflex arc pattern

Humans have many kinds of reflex, which can be roughly divided into two categories, namely the unconditioned reflex[3] and the conditioned reflex[4]. An unconditioned response is the unlearned response that occurs naturally in reaction to the unconditioned stimulus. Such as sucking reflex, swallowing reflex, pupillary light reflex, flexion reflex. The best–known and most thorough early work on classical conditioned reflex was done by Ivan Pavlov. Classical conditioned reflex occurs when a conditioned stimulus is paired with an unconditioned stimulus. Usually, the conditioned stimulus is a neutral stimulus, the unconditioned stimulus is biologically potent and the unconditioned response to the unconditioned stimulus is an unlearned reflex response. After pairing is repeated, the organism exhibits a conditioned response to the conditioned stimulus when the conditioned stimulus is presented alone. The conditioned response is usually similar to the unconditioned response, but unlike the unconditioned response, it must be acquired through experience and is relatively impermanent. The advantage of condi-

[1] 反射弧。

[2] 反射弧包括五个成分：感受器、传入神经、中枢、传出神经和效应器。

[3] 非条件反射。

[4] 条件反射。

tional reflex is that it can make a large number of irrelevant stimuli become some kind of environmental changes in the upcoming signal, so that the body can adjust the relevant functional activities in advance. Therefore, the conditional reflex has greater predictability, adaptability, flexibility, greatly improving the body's ability to adapt to the environment. The nervous system provides for rapid communication between body parts, with conduction times measured in milliseconds.

In conclusion, the nervous regulation is characterized by rapid response, precise, limited and transient[1]. Many reflexes function in a homeostatic manner to keep a physical or chemical variable of the body relatively constant.

2 Humoral regulation

In addition to reflexes, another group of biological responses, called humoral regulation responses, is of great importance for homeostasis. Humoral regulation concerned with the description and characterization of processes involved in the regulation and integration of cells and organ systems by a group of specialized chemical substances called hormones[2]. It is the slower than neural regulation. However, its the more stable controller in maintaining long term healthy life. Hormones serve as regulators and coordinators of various biological functions in the animals, and they are chemical substances that secreted by endocrine glands located in the body. Hormones are transported in the extracellular fluid to all parts of the body to help regulate cellular function. The humoral regulation is a system of regulation that complements the nervous system. The nervous system regulates mainly muscular and secretory activities of the body, whereas the hormonal system regulates many metabolic functions. There are three categories of hormones: endocrine, paracrine and autocrine agents[3].

2.1 Endocrine agents

A hormone functions as a chemical messenger that enables the hormone–secreting cell to communicate with cells acted upon by the hormone—its target cells—with the blood acting as the delivery system. These endocrine hormones are carried by the circulatory system to tissues and cells throughout the body, where they bind with receptors and initiate many reactions. Some endocrine hormones influence many different types of cells; for example, growth hormone causes growth in most parts of the body, and insulin (from the pancreas) increases the

[1] 神经调节的特点是反应迅速、精确，作用局限而短暂。

[2] 激素。

[3] 激素可分为三种类型：远距离分泌激素、旁分泌激素和自分泌激素。

rate of glucose uptake in almost all the body's cells. Other hormones affect only specific target tissues, because only these tissues have receptors for the hormone. For example, calcitonin[1] from the thyroid C cells specifically stimulates the osteoblast[2] to promote bone formation, and the adrenocorticotropic hormone (ACTH) from the anterior pituitary gland specifically stimulates the adrenal cortex, causing it to secrete adrenocortical hormones.

2.2 Paracrine agents

Chemical messengers involved in local communication between cells are known as paracrine agents. Paracrine agents are synthesized by cells and released, once given the appropriate stimulus, into the extracellular fluid. They then diffuse to neighboring cells, some of which are their target cells. For example IL–2.

2.3 Autocrine agents

There is one category of local chemical messengers that are not intercellular messengers——that is, they do not communicate between cells. Rather, the chemical is secreted by a cell into the extracellular fluid and then acts upon the very cell that secreted it. Such messengers are termed autocrine agents. Frequently a messenger may serve both paracrine and autocrine functions simultaneously——that is, molecules of the messenger released by a cell may act locally on adjacent cells as well as on the same cell that released the messenger.

The humoral regulation provides for slower and more diffuse communication. The hormonal system produces hormones in response to a variety of stimuli. In contrast to the effects of nervous system stimulation, responses to hormones are much slower (seconds to hours) in onset, and the effects often last longer. Hormones are carried to all parts of the body by the bloodstream. A particular cell can respond to a hormone only if it possesses the specific receptor for the hormone. Hormonal effects may be discrete. Hormones play a critical role in controlling such body functions as growth, metabolism, and reproduction.

3 Autoregulation

Autoregulation is that some organizations or organs do not rely on neuroregulation or humoral regulation, while when the internal or external environment changed, they can make some adaptive response by themselves. For example, in an in vitro artificial perfusion cardiac experiment, we can be observed that in a certain range, when the perfusion fluid is increased,

[1] 降钙素。

[2] 成骨细胞。

the cardiac contractility is strengthened, and the perfusion fluid discharged from the ventricle is correspondingly increased, so that the cardiac output and the input quantity are kept relatively balanced.

The range of autoregulation is limited, and the sensitivity of the stimulus is low. It is an auxiliary way to regulate the body in addition to two vital regulators discussed above.

Section 5 Automatic control principle of the body function

Cybernetics [1] is the theory of information exchange and control processes. According to this theory, an organized system is continuously controlled and adjusted according to the changes of internal and external conditions, so as to overcome the inaccuracy of the system and make the system reach a certain state for the optimum functions. When applying the principle of cybernetics to the analysis of the regulation of the function of the human body, it is found that there are many kinds of automatic control systems in the human body. The control system can be divided into two types: feedback control system and feedforward control system [2].

Each control system is a closed loop system, composed of the controller part [3] and the controlled part[4]. There is a two-way association between the controller part (the central or endocrine gland) and the controlled part (effector, target organ or target cell). That is, the control part has control information (adjustment information) to reach the controlled part, while the controlled part will continue to have feedback information back to the control part. The process of sending information back to the control part from the controlled part is called feedback [5]. In the control system, the form of transmission of information can be different, but mainly are electrical signals (nerve impulses) and chemical signals (hormones or bioactive substances).

Therefore, the coordination of body movements and the regulation of homeostasis, in addition to the fundamentals of the neural–, humoral– and auto– regulations, also requires feedback information to modify and adjust the contrl's output singnals in order to achieve a more precise regulations.

---

[1] 控制论。

[2] 控制系统可分为反馈控制系统和前馈控制系统。

[3] 控制器部分。

[4] 控制部分。

[5] 反馈。

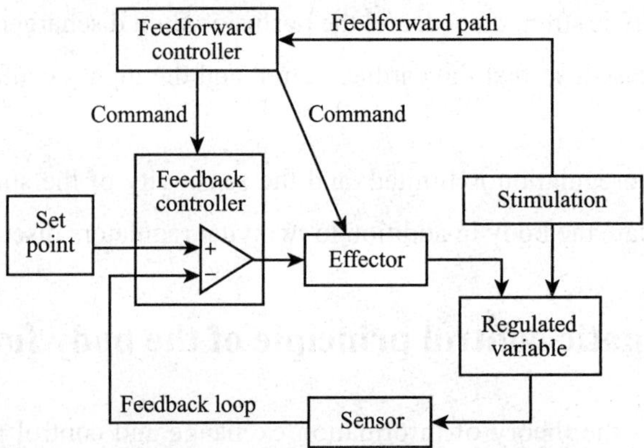

Figure 1–3 Feedback control system pattern

1 Feedback

Feedback, a term borrowed from engineering, is a fundamental feature of homeostasis. Without feedback, oscillations like some of those examples described in this Section would be much greater (i.e., the variability in a given system would increase). In simpler terms, it's the relationship between the inputs and outputs in a closed loop system of response.

Feedback also prevents the compensatory responses to a loss of homeostasis from continuing unabated. For example, one major compensatory response that is common to a loss of homeostasis in many variables is a rise in the blood level of a hormone called cortisol. Cortisol, which is produced in the adrenal glands, is normally secreted into the blood whenever the body is placed under physiological stress. The effects of cortisol are widespread, encompassing metabolic, cardiovascular, respiratory, renal, and immune activities. These actions tend to restore homeostasis (e. g., help restore blood glucose levels if glucose falls below normal). Although vital and often life–saving, too much cortisol can be dangerous. Prolonged exposure to cortisol may produce a variety of problems; in the previous example, too much cortisol would cause blood glucose levels to rise above the normal range. Thus, it is crucial that once cortisol has done its job, it is removed from the circulation and returned to normal levels. This is accomplished by the process of negative feedback inhibition. In this case, cortisol inhibits the production of those blood–borne signals that stimulate the production of cortisol in the first place.

Feedback can occur at multiple levels of organization, and it can be either negative or positive, with the former by far the more common.

1.1 Negative feedback [1]

This mechanism allows the effectors to oppose any deviation from the normal set

[1] 负反馈。

points-baseline ranges of any parameters. It brings back the status quo in our body system.

With negative feedback, the regulated variable is sensed, and information about its level is fed back to a feedback controller, which compares it to a desired value. If there is a difference, an error signal is generated, which drives the effectors to bring the regulated variable closer to the desired value. The thermoregulatory system is an example of a negative feedback system, in which an increase or decrease in the variable being regulated brings about responses that tend to move the variable in the direction opposite ("negative") to the direction of the original change. Thus, a decrease in body temperature leads to responses that tend to increase the body temperature—that is, move it toward its original value. The negative feedback control system is the most common in the body. As it has a two-way effect of strengthening or weakening, its important role is to maintain the body homeostasis in the opposite direction to the stimulus.

1.2 Positive feedback [1]

This mechanism allows the effectors to deviate from the normal set points-baseline ranges of any parameters. It destabilizes the status quo of the homeostasis for the better or worse!

Not all forms of feedback are negative, however, in some cases, positive feedback may actually accelerate a process, leading to an "explosive" system. In other words, the initiating stimulus causes more of the same, which is a positive feedback. Positive feedback is less common in nature than negative feedback. Though positive feedback is better known as a "vicious cycle [2]", in some instances, the body uses positive feedback to its advantage. One well-described example is the process of parturition. As the uterine muscles contract and its walls are stretched during labor, signals from the uterus are relayed via nerves to a gland at the base of the brain called the posterior pituitary gland. This gland responds by secreting the hormone oxytocin, which is a potent stimulator of further uterine contractions. As the uterus contracts ever harder in response to oxytocin, more stretch occurs in the walls of the uterus, and more signals are sent to the pituitary, resulting in yet more oxytocin secretion. This self-perpetuating cycle continues until finally the baby is born.

Another example of positive feedback is calcium-induced calcium release, which occurs with each heartbeat. Depolarization of the cardiac muscle plasma membrane leads to a small influx of calcium through membrane calcium channels. This leads to an explosive release of calcium from the muscle's sarcoplasmic reticulum[3], which rapidly increases the cytosolic calcium level and activates the contractile machinery.

Positive feedback refers to the feedback from the controlled part will promote or strength-

[1] 正反馈。

[2] 恶性循环。

[3] 肌浆网（终池）。

en the activities of the control part. Therefore, the control information and feedback information repeated exchanges, so that the activities of the controlled part are gradually strengthened until the completion of all activities. It can be seen that the effect of positive feedback is not to maintain the homeostasis, but to make the whole control system in a state of constant repetition and strengthening, and totally to complete a physiological activity.

2 Feedforward [1]

Another type of regulatory process often used in conjunction with feedback systems is feedforward. Feedforward control is another strategy for regulating systems in the body, particularly when a change with time is desired. In this case, a command signal is generated, which specifies the target or goal. The moment–to–moment operation of the controller is "open loop"; that is, the regulated variable itself is not sensed. Feedforward control mechanisms often sense a disturbance and can, therefore, take corrective action that anticipates change. For example, the smell of food triggers nerve responses from smell receptors in the nose to the cells of the gastrointestinal system. This prepares the stomach and intestines for the process of digestion. Thus, the stomach begins to churn and produce acid even before we actually consume any food. Thus, feedforward regulation anticipates changes in regulated variables such as internal body temperature or fuel availability, improves the speed of the body's homeostatic responses, and minimizes fluctuations in the level of the variable being regulated—that is, it reduces the amount of deviation from the set point. Another example is heart rate and breathing increase even before a person has begun to exercise.

In these examples, feedforward control utilizes a set of external or internal environmental detectors. It is likely, however, that many examples of feedforward control are the result of a different phenomenon—learning. The first time they occur, early in life, perturbations in the external environment probably cause relatively large changes in regulating internal environmental factors, and in responding to these changes in the central nervous system learns to anticipate them and resist them more effectively. The role of the feedforward control system is to pre–monitor the interference, to prevent interference disturbances, or advanced insight into the cause, to make adaptive responses in a timely manner. However, the reaction caused by feedforward control may be faulty. For example, if the animal seeing food but it did not eat the food, the secretion of saliva is a kind of mistake. The feedforward control system is more predictable than the negative feedback control system. It can make an adaptive response in advance, preventing interference and closed loop system namely negative feedback acts as a complimentary to precise the feedforward actions.

---

[1] 前馈。

Chapter 2 BASIC FUNCTIONS OF CELLS

Section 1 The basic structure of cell membrane and transmembrane transport

The basic living unit of the body is the cell and each organ is actually all aggregation of many different cells held together by intercellular supporting structures. Although different cell has different shape and functions, most cells have common characters in shape and function, such as the transportation of cell membrane and excitability[1].

The cells are separated from the surrounding fluids by the cell membrane. Transport across cell membranes is accomplished primarily by movement through ion channels, primary and secondary active transport, exocytosis and endocytosis[2]. The method of substances across cell membrane depends on the characteristics of the substances themselves and the membrane structure.

1 Membrane structure and chemical composition

The cell membrane, which envelops the cell, is a thin, pliable, elastic structure only 7.5 to 10 nanometers thick. It is composed almost entirely of proteins and lipids. The approximate composition is proteins, 55%; phospholipids, 25%; cholesterol, 13 per cent; other lipids, 4 per cent; and carbohydrates, 3 per cent (Figure 2–1).

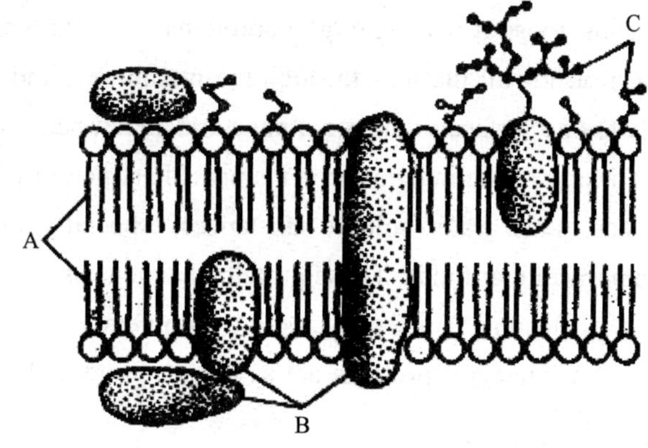

A: lipid bilayer B: membrane protein C: carbohydrate chain

Figure 2–1 The cell membrane

[1] 兴奋性。

[2] 离子通道，原发和继发性主动转运及出胞和入胞。

1.1 The lipid bilayer

The cellular basic structure is a lipid bilayer[1], which is a thin, double-layered film of lipids-each layer only one molecule thick that is continuous over the entire cell surface. The basic lipid bilayer is composed of phospholipid[2] molecules. One end of each phospholipid molecule is soluble in water. The other end is soluble only in fats. The phosphate end of the phospholipid is hydrophilic[3], and the fatty acid portion is hydrophobic[4]. Because the hydrophobic portions of the phospholipid molecules are repelled by water but are mutually attracted to one another, they have a natural tendency to attach to one another in the middle of the membrane, as shown in Figure 2-1. The hydrophilic phosphate portions then constitute the two surfaces of the complete cell membrane, in contact with intracellular water on the inside of the membrane and extracellular water on the outside surface.

The lipid layer in the middle of the membrane is impermeable to the usual water-soluble substances, such as ions, glucose, and urea. Conversely, fat-soluble substances, such as oxygen, carbon dioxide, and alcohol, can penetrate this portion of the membrane with ease. The cholesterol molecules in the membrane are also lipid in nature because their steroid nucleus is highly fat-soluble. These molecules, in a sense, are dissolved in the bilayer of the membrane. They mainly help determine the degree of permeability (or impermeability) of the bilayer to water-soluble constituents of body fluids. Cholesterol controls much of the fluidity of the membrane as well.

1.2 Cell membrane proteins

Figure 2-1 also shows globular masses floating in the lipid bilayer. These are membrane proteins, most of which are glycoproteins[5]. Two types of protein occur: ① integral proteins that protrude all the way through the membrane, and ② peripheral proteins that are attached only to one surface of the membrane and do not penetrate all the way through.

Many of the integral proteins provide structural channels (or pores) through which water molecules and water-soluble substances, especially ions, can diffuse between the extracellular and intracellular fluids. These protein channels also have selective properties that allow preferential diffusion of some substances over others.

Other integral proteins act as carrier proteins for transporting substances that otherwise

[1] 脂质双分子层。

[2] 磷脂。

[3] 亲水的。

[4] 疏水的。

[5] 糖蛋白。

could not penetrate the lipid bilayer. Sometimes these even transport substances in the direction opposite to their natural direction of diffusion, which is called "active transport."

Integral membrane proteins can also serve as receptors for water–soluble chemicals, provide a means of conveying information about the environment to the cell interior. Peripheral protein molecules are often attached to the integral proteins. These peripheral proteins function almost entirely as enzymes or as controllers of transport of substances through the cell membrane "pores."

1.3 Membrane carbohydrates – the cell "glycocalyx"

Membrane carbohydrates occur almost invariably in combination with proteins or lipids in the form of glycoproteins or glycolipids[1]. In fact, most of the integral proteins are glycoproteins, and about one tenth of the membrane lipid molecules are glycolipids. The "glyco" portions of these molecules almost invariably protrude to the outside of the cell, dangling outward from the cell surface. Many other carbohydrate compounds, called proteoglycans – which are mainly carbohydrate substances bound to small protein cores – are loosely attached to the outer surface of the cell as well. Thus, the entire outside surface of the cell often has a loose carbohydrate coat called the glycocalyx.

The carbohydrate moieties attached to the outer surface of the cell have several important functions: ① Many of them have a negative electrical charge, which gives most cells an overall negative surface charge that repels other negative objects. ② The glycocalyx of some cells attaches to the glycocalyx of other cells, thus attaching cells to one another. ③ Many of the carbohydrates act as receptor substances for binding hormones, such as insulin; when bound, this combination activates attached internal proteins that, in turn, activate a cascade of intracellular enzymes. ④ Some carbohydrate moieties enter into immune reactions.

2 Membrane transport

It is one of the basic process of the cell through which metabolite of the cell can leave the cell and nutritional substance can enter the cell through this process. Ion concentration can keep the stable difference between intra– and extracellular fluid. Different substances are transported through the cell membrane by different processes. It includes passive, active transport, and exocytosis and endocytosis.

2.1 Passive transport

Diffusion is the process by which a gas or a substance moving from low concentration area to high concentration area. The diffusing rate is directly proportionate to the diffusing area

---

[1] 糖脂。

and the concentration gradient, or chemical gradient, which is the difference in concentration of the diffusing substance. And also, the conductance of an ion, a measure of the membrane permeability to that ion, is an important factor influencing diffusion. There are two kinds of passive transport, simple diffusion[1] and facilitated diffusion[2].

2.1.1 Simple diffusion Substances that are soluble in lipids such as oxygen, carbon dioxide, alcohol, etc, can dissolve in the cell membrane and diffuse across it from areas of high concentration to areas of low concentration. Only lipid soluble substance can do like this.

2.1.2 Facilitated diffusion Some substances which are insoluble in lipids, such as Na^+, K^+, glucose, amino acids, pass through the cell membrane by facilitated diffusion. Substances are transported in the direction of their chemical and/or electrical gradients (electrochemical gradient[3]), and no energy input is required. There are two kinds of facilitated diffusion according to the different membrane proteins involved: channel mediated diffusion and carrier mediated diffusion.

In the channel mediated diffusion, the relative transport proteins are simple aqueous ion channels. Some of these are continuously open, whereas others are gated; i.e., they have gates that open or close. Some are gated by alterations in membrane potential, which are called voltage-gated channels[4], whereas others are opened or closed when they bind a ligand, which are called ligand-gated channels[5]. The ligand is often external, e.g., a neurotransmitter[6] or a hormone. However, it can also be internal, intracellular Ca^{2+}, cyclic AMP (cAMP), or one of the G proteins produced in cells can bind directly to channels and activate them. A typical voltage-gated channel is the Na^+ channel, and a typical ligand-gated channel is the acetylcholine receptor. Some channels are also opened by mechanical stretch, and these mechanosensitive channels[7] play an important role in cell movement.

In the carrier mediated diffusion, transport proteins are carriers that bind ions and other molecules and then change their configuration, moving the bound molecule from one side of the cell membrane to the other. Molecules move from area of high concentration to areas of low concentration (down their chemical gradient), and cations move to negatively charged areas whereas anions move to positively charged areas (down their electrical gradient). It has such characteristics: high specificity, meaning one kind of carriers only transporting one kind

[1] 单纯扩散。

[2] 易化扩散。

[3] 电化学梯度。

[4] 电压门控通道。

[5] 配基门控通道。

[6] 神经递质。

[7] 机械敏感通道。

of substances; saturated phenomenon, meaning that transportation velocity will not increasing with the substance concentration after all carriers having combined with substances; competitive inhibition, meaning substance concentration is the determining factor which substance can be transported first from several transported substances of the carrier.

Moreover, water can move across the cell membrane in two ways. First, since the lipid part of the plasma membrane is very hydrophobic, the movement of water across it is too slow to explain the speed at which water can move in and out of the cells. Secondly, Specific membrane proteins that function as water channels explain the rapid movement of water across the plasma membrane. These water channels are small (molecular weight about 30 kDa) integral membrane proteins known as aquaporins(AQPs)[1]. Ten different forms have been discovered so far in mammals. At least six forms are expressed in cells in the kidney and seven forms in the gastrointestinal tract, tissues where water movement acsoss cell membranes is particularly rapid.

2.2 Active transport

Active transport is the movement of substances across the membrane occurs against the electrochemical gradient with the necessity of consumption of metabolic energy. Active transport can be divided into primary active transport, in which cellular energy is consumed directly, and secondary active transport, in which cellular energy is consumed indirectly.

2.2.1 Primary active transport Solutes e.g. molecules or ions of some substance are transported from a dilute solution to concentrated solution through the cell membrane. This process of moving molecules uphill against a concentration gradient is often called a "pump", such as Na^+–K^+ pump[2].

Na^+–K^+ pump is a heterodimer made up of an α subunit with a molecular weight of approximately 100,000 and a β subunit with a molecular weight of approximately 55,000. Both extend through the cell membrane. Separation of the subunits eliminates activity. However, the β subunit is a glycoprotein, whereas Na^+ and K^+ transport occur through the α subunit. The β subunit has a single membrane–spanning domain and three extracellular glycosylation sites, all of which appear to have attached carbohydrate residues. These residues account for one–third of its molecular weight. The α subunit probably spans the cell membrane 10 times, with the amino and carboxylic terminals both located intracellularly. This subunit has intracellular Na^+ and ATP–binding sites and a phosphorylation site; it also has extracellular binding sites for K^+ and ouabain[3].

---

[1] 水通道蛋白。

[2] 钠 – 钾泵。

[3] 哇巴因。

The possible mechanism of Na^+–K^+ pump is that when 3 Na^+ ions bind to the α subunit, ATP also binds and is converted to ADP, with a phosphate being transferred to Asp376, the phosphorylation site (Figure2–2). This causes a change in the configuration of the protein, extruding Na^+ into the extracelluar fluid (ECF). Na^+–K^+ pump then binds to $2K^+$ ions extracellulary. Dephosphorylating α subunit, which returns to its previous conformation, releasing K^+ into the cytoplasm (Figure 2–2). Because Na^+–K^+ pump can hydrolyze ATP to ADP, it is also called Na^+–K^+ ATPase [1]. Active transport of Na^+ and K^+ is one of the major energy–using processes in the body. On the average, it accounts for about 24% of the energy utilized by cells, and in neurons it accounts for 70%. Thus, it accounts for a large part of the basal metabolism [2].

Na^+–K^+ pump can function in many sections: to establish Na^+ and K^+ concentration gradients across the plasma membrane of all cells, which are critically important in the ability of nerve and muscle cells to generate electrical impulses essential to their functioning; to help regulate cell volume by controlling the concentrations of solutes inside the cell and thus minimizing osmotic effects that would induce swelling or shrinking of the cell; the energy derived from Na^+–K^+ pump also indirectly serves as the energy source for the cotransport [3] of glucose and amino acids across intestinal and kidney cells.

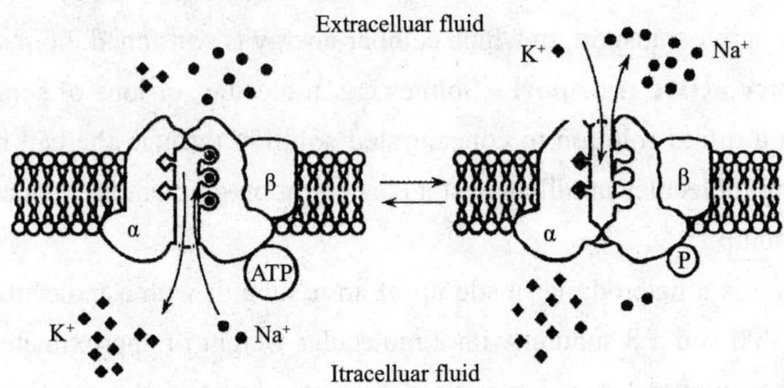

Figure 2–2 The mechanism of the Na^+ – K^+ pump

2.2.2 Secondary active transport In many situations, the active transport of Na^+ is coupled to the transport of some nutrient molecules, such as glucoses and amino acids, which is secondary active transport, or cotransport. For example, there are carrier in the luminal membranes of the small intestine and renal tubule, which have two binding sites, one for Na^+ and one for the nutrient molecule, for instance, glucose. Binding of luminal Na^+ to the carrier

[1] 钠 – 钾 ATP 酶。

[2] 基础代谢。

[3] 协同转运。

can increase the carrier's affinity for glucose. And there are Na^+–K^+ pumps in the basolateral membrane of these cells. When both Na^+ and glucose bind to the carrier, the carrier undergoes a conformational change[1], causing Na^+ and glucose to be released into the cell. The Na^+ movement is passive because intracellular Na^+ concentration is low, but the glucose movement is active because glucose becomes concentrated in the cell. The released Na^+ is quickly pumped out through basolateral membrane by Na^+–K^+ pump, keeping the level of intracellular Na^+ low. The energy expended in this process is helpful for glucose moving into the cell again concentration difference.

2.3 Exocytosis and endocytosis

Particles that are secreted by cell move from the endoplastic reticulum to the Golgi complex where they are packaged in secretary granules or vesicles. These granules or vesicles move to the cell membrane. The granule membrane and cell membrane then fuse and the area of fusion breaks down, leaving the contents of the granule outside the cell and the cell membrane intact. This process is called exocytosis.

Endocytosis is the reverse of exocytosis. One form of endocytosis called phagocytosis, or cell eating, is the process by which bacteria, dead tissue of other bits of material visible under the microscope are engulfed by cell such as the polymorphonuclear leukocytes of the blood. The material makes contact with the cell membrane, which then invaginates. The invagination is pinched off, leaving the engulfed material in the membrane–enclosed vacuole and the cell membrane intact. Another form of endocytosis is pinocytosis, or cell drink, is essentially the same process, the only difference being that substances ingested are in solution and hence not visible by the microscope.

Section 2 Transmembrane signaling transduction

First action of most chemical messenger (hormone, neurotransmitter, or cytokine) is to bind to the extracellular domain of the specific protein receptors in the plasma membrane of the target cells, and then to exert their effects on cells via signal–transduction pathways[2]. A discussion of signal–transduction pathways is a comprehensive subject. Therefore only certain transmembrane signal–transduction pathways are described.

1 G protein coupled receptor mediated signal transduction

Many hormones, neuro-modulators, and other regulatory molecules that alter cellular pro-

[1] 变构。

[2] 信号转导途径。

cesses do so by signal–transduction pathways involving heterotrimeric GTP–binding proteins, also called simply G proteins. A G protein is a molecular switch (Figure 2–3) that can exist in two states. In its activated state, a G protein has a higher affinity for GTP. The inactivated G protein preferentially binds GDP. When certain membrane receptors have agonist[1] molecules bound to them, they interact with specific G proteins to promote the conversion of proteins to their activated state by binding GTP. An activated G protein can then interact with many effector proteins, most notably enzymes or ion channels, to alter their activities. The activated G protein has GTPase activity, so eventually the bound GTP is hydrolyzed to GDP, and the G protein reverts to its inactive stare (Figure 2–3).

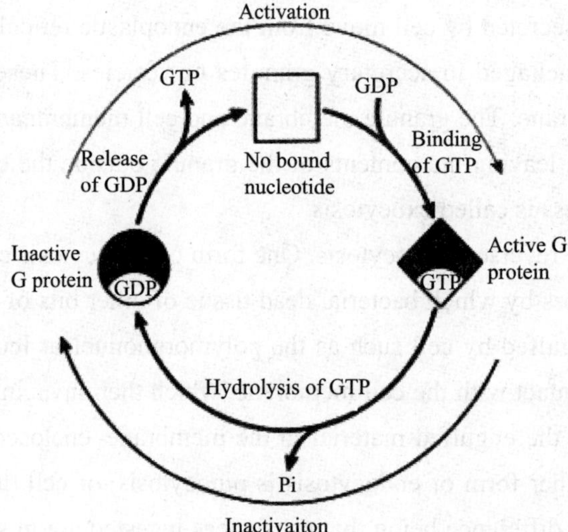

Figure 2–3 Activity cycle of a GTP–binding protein

Among the most important targets of activated G proteins are molecules that change the cellular concentrations of the second messengers cyclic AMP, cyclic GMP, Ca^{2+}, IP_3, and diacylglycerol (Figure 2–3). Adenylyl cyclase and cyclic GMP phosphodiesterase, the enzymes responsible for the synthesis of cyclic AMP and the breakdown of cyclic GMP, respectively, are powerfully modulated by G protein–mediated mechanisms. Ca^{2+} channels may be modulated directly by G proteins or indirectly by second messenger–dependent protein kinases. Other effectors that are modulated by G proteins include certain K^+ channels and phospholipases C, A_2, and D.

In general, a G protein–protein kinase–mediated signal–transduction pathway involves the following events (Figure 2–4): ① A hormone or other agonist binds to its plasma membrane receptor. ② The ligand–bearing receptor interacts with a G protein and activates it,

[1] 激动剂。

the activated G protein binds GTP. ③ The activated G protein interacts with one or more of the following effectors to activate or inhibit them: adenylyl cyclase, cyclic GMP phosphodiesterase, Ca^{2+} or K^{+} channels, or phospholipases C, A_2, or D. ④ The cellular level of one or more of the following second messengers increases or decreases: cyclic AMP, cyclic GMP, Ca^{2+}, IP_3, or diacylglycerol. ⑤ The increase or decrease of the concentration of a second messenger changes the activity of one or more of the second messenger–dependent protein kinases: cyclic AMP–dependent protein kinase, cyclic GMP–dependent protein kinase, calmodulin–dependent protein kinase, or protein kinase C. It can also activate an ion channel. ⑥ The level of phosphorylation of an enzyme or an ion channel is altered, or an ion channel activity changes because of interaction with an activated G protein and causes the final cellular response.

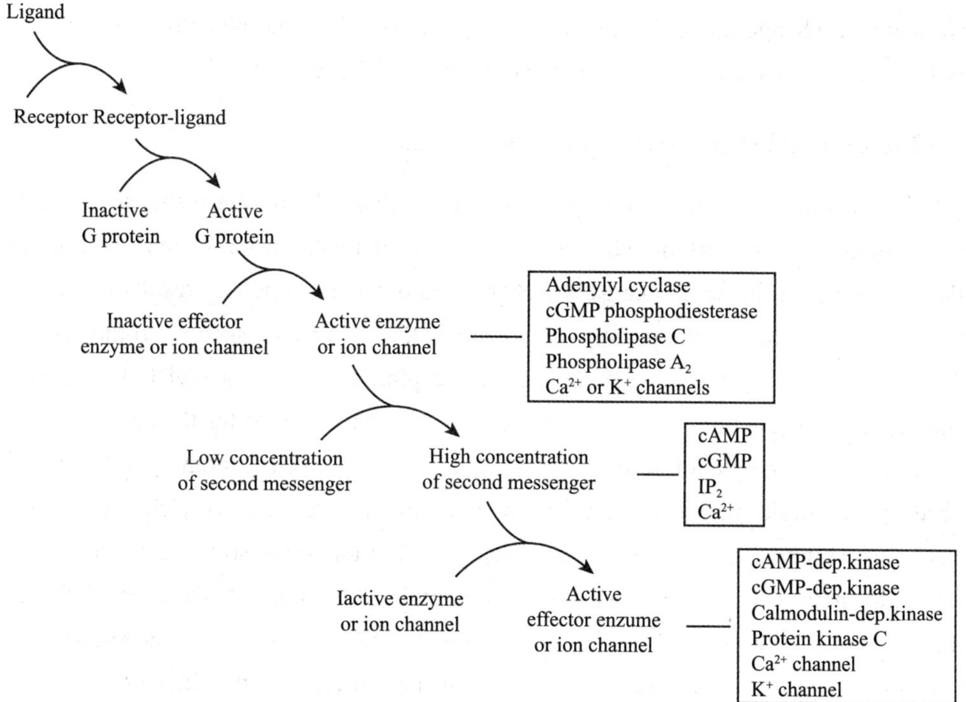

Figure 2–4 G protein–protein kinase–mediated signal–transduction pathway

2 Enzyme coupled receptor mediated signal transduction

The receptors for certain peptide hormones [1] and growth factors are proteins with a glycosylated extracellular domain, a single transmembrane sequence, and an intracellular domain with protein–tyrosine kinase activity. Members of this superfamily of peptide receptors include

[1] 肽类激素。

the receptors for insulin and related growth factors, epidermal growth factor, nerve growth factor, platelet-derived growth factor, colony-stimulating factor, fibroblast growth factor, and hepatocyte growth factor. The binding of hormone or growth factor to its receptor triggers multiple cellular responses, including Ca^{2+} influx, increased Na^+–H^+ exchange, stimulation of the uptake of sugars and amino acids, and stimulation of phospholipase Cβ to hydrolyze phosphatidylinositol 4,5-bisphosphate.

The known protein-tyrosine kinase receptors[1] fall into eight subfamilies. The binding of ligand to the receptor results in dimerization of the receptor-ligand complexes. The dimerization enhances binding affinity and activates the protein-tyrosine kinase activity. Each monomer in a dimer phosphorylates the other monomer on multiple tyrosine residues. In subclass 11 receptors, the insulin receptor family, the non-coordination receptor exists as a disulfide-linked dimer, and binding of insulin results in a conformational change of both "monomers". This conformational change enhances insulin binding and activates the receptor's tyrosine kinase activity, which leads to enhanced autophosphorylation of the receptor.

3 Ion channel mediated signal transduction

Some membrane receptors are ligand-gated ion channel, and the response of the cell is a ligand-induced ionic current. The receptor itself constitutes an ion channel,and activation of the receptor by a messenger cause the channel to open. The opening results in an increase in the net diffusion across the plasma membrane of the ion or ions specific to the channel. In such cases the ligand-gated ion channel-linked receptor, such as the acetylcholine receptor of the neuromuscular junction[2], is both the receptor and the effector for the action of the neurotransmitter. The acetylcholine receptor protein is an integral membrane protein that spans the hydrophobic lipid matrix of the post junctional membrane. The acetylcholine receptor of five subunits (Figure2-5), two of which (αsubunits) are identical, so there are four different polypeptide chains (i.e.,α,β,δ,γ).Each α subunit contains a binding site for acetylcholine: both αsubunits must bind acetylcholine to open the ion channel. The binding of acetycholine to an acetycoline receptor causes a transient opening of the ion channel that increases the conductance of the postjunctional membrane[3] to Na^+ and K^+.

[1] 蛋白－酪氨酸激酶受体。

[2] 神经－骨骼肌接头。

[3] 接头后膜。

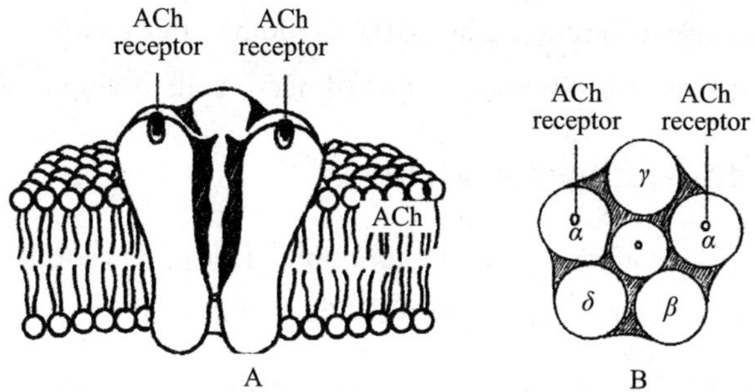

Figure 2–5 Structure of a nicotinic acetylcholine receptor protein

Section 3 Cell bioelectrical phenomenon

Nerve, muscle and glandular cells are excitable cells[1]. As excitable cells,there are obvious potential differences across membrane of nerve, muscle and glandular cells at rest, and the membrane potential differences at rest change markedly when they are excited.This phenomenon is called bioelectricity[2].In this section, mainly two membrane potentials that influence the cellular states, resting membrane potential[3] and action potential[4], are explained.

1 Resting potential

1.1 Recording of resting potential

When two electrodes are connected through a suitable amplifier to a cathode ray oscilloscope (CRO)[5] and placed on the surface of a single axon, no potential difference is observed. However, if one electrode is inserted into the interior of the cell, a constant potential difference is observed, with the inside negative relative to the outside of the cell at rest. This resting membrane potential is found in almost all cells. The membrane potential of large nerve fibers when they are not transmitting nerve signals, that is, when they are in the so–called "resting" state, is about –90 millivolt (mV). That is, the potential inside the fiber is 90 mV more negative than the potential in the interstitial fluid on the outside of the fiber, which is polarization[6]. And this potential is called resting membrane potential, or resting potential (RP).The resting potential

[1] 可兴奋细胞。

[2] 生物电。

[3] 静息电位。

[4] 动作电位。

[5] 阴极射线示波器。

[6] 极化。

levels of different cells are different, about –10 ~ –100mV. For example, the resting potential of skeletal muscle cells is about –90mV, and that of nerve cells is about –70mV.

1.2 Genesis of the resting potential

The distribution of ions across the cell membrane (Table 2–1) and the nature of this membrane provide the explanation for the resting membrane potential.

Table 2–1 Concentration of ions inside and outside mammalian spinal motor neurons

Ion	Concentration (mmol/L of H_2O)	
	Intracellular	Extracellular
Na^+	15.0	150.0
K^+	150.0	5.5
Cl^-	9.0	125.0

The concentration gradient for K^+ facilitates its movement out of the cell via K^+ channels, but its electrical gradient is in the opposite (inward) direction. Consequently, an equilibrium is reached in which the tendency of K^+ to move out of the cell is balanced by its tendency to move into the cell, and at that equilibrium there is a slight excess of cations on the outside and anions on the inside. This condition is maintained by Na^+– K^+ ATPase, which pumps K^+ back into the cell and keeps the intracellular concentration of Na^+ low.

Its magnitude can be calculated from the Nernst equation, as follows:

$$E_K = \frac{RT}{FZ}\ln\frac{[K^+]_0}{[K^+]_i}$$

where

E_K= equilibrium potential for K^+

R= gas constant

T= absolute temperature

F= the faraday (number of coulombs per mole of charge)

Z= valence of ion

$[K^+]_o$=K^+ concentration outside the cell

$[K^+]_i$=K^+ concentration inside the cell

The Na^+–K^+ pump is also electrogenic[1], because it pumps 2 K^+ ions into the cell, and 3 Na^+ions out of the cell every time; thus, it also contributes a small amount to the membrane potential by itself. It should be emphasized that the number of ions responsible for the membrane potential is a minute fraction of the total number present and that the total concentrations of

[1] 生电性。

positive and negative ions are equal everywhere except along the membrane. Na^+ influx does not compensate for the K^+ efflux because the K^+ channels make the membrane more permeable to K^+ than to Na^+ at rest.

2 Action potential

2.1 Recording of action potential

If the axon is stimulated and a conducted impulse occurs, a characteristic series of potential changes known as the action potential (AP) is observed as the impulse passes the external electrode (Figure 2–6). When the stimulus is applied, there is a brief irregular deflection of the baseline[1], the stimulus artifact. This artifact is due to current leakage from the stimulating electrodes to the recording electrodes. It usually occurs despite careful shielding, but it is of value because it marks on the cathode ray screen the point at which the stimulus was applied. The stimulus artifact[2] is followed by an isopotential interval (latent period) that ends with the start of a potential change that can be conducted, which is called action potential and corresponds to the time it takes the impulse to travel along the axon from the site of stimulation to recording electrodes. Its duration is proportionate to the distance between the stimulating and recording electrodes and inversely proportionate to the speed of conduction.

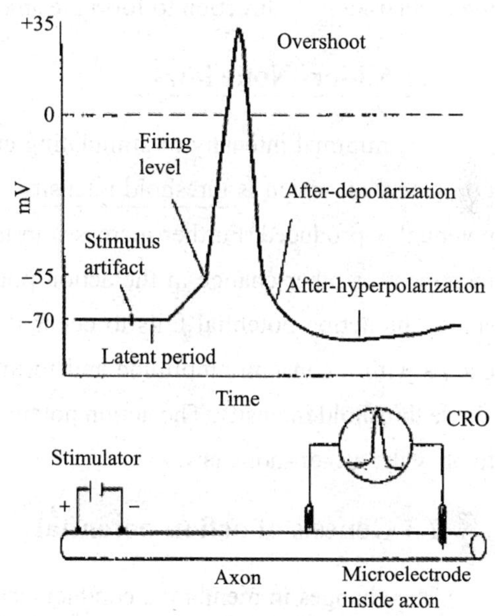

Figure 2–6 Action potential in a neuron recorded with one electrode inside the cell

The first manifestation of the approaching action potential is an initial increase in the intracellular potential on the basis of resting potential, which is called depolarization[3]. After an initial 15mV of depolarization, the rate of depolarization increases. The point at which this change in rate occurs is called the firing level or the threshold potential[4]. Thereafter, the trac-

[1] 基线。

[2] 刺激伪迹。

[3] 去极化。

[4] 阈电位。

ing on the oscilloscope rapidly reaches and overshoots[1] the isopotential (zero potential) line[2] to approximately +35 mV, which is also called reverse polarization[3]. It then reverses and falls rapidly toward the resting level, which is called repolarization[4]. When repolarization is about 70% completed, the rate of repolarization decreases and the tracing approaches the resting level more slowly. The sharp rise and rapid fall are the spike potential[5] of the axon,which are also seen in skeletal muscle cells, and the slower fall at the end of the process are the after–depolarization[6]. After reaching the previous resting level, the tracing overshoots slightly in the hyperpolarizing[7] direction to form the small but prolonged after–hyperpolarization[8].

2.2 All–or–None law[9]

The minimal intensity of stimulating current acting for a given duration can cause an action potential, which is threshold intensity[10]. When threshold intensity is reached, an action potential is produced. Further increases in the intensity of a threshold stimulus[11] produce no increment or other change in the action potential as long as the other conditions remain constant. The action potential fails to occur if the stimulus is subthreshold in magnitude, and it occurs with a constant amplitude and form regardless of the stimulus if the stimulus is at or above threshold intensity. The action potential is therefore "all or none" in character and is said to obey the all–or–none law.

2.3 Genesis of action potential

The changes in membrane conductance of Na^+ and K^+ that occur during the action potentials are shown in Figure 2–6. When depolarization exceeds 7mV, the voltage–gated Na^+ channels[12] start to open at an increased rate (Na^+ channel activation[13]), and when the firing level is

[1] 超射。
[2] 等电位线。
[3] 反极化。
[4] 复极化。
[5] 峰电位。
[6] 后去极化电位（负后电位）。
[7] 超极化
[8] 后超极化电位（正后电位）。
[9] 全或无定律。
[10] 阈强度。
[11] 阈刺激。
[12] 电压门控钠通道。
[13] 激活。

reached, the influx of Na^+ along its inwardly directed concentration and electrical gradients is so great that it temporarily swamps the repolarization forces.

The equilibrium potential for Na^+ in mammalian neurons, calculated by using the Nernst equation, is about +60 mV. The membrane potential moves toward this value but does not reach it during the action potential, primarily because the increase in Na^+ conductance is short–lived. The Na^+ channels rapidly enter a closed state called the inactivated state[1] and remain in this state for a few milliseconds before returning to the resting state[2]. In addition, the direction of the electrical gradient for Na^+ is reversed during the overshoot because the membrane potential is reversed, and this limits Na^+ influx.

A third factor producing repolarization[3] is the opening of voltage–gated K^+ channels[4]. This opening is slower and more prolonged than the opening of the Na^+ channels, and consequently, much of the increase in K^+ conductance comes after the increase in Na^+ conductance. The net movement of positive charge out of the cell due to K^+ efflux at this time helps complete the process of repolarization. The slow return of the K^+ channels to the closed state also explains the after–hyperpolarization.

3 Local potential and the cause and conduction of excitation on the same cell

3.1 Action potential transport along the nerve fiber

If the nerve fiber is surrounded with myelin sheath[5], it is called myelinated nerve fiber[6], without myelin sheath, it is called unmyelinated nerve fiber[7]. The myelin sheath can increase the resistance to ion flow. In unmyelinated nerve fiber, ions can flow free through the cellular membrane. This leads to the low velocity of the myelinated nerve fiber conducting impulses because action potentials must spread all the cell membrane, which is called local current[8].

Although ions cannot flow significantly through the thick myelin sheaths of myelinated nerves, they can flow with considerable ease through the nodes of Ranvier where no sheath exists. Therefore, action potentials can occur only at the nodes. Yet, the action potentials are

---

[1] 失活状态。

[2] 静息状态。

[3] 复极化。

[4] 电压门控钾通道。

[5] 髓鞘。

[6] 有髓神经纤维。

[7] 无髓神经纤维。

[8] 局部电流。

conducted from node to node, as illustrated in Figure 2–7, this is called saltatory conduction[1]. Saltatory conduction is of value for two reasons: First, by causing the depolarization process to jump long intervals along axis of the nerve fiber, this mechanism increases the velocity of nerve transmission in myelinated fibers an average of five– to sevenfold. Second, saltatory conduction conserves energy for the axon, for only the nodes depolarize, allowing perhaps a hundred times smaller loss of ions than would otherwise be necessary and therefore requiring little extra metabolism for re–establishing the sodium and potassium concentration differences across the membrane after a series of nerve impulses.

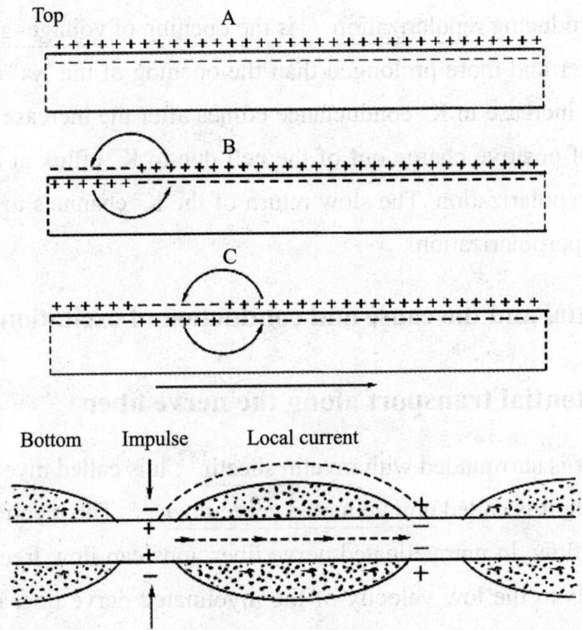

Figure 2–7 Local current flow (movement of positive charges) around an impulse in an axon. Top: unmyelinated axon. Bottom: myelinated axon

3.2 Stimulus and excitation

The appearance of action potential of excitatory cells indicates that stimulus[2] causes them excited. But not all stimuli can cause excitation.

3.2.1 Conditions of effective stimulus

One of the widest used stimulation is electrical stimulus, for its parameters can be easily controlled and the damage to the cells is not severe, and also the stimuli can be repeated when necessary.

[1] 跳跃式传导。

[2] 刺激。

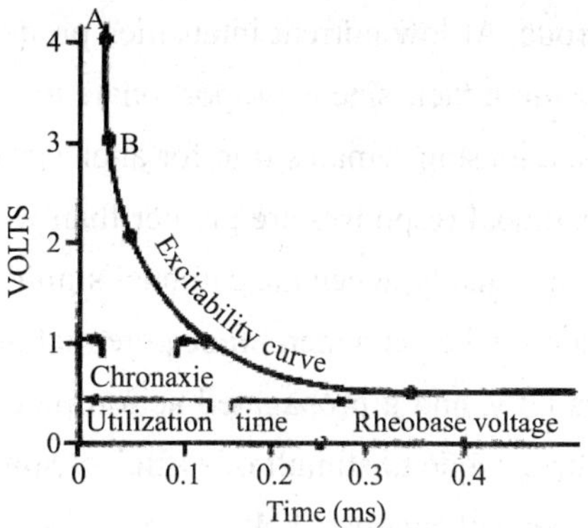

Figure 2–8 Excitability of large myelinated nerve fiber

Stimulus intensity, duration and the ratio of strength–duration[1] are three needed conditions if the stimulus can excite the cell (Figure 2–8). To obtain this curve a high voltage electrical stimulus (4 volts, in this instance) is applied to the fiber, and the minimum duration of stimulus required to excite the fiber is found. The voltage and duration are plotted as point A. Then a stimulus voltage of 3 volts is applied, and the duration required is again determined; the results are plotted as point B. The same is repeated at 2 volts, 1 volt, 0.5 volt, and so forth, until the least voltage possible at which the membrane is stimulated has been reached. On connection of these points, the excitability curve is generated.

The least possible voltage at which it will fire is called the rheobase[2], and the time required for this least voltage to stimulate the fiber is called the utilization time[3]. Then, if the voltage is increased to twice the rheobase voltage, the time required to stimulate the fiber is called the chronaxie[4]. The chronaxie is often used as a means of expressing relative excitabily of different tissues.

3.2.2 Electrotonic potentials, local response and firing level

Although subthreshold stimuli[5] do not produce an action potential, they do have an effect on the membrane potential. This can be demonstrated by placing recording electrodes within a few millimeters of a stimulating electrode and applying subthreshold stimuli of fixed duration. Application of such currents with a cathode leads to a localized depolarization potential change that rises sharply and decays exponentially with time. The magnitude of this response drops off rapidly as the distance between the stimulating and recording electrodes is increased. Conversely, an anodal current produces a hyperpolarization potential change of similar duration. These potential changes are called electrotonic potentials[6], those produced at a cathode being catelectrotonic and those at an anode anelectrotonic. They are passive changes in membrane polarization caused by addition or subtraction of charge by the particular elec

[1] 刺激强度、刺激时间和强度 – 时间变化率。

[2] 基强度。

[3] 利用时。

[4] 时值。

[5] 阈下刺激。

[6] 电紧张电位。

trode. At low current intensities producing up to about 7 mV of depolarization or hyperpolarization, their size is proportionate to the magnitude of the stimulus. With stronger stimuli, this relationship remains true for anelectrotonic responses but not for responses at the cathode; the cathodal responses are greater than would be expected from the magnitude of the applied current. Finally, when the cathodal stimulation is great enough to produce about 15mV of depolarization, i.e., at a membrane potential of –55mV, the membrane potential suddenly begins to fall rapidly, and a propagated action potential occurs. The disproportionately greater response at the cathode to stimuli of sufficient strength to produce 7 ~ 15mV of depolarization is produced when voltage-gated Na^+ channels begin to open and is called the local response[1] (Figure 2–9).

Thus, cathodal currents that produce up to 7mV of depolarization have a purely passive charges. Those producing 7 ~ 15mV of depolarization also initiate a slight active contribution to the depolarization process. However, the repolarization forces are still stronger than the depolarization forces, and the potential decays. At 15mV of depolarization, the depolarization forces are strong enough to overwhelm the repolarization processes, and an action potential results.

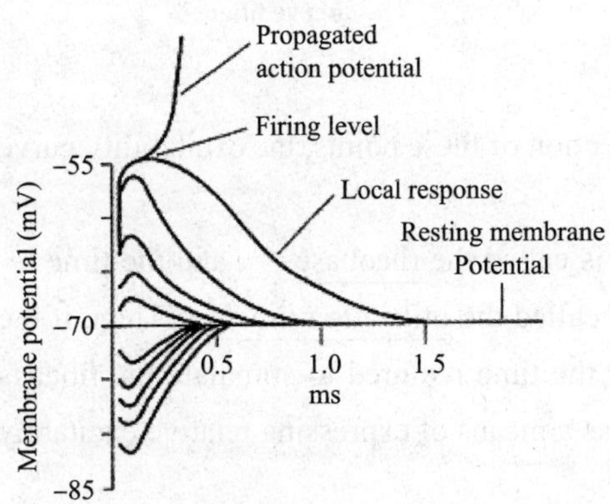

Figure 2–9 Electrotonic potentials and local response

Stimulation normally occurs at the cathode, because cathodal stimuli are depolarization. Anodal currents, by taking the membrane potential farther away from the firing level, inhibit impulse formation. However, cessation of an anodal current may lead to an overshoot of the membrane potential in the depolarization direction. This rebound is sometimes large enough to cause the nerve to fire at the end of an anodal stimulus.

3.2.3 Changes in excitability during electrotonic potentials

During the action potential as well as during catelectrotonic and anelectrotonic potentials and the local response, there are changes in the threshold of the neuron to stimulation. Hyperpolarizing an electrotonic responses elevate the threshold and depolarizing catelectrotonic potentials lower it as they move the membrane potential closer to the firing level. During the local response, the threshold is lowered, but during the rising and much of the falling phases of

[1] 局部反应。

the spike potential, the neuron is refractory to stimulation. This refractory period [1] is divided into an absolute refractory period [2], corresponding to the period from the time the firing level is reached until repolarization is about one-third complete, and a relative refractory period [3], lasting from this point to the start of after-depolarization. During the absolute refractory period, no stimulus, no matter how strong, will excite the nerve, but during the relative refractory period, stronger than normal stimuli can cause excitation. During after-depolarization, the threshold is again decreased, and during after-hyperpolarization, it is increased. These changes in threshold are correlated with the phases of the action potential in Figure 2-10.

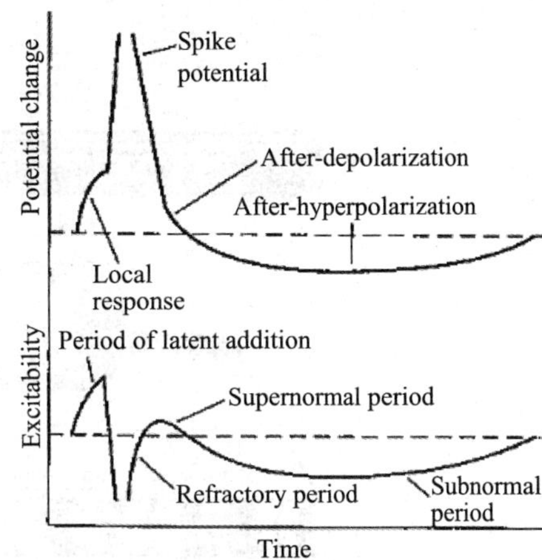

Figure 2-10 Relative changes in excitability of a nerve cell membrane during the passage of an impulse

Section 4 Contraction of muscle cells

Approximately 40% of the body is skeletal muscle and almost another 10% is smooth and cardiac muscle, and skeletal muscles and cardiac muscles are called striated muscles [4]. Many of the same principles of contraction apply to these different types of muscle, but here the function of skeletal muscles is considered mainly.

1 Striated muscle

1.1 Physiologic anatomy of striated muscle

Striated muscles are made of numerous fibers. Each of these fibers in turn is made up of successively smaller subunits which is illustrated in Figure 2-11.

[1] 不应期。

[2] 绝对不应期。

[3] 相对不应期。

[4] 横纹肌。

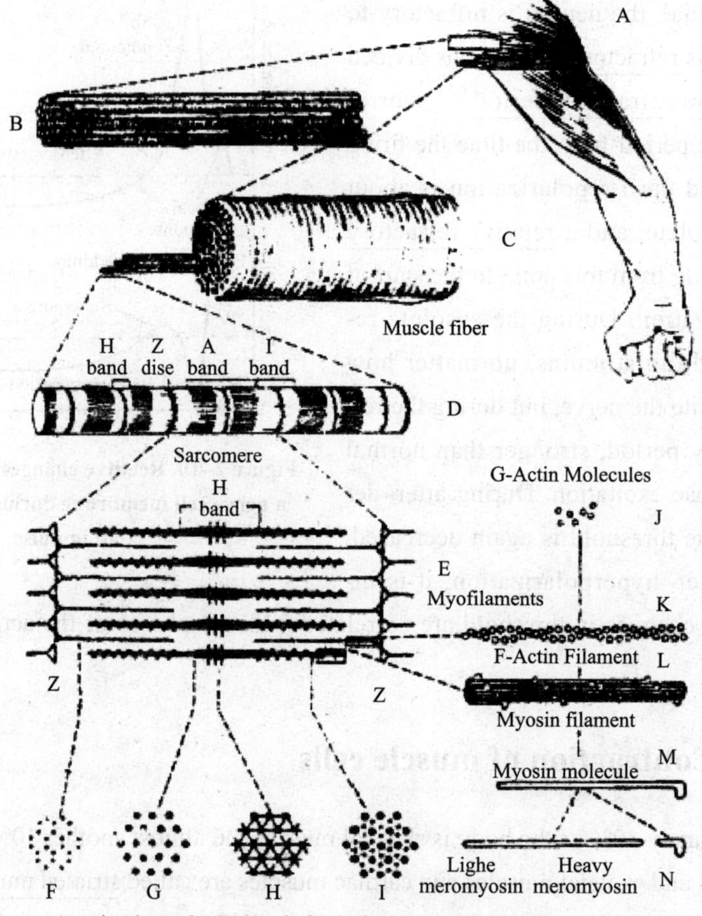

A, striated muscle; B, muscle fasciculus; C, muscle fiber, D, myofibril;
E, sarcomere; F, G, H and I are cross-sections at the levels

Figure 2-11 Organization of the striated muscle from the gross to the molecular.

1.1.1 Myofibrils and sarcomere

Each muscle fiber contains several hundred to several thousand myofibrils [1]. Each myofibril in turn has, lying side-by-side, about 1,500 myosin [2] filaments and 3,000 actin [3] filaments. These are represented diagrammatically in Figure 2-11 E. The thick filaments [4] are myosin and thin filaments [5] are mainly actin. Note that the myosin and actin partially interdigitate and thus cause the myofibrils to have alternate light and dark bands. The light bands, which contain only actin filaments, are called I bands because they are mainly isotropic to

[1] 肌原纤维。

[2] 肌球蛋白。

[3] 肌动蛋白。

[4] 粗肌丝。

[5] 细肌丝。

polarized light. The dark bands, which contain the myosin filaments as well as the end of the actin filaments where they overlap the myosin, are called A bands because they are anisotropic to polarized, light.

Figure 2–11 E also shows that the actin filaments are attached to the so-called Z disc [1], and the filaments extend on either side of the Z disc to interdigitate with the myosin filaments. The Z disc also passes from myofibril to myofibril, attaching the myofibrils to each other all the way across the muscle fiber. Therefore, the entire muscle fiber has light and dark bands, as is also true of the individual myofibrils. These bands give skeletal and cardiac muscle their striated appearance.

The portion of a myofibril that lies between two successive Z discs is called a sarcomere [2]. It is the basic unit of contraction.

1.1.2 Molecular structure of the myofibril

1.1.2.1 The myosin filament

The myosin filament is made up of about 200 individual myosin molecules. Figure 2–12 A illustrates an individual molecule. The myosin molecule is comprised of six polypeptide chains, two heavy chains and four light chains. The two heavy chains coil around each other to form a double helix. However, one end of each of these chains is folded into a globular protein mass called the myosin head. The myosin head can function as an ATPase enzyme. This allows the head to hydrolyze ATP and to use the energy derived from the ATP energize the contraction process.

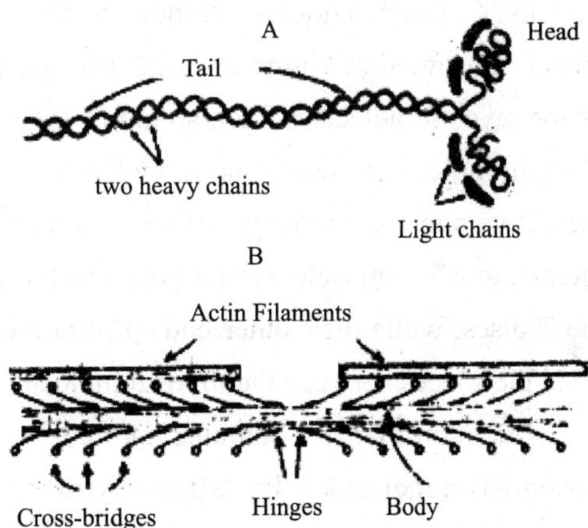

A, the myosin molecule. B, combination of many myosin molecules to form a myosin filament.

Figure 2–12 The myosin structure and its combination with actin.

There at two free heads lying side by side at one end of the double helix myosin molecule; the other end of the coiled helix is called the tail. The four light chains are also parts of the myosin heads, two to each head. These light chains help control the function of the head during the process of muscle contraction.

The central portion of one of these filaments is illustrated in Figure 2–12 B, showing the tails of the myosin molecules bundled together to form the body of the filament, while many heads of the molecules hang outward to the sides of the body. Also, part of the helix portion

[1] Z线（盘）。

[2] 肌节。

of each myosin molecule extends to the side along with the head, thus providing an arm that extends the head outward from the body. The protruding arms and heads together are called cross–bridges[1], and each of these is believed to be flexible at two points called hinges, one where the arm leaves the body of the myosin filament and the other where the two heads attach to the arm. The hinged arms allow the heads to be extended either far outward from the body of the myosin filament or to be brought close to the body. The hinged heads are believed to participate in the actual contraction process.

The myosin filaments itself is twisted so that each successive set of cross–bridges is axially displaced from the previous set by 120 degrees. This insures that the cross–bridges extend in all directions around the filament.

1.1.2.2 The thin filament

The thin filament is composed of three different components: actin, tropomyosin[2] and troponin[3]. Actin, a double–stranded F–actin protein molecule, is the backbone of the actin filament, illustrated in Figure 2–12 A. The two strands are wound in a helix in the same manner as the myosin molecule. Each strand of the double F–actin helix is composed of polymerized G–actin molecules. The G–actin molecule is one molecule of ADP. These ADP molecules are the active sites on the actin filaments with which the cross–bridges of the myosin filaments interact to cause muscle contraction. The bases of the actin filaments are inserted strongly into the Z discs, while their other ends protrude in both directions into the adjacent sarcomeres to lie in the spaces between the myosin molecules.

The actin filament contains another two additional protein strands that are polymers of tropomyosin molecules. Each tropomyosin strand is loosely attached to an F–actin strand and that in the resting state it physically covers the active sites of the actin strands so that interaction cannot occur between the actin and myosin to cause contraction.

Attached approximately two thirds distance along each tropomyosin molecule is a complex of three globular protein molecules called troponin. One of the globular proteins (troponin I) has a strong affinity for actin, another (troponin T) for tropomyosin, and a third (troponin C) for calcium ions. This complex attaches to the tropomyosin to the actin (Figure 2–13 A).

In resting muscle, troponin I is tightly bound to actin and tropomyosin covers the sites where myosin heads bind to actin. Thus, the troponin – tropomyosin complex constitutes a "relaxing protein" that inhibits the interaction between actin and myosin. When Ca^{2+} binds to troponin C, the binding of troponin I to actin is presumably weakened, and this permits the tropomyosin to move laterally (Figure 2–13 B). This movement uncovers binding sites for the

---

[1] 横桥。

[2] 原肌球蛋白。

[3] 肌钙蛋白。

myosin heads. ATP is then split and contraction occurs. Seven myosin–binding sites are uncovered for each molecule of troponin that binds a calcium ion.

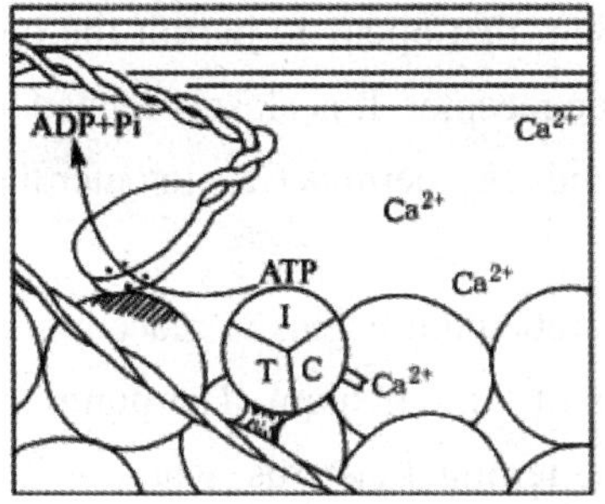

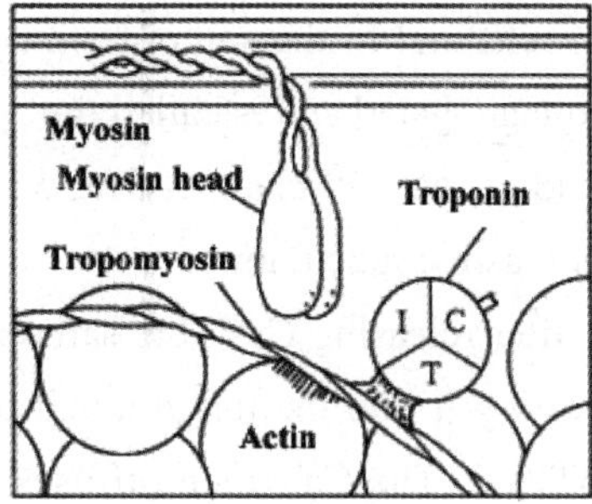

Figure 2–13 Initiation of muscle contraction by Ca^{2+}

When Ca^{2+} binds to troponin C, tropomyosin is displaced laterally, exposing the binding site for myosin actin (dark area). The myosin head then binds, ATP is hydrolyzed, and the configuration of the head and neck region of myosin changes.

1.1.3 Sarcotubular system

The muscle fibrils are surrounded by structures made up of the sarcotubular system[1], which is made up of a T system and a sarcoplasmic reticulum (Figure 2–14). The T system of transverse tubules (T tubules), which is continuous with sarcolemma[2], forms a grid perforated by the individual muscle fibrils. The space in the T system is an extension of the extracellular space. The sarcoplasmic reticulum, which forms an irregular curtain around each of the fibrils, has enlarged terminal cisterns[3] in close contact with the T system at the junctions between the A and I bands. At these points of contact, the arrangement of the central T system with two cisterns of the sarcoplasmic reticulum on both sides is called triad[4].

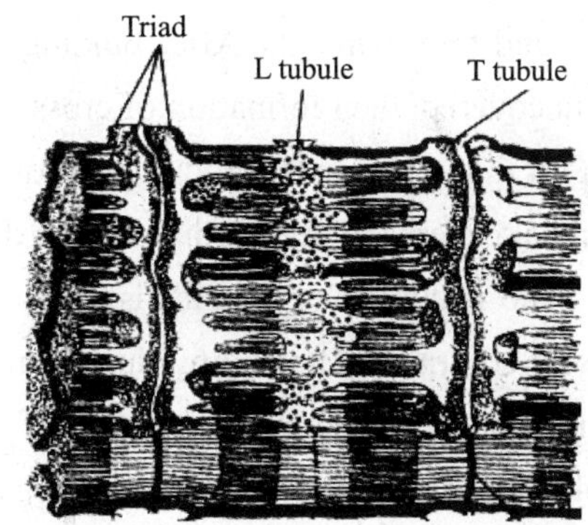

Figure 2–14 Sarcotubular system of the skeletal muscle

The function of the T system is the rapid transmission of the action potential from the cell membrane to all the fibrils in the muscle. Depolarization of the T tubule membrane activates

[1] 肌管系统。

[2] 肌膜。

[3] 终池。

[4] 三联管。

the sarcoplasmic reticulum via dihydropyridine receptors, which are voltage–gated Ca^{2+} channels in the T tubule membrane. The dihydropyridine receptor serves as the voltage sensor and trigger that unlocks release of Ca^{2+} from the nearby sarcoplasmic reticulum.

The Ca^{2+} channel in the sarcoplasmic reticulum that opens to permit the outpouring of Ca^{2+} is not voltage–gated and is called the ryanodine receptor. It is closely related to the IP_3 receptor, a ligand–gated Ca^{2+} channel that, when it binds IP_3, permits Ca^{2+} to enter the cytoplasm from the endoplasmic reticulum.

Shortly after releasing Ca^{2+}, the sarcoplasmic reticulum begins to reaccumulate it by actively transporting it into the longitudinal portions of the reticulum. The pump involved is a Ca^{2+}–Mg^{2+} ATPase. The Ca^{2+} then diffuses into the terminal cisterns, where it is stored until released by the next action potential.

1.2 Molecular mechanism of contraction

The process by which depolarization of the muscle fiber initiates contraction is called excitation–contraction coupling[1]. The action potential is transmitted to all the fibrils in the fiber via the T system. It triggers the release of Ca^{2+} from the terminal cisterns and Ca^{2+} diffuse to thick and thin filaments. After binding of Ca^{2+} to troponin C, myosin–binding sites on actins are uncovered, then formation of cross–linkages between actin and myosin cause the sliding of thin on thick filaments, producing shortening. However, the mechanism of Ca^{2+} release from terminal cisterns in myocardial cells is different from that in skeletal cells.

The width of the A bands is constant, whereas the Z lines move closer together when the muscle contracts. The sliding during muscle contraction occurs when the myosin heads bind firmly to actin, bend at the junction of the head with the neck, and then detach. This "power stroke" depends on the simultaneous hydrolysis of ATP. There is still debate about the exact details. The myosin head detaches from actin, moves several nm along the actin strand, and reattaches. Many heads cycle at or near the same time, and they cycle repeatedly, producing gross muscle contraction. Each power stroke shortens the sarcomere about 10 nm. Each thick filament has about 500 myosin heads, and each of these cycles about five times per second during a rapid contraction.

To end contraction, Ca^{2+} must be actively transported into the longitudinal portions of the reticulum by Ca^{2+}–Mg^{2+} –ATPases. Once the Ca^{2+} concentration outside the reticulum has been lowered sufficiently, chemical interaction between myosin and actin ceases and the muscle relaxes. Note that ATP provides the energy for both contraction and relaxation. If transport of Ca^{2+} into the reticulum is inhibited, relaxation does not occur even though there are no more action potentials. The resulting sustained contraction is called a contracture.

---

[1] 兴奋－收缩耦联。

1.3 Single twitch and tetanus of skeletal muscle

A single action potential causes a brief contraction which is called a single twitch[1] with rapidly repetitive stimulation, the contractile mechanism is continuously activated and individual responses fuse into a continuous contraction which is known as a tetanus[2] or a tetanic contraction. It is a complete tetanus when there is no relaxation between contractions. It is an incomplete tetanus when there are periods of incomplete relaxation between contractions.

Muscular contraction involves shortening of the contractile elements, but because muscles have elastic and viscous elements in series with the contractile mechanism, it is possible for contraction to occur without an appreciable decrease in the length of the whole muscle. Such a contraction is called isometric contraction[3]. Contraction against a constant load,with approximation of the ends of the muscle,is isotonic contraction[4].

A single action potential causes a brief contraction followed by relaxation. This response is called a muscle twitch. Because the contractile mechanism does not have a refractory period, repeated stimulation before relaxation produces additional activation of the contractile elements. This phenomenon is known as summation of contractions. It can be categorized into based on the time interval of the stimulus given. The tension developed during summation is considerably greater than that during the single muscle twitch. With rapidly repeated stimulation activation of the contractile mechanism occurs repeatedly before any relaxation has occurred, and the individual responses fuse into one continuous contraction. Such a response is called a tetanus. It is a complete tetanus[5] when there is no relaxation between stimuli and an incomplete tetanus[6] when there are periods of incomplete relaxation between the summated stimuli.

The stimulation frequency at which summation of contractions occurs is determined by the twitch duration of the particular muscle being studied. When a series of maximal stimuli is delivered to skeletal muscle at a frequency just below the tetanizing frequency, there is an increase in the tension developed during each twitch until after several contractions, a uniform tension per contraction is reached. This phenomenon is known as treppe,or the "staircase" phenomenon. Treppe is believed to be due to increased availability of Ca^{2+} for binding to troponin C.

---

[1] 单收缩。

[2] 强直收缩。

[3] 等长收缩。

[4] 等张收缩。

[5] 完全强直收缩。

[6] 不完全强直收缩。

1.4 Factors influencing contractionefficiency of striated muscles

1.4.1 Effect of preload

Preload [1] is the load given to the muscle before its contraction. Preload elongates the muscle thus enabling it to contract in a pre–stretched state. Every muscle has its adequate pre-load or adequate initial length [2]. The initial length of a muscle has a strong influence on its contraction. A pre–loading muscle performs better than an after–loading or unloading muscle. The length of many of the muscles in the body at rest is the length at which they develop the maximal tension. At the resting length of a muscle (with a sarcomere spacing of 2.0 ~ 2.2μm), the maximum number of cross–bridges is utilized so that the force generated is maximal at this length.

1.4.2 Effect of afterload

Afterload [3] is the load given to the muscle after the beginning of contraction. When the afterload is zero, i. e., the muscle contracts freely without load, the velocity of contraction is at its maximum and is called V_{max}. It reflects the efficiency (or velocity) of the mechanical energy released by a single active crossbridge. It has been suggested that V_{max} be used as the index of contractility [4]. The muscle performs no work when the load is zero. When the afterload is above a certain level and the muscle is incapable of lifting it, the contraction is isometric. The tension developed during isometric contraction is the maximum that a muscle is capable of producing.Power is proportional to the number of active corss–bridges.The muscle performs no work during isometric contraction. When the afterload is below a certain level and the muscle is capable of lifting it, the contraction is isotonic. The muscle performs work during isotonic contraction, and the load at which maximum work is done per contraction is known as the optimum load. It is generally found to be approximately 40% of that which the muscle just cannot lift. As a rule, with the same strength of stimulus, a fairly well–loaded muscle does more work than one under–load or overloaded.

2 Smooth muscle

Smooth muscle can generally be divided into two major types: single–unit smooth muscle and multi–unit smooth muscle.The basic mechanism of contraction of smooth muscles is similar to that of skeletal muscles, but troponin has not been isolated. It appears that regulation of smooth muscle activity by calcium is mediated by calmodulin (with an amino acid sequence

[1] 前负荷。
[2] 初长度。
[3] 后负荷。
[4] 收缩性。

very similar to that of troponin C).

2.1 Singe–unit smooth muscle

Single–unit muscle cells, also called visceral smooth muscle, are usually arranged in sheets or bundles and the cell membranes contact each other at multiple points to form many gap junctions. Thus the fibers form a functional syncytium that usually contracts in large areas at once. This type of muscles is found in most of the organs of the body, especially in the walls of the gut, the bile ducts, the ureters, the uterus, and so forth. For this reason, this type of smooth muscle is also known as visceral smooth muscle. Many single–unit smooth muscles contract spontaneously and rhythmically. Single–unit smooth muscles are sensitive to stretch and respond with a depolarization of the cell membrane. The stretch sensitivity is a property of the smooth muscle cell itself and does not depend on the nervous elements within the tissue. Single–unit smooth muscles are innervated by autonomic nerves.

2.2 Multi–unit smooth muscle

This type of smooth muscle is composed of discrete smooth muscle fibers. Each fiber operates entirely independently of the others and is often innervated by a single nerve ending, resembling skeletal muscle fibers. Some examples of multi–unit smooth muscles found in the body are the smooth muscle fibers of the ciliary muscle of the eye, the iris of the eye, the pilo-erector muscles and the smooth muscle of many of the larger blood vessels.

The most important characteristic of multi–unit smooth muscle fibers is that their control is exerted almost entirely by nerve signals and very little by other stimuli such as local tissue factors. This is in contrast to a major share of the control of single–unit smooth muscle by non–nervous stimuli. An additional characteristic is that they rarely exhibit spontaneous contractions.

Chapter 3 BlOOD

The blood is an opaque, red liquid consisting of several types of cells suspended in a complex, amber fluid known as the plasma.[1] The whole blood belongs histologically to connective tissue[2] because its composition is similar to the typical characteristics of connective tissue, composed of fewer cells and larger amount of intercellular substance[3]. In the cardiovascular system, the constant flow of the blood keeps all the cells well dispersed throughout the plasma. The blood has multiple functions closely connected with its components and with the vascular system. The main function of the circulating blood is to carry oxygen and nutrients to the tissues and to remove carbon dioxide and waste products from the tissues. In addition, the blood transports other substances, such as hormones, from their sites of production to their sites of action. The blood also plays an important role in the distribution of water, solutes, and heat, and thus it contributes to homeostasis[4].

Section 1 The blood composition and physical and chemical properties

1 Blood composition and blood volume

Blood is composed of the plasma and blood cells. The cells are the red blood cells (RBC, erythrocytes), the white blood cells (WBC, leukocytes), and the platelets[5] (thrombocytes), which are not complete cells but cell fragments.

1.1 Hematocrit

The hematocrit is defined as the percentage of blood volume that is occupied by the blood

[1] 血液是一种不透明的红色的流体组织，由淡黄色的血浆和悬浮于其中的多种细胞组成。

[2] 结缔组织。

[3] 细胞间质。

[4] 稳态。

[5] 血小板。

cells[1]. It is measured by centrifuging (spinning at high speed) a sample of anticoagulated[2] blood. The red blood cells are forced to the bottom of the centrifuge tube, the plasma remains on top, and the white blood cells and platelets form a very thin interface between them, called buffy coat[3]. Hematocrit values of the blood of healthy adults are 40% ~ 50% for men and 37% ~ 48% for women. The hematocrit is an index of the relative amount of the red blood cells in the blood.[4]

1.2 Blood volume

The blood is normally confined to the circulation, including the heart and the pulmonary and systemic blood vessels. The total circulating blood volume accounts for 7% to 8% of the body weight of a healthy adult. It is normally 5.0 to 6.0 liters in men and 4.5 to 5.5 liters in women, depending on individual size.

The blood volume[5] is kept fairly constant. Obviously, there must initially be a balance between fluid intake and fluid output by urine, sweat, and the insensible loss of fluid through skin and lungs. It is of great significance for human body to maintain the stability of the total blood volume. The effects of blood loss depend on the amount and the rate of bleeding.[6] If blood loss is less than 10% of the total blood volume, blood volume can be recovered rapidly. If blood loss reaches 20%, blood pressure will decrease and organ ischemia[7] occurs. If blood loss is over 30%, shock[8] may develop.

2 The main components of plasma

The plasma is the liquid part of blood and is approximately 91% water. Plasma consists of a large number of organic and inorganic substances dissolved in water, including proteins, lipids (fats), carbohydrates, amino acids, vitamins, minerals, hormones, wastes, cofactors, gases, and electrolytes. The solutes in plasma play crucial roles in homeostasis, such as maintaining

---

[1] 血细胞比容是指血细胞在全血中所占的容积百分比。

[2] 抗凝的。

[3] 棕黄色的覆盖层。

[4] 血细胞比容主要反映血液中红细胞数量的相对值。

[5] 血量：机体内血液的总量。正常成人血量相当于自身体重的 7% ~ 8%。

[6] 失血对机体的影响取决于失血量和失血速度。

[7] 器官缺血。

[8] 休克：机体遭受强烈的致病因素侵袭后，由于有效循环血量锐减，机体失去代偿，组织缺血缺氧，神经 - 体液因子失调的一种临床症候群。其主要特点是：重要脏器组织中的微循环灌流不足，代谢紊乱和全身各系统的机能障碍。

normal plasma pH and osmolarity[1].

The plasma proteins (also termed colloids) constitute most of the plasma solutes, by weight[2]. According to salting out, they can be classified into three broad groups: the albumins, the globulins, and the fibrinogen[3]. The albumins are the most abundant of the three plasma protein groups and are synthesized by the liver. The globulins can also be divided into the alpha, beta and gamma globulins through electrophoresis. The alpha and beta globulins are also synthesized by the liver and act as carriers for molecules such as fats. The gamma globulins are antibodies produced by lymphocytes. Antibodies initiate the destruction of pathogens and provide us with immunity. In normal adult, the ratio of albumin to globulin is 1.5 ~ 2.0. Plasma proteins play several important roles, including transportation, immunity, maintenance of plasma colloid osmotic pressure, clotting function, buffering[4] and nutrition.

In addition to the organic solutes, including proteins, nutrients, metabolic wastes, the plasma contains a variety of mineral electrolytes. These ions contribute much less to the weight of the plasma than do the proteins, but in most cases they have much higher molar concentrations[5].This is because the molarity is a measure not of weight but of number of molecules or ions per unit volume[6]. Thus, there are many more ions than protein molecules, but the protein molecules are so large that a very small number of them greatly outweigh the much larger number of ions.

3 Blood physical and chemical properties

3.1 Density

The density (or specific gravity) of the blood is 1.050–1.060 g/mL, determined by the number of the red blood cells present. The density of the plasma is 1.025–1.030 g/mL, determined by the content of the plasma proteins.

3.2 Viscosity[7]

This means thickness or resistance to flow. While the blood is only slightly heavier than water, it is certainly much thicker. The viscosity of the blood is 3 to 4 times that of water,

---

[1] 渗透压。

[2] 血浆蛋白，又称为胶体物质，在质量上占血浆中溶质的大多数。

[3] 血浆蛋白分为三类：白蛋白、球蛋白和纤维蛋白原。

[4] 缓冲。

[5] 血浆中离子质量上少于血浆蛋白，但却有更高的摩尔浓度。

[6] 摩尔浓度测量的不是单位容积的分子或离子质量，而是数量。

[7] 黏滞性

whereas the viscosity of the plasma is 1.6 to 2.4 times that of water. Blood's viscosity increases as the total number of blood cells present increases and when the concentration of large molecules (macromolecules), mainly the plasma proteins, in the plasma increases [1].

3.3 Osmotic pressure

3.3.1 Osmosis and osmotic pressure

Osmosis is the net diffusion of solvent molecules (mainly water) across a selectively permeable membrane from a region of high water concentration to one that has a lower water concentration [2]. Cell membranes are relatively impermeable to most solutes but highly permeable to water (i.e., selectively permeable). When a solute is added to pure water, the concentration of water in the mixture is reduced. Thus, the higher the solute concentration in a solution, the lower the water concentration. Further, water diffuses from a region of low solute concentration (high water concentration) to one with a high solute concentration (low water concentration).

When a solution containing nonpenetrating solutes is separated from pure water by a membrane, the pressure that must be applied to the solution to prevent the net flow of water into the solution is termed the osmotic pressure of the solution [3]. The osmotic pressure exerted by the particles in a solution, whether they are molecules or ions, is determined by the number of the particles per unit volume of fluid, not by the mass or type of the particles [4]. Consequently, the factor that determines the osmotic pressure of a solution is the concentration of the solution. The total solute concentration of a solution is known as its osmolarity. The unit called the osmole is used to express the concentration of a solution in terms of numbers of particles [5]. One osmole (osm) is equal to 1 mole (mol) (6.02×10^{23}) of solute particles. Therefore, a solution containing 1 mole of glucose in each liter has a concentration of 1 osm/L. If a molecule dissociates into two ions (giving two particles), such as sodium chloride ionizing to give chloride and sodium ions, then a solution containing 1 mol/L will have an osmolar concentration of 2 osm/L. Thus, the term osmole refers to the number of permeable particles in a solution rather than to the molar concentration. The osmole is too large a unit for expressing osmotic activity of solutes in the body fluids. The unit milliosmole (mOsm), which equals 1/1000 osmole, is commonly used.

---

[1] 当血细胞数量增多和血浆中大分子物质（主要是血浆蛋白）浓度升高时，血液黏滞性增大。

[2] 渗透是指水等溶剂分子通过半透膜由高水浓度一侧向低水浓度一侧的扩散过程。

[3] 渗透压是指溶液中溶质颗粒所具有的吸引水分子透过半透膜的力量。

[4] 渗透压的大小与溶质颗粒数目的多少呈正比，而与溶质颗粒的大小和种类无关。

[5] 根据溶液中所含溶质颗粒的数量，采用渗作为单位来表示溶液的浓度。

3.3.2 Plasma osmotic pressure

The plasma osmotic pressure is normally about 300 mOsm/L. Low-molecular-weight solutes (also termed crystalloids[1]) in the plasma, which mostly are sodium and chloride, form the crystal osmotic pressure, accounting for about 99.6% of the plasma osmotic pressure because of large quantities. High-molecular-weight solutes known as the plasma proteins, especially the albumins, form the plasma colloid osmotic pressure[2] (also called oncotic pressure), which is about 1.3 mOsm/L.

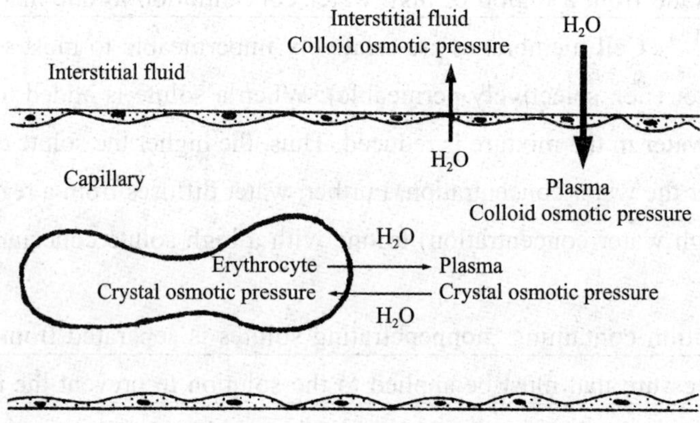

Figure 3-1 Plasma osmotic pressure

The plasma osmotic pressure includes the crystal osmotic pressure and the colloid osmotic pressure. Crystal osmotic pressure mainly regulates water distribution between intracellular and extracellular compartments; colloid osmotic pressure primarily controls intravascular and extravascular fluid distribution.

3.3.2.1 Crystal osmotic pressure

Since the capillary lining is highly permeable to all these crystalloids and water, their concentrations in the plasma and the interstitial fluid are essentially identical. Accordingly, there is no significant difference in the crystal osmotic pressure in the plasma and the interstitial fluid[3]. Because cell membranes are relatively impermeable to most solutes but highly permeable to water (i.e., selectively permeable), whenever there is a higher concentration of solute on one side of the cell membrane, water diffuses across the membrane toward the region of higher solute concentration. Thus, the distribution of fluid between intracellular and extracellular compartments is determined mainly by the crystal osmotic pressure (Figure 3-1)[4].

[1] 晶体。

[2] 血浆胶体渗透压。

[3] 晶体渗透压在血管内外没有明显的差别。

[4] 晶体渗透压主要调节细胞内外水分交换。

3.3.2.2 Colloid osmotic pressure

In contrast, the plasma proteins, being essentially non–permeating through the capillary, have a very low concentration in the interstitial fluid. The difference in protein concentration between the plasma and interstitial fluid means that the water concentration of the plasma is very slightly lower than that of interstitial fluid, inducing an osmotic flow of water from the interstitial compartment into the capillary. Therefore, the relative amounts of extracellular fluid distributed between the plasma and interstitial compartments are determined mainly by the balance of the colloid osmotic forces across the capillary membranes (Figure 3–1). [1]

3.3.3 Isotonic, hypotonic, and hypertonic fluids

If a cell is placed in a solution with solutes can not permeate the cellmembrane having an osmolarity of 282 mOsm/L, the cells will not shrink or swell because the water concentration in the intracellular and extracellular fluids is equal and the solutes cannot enter or leave the cell. Such a solution is said to be isotonic because it neither shrinks nor swells the cells. [2] Examples of isotonic solutions include a 0.9% solution of sodium chloride or a 5% glucose solution. [3] Solutions of sodium chloride with a concentration of less than 0.9% cent are hypotonic and cause cells to swell. Sodium chloride solutions of greater than 0.9% cent are hypertonic and cause cells to shrink.

Solutions with an osmolarity the same as the cell are called isosmotic [4], regardless of whether the solute can penetrate the cell membrane. The terms isotonic, hypotonic, and hypertonic refer to whether solutions will cause a change in cell volume. The tonicity of solutions depends on the concentration of impermeable solutes. [5] Some solutes, however, can permeate the cell membrane. Highly permeating substances, such as urea, can cause transient shifts in fluid volume between the intracellular and extracellular fluids, but given enough time, the concentrations of these substances eventually become equal in the two compartments and have little effect on intracellular volume under steady–state conditions.

3.4 Plasma pH

The normal pH range of the blood is 7.35 to 7.45, which is slightly alkaline. The main system that regulates the H^+ concentration in the body fluids is the chemical acid–base buffer systems [6] of the body fluids, which immediately combine with acid or base to prevent exces-

[1] 胶体渗透压主要调节毛细血管内外水分交换。

[2] 等张溶液是指能使悬浮于其中的细胞保持正常体积和形状的溶液。

[3] 0.9% 氯化钠溶液和 5% 葡萄糖溶液属于等张溶液。

[4] 等渗溶液是指渗透压与细胞内液渗透压相等的溶液。

[5] 张力大小取决于溶液中不能透过细胞膜的溶质颗粒的浓度。

[6] 酸碱缓冲对。

sive changes in H^+ concentration. The most important buffer system is the bicarbonate buffer system. This system consists of a water solution that contains two ingredients: a weak acid, H_2CO_3, and a bicarbonate salt, such as $NaHCO_3$. The phosphate buffer system and proteins are all play a major role in buffering. Venous blood normally has a lower pH than does arterial blood because of the presence of more carbon dioxide.

Section 2 Blood cell physiology

1 Red blood cell

1.1 The morphology and number of red blood cells

Normal human erythrocytes are round, biconcave–disk–shaped [1] and anuclear [2] structures with an average diameter of 7.5 μm and a thickness of 2μm at the edges and of 1μm or less in the middle. This shape gives them an optimal surface to volume ratio [3], favoring oxygen uptake and release (through short diffusion distances) and facilitating passive deformation during passage through narrow capillaries. The normal red cell count in a man is about $(4.5 \sim 5.5)\times10^{12}$/L, while in a woman it is $(3.8 \sim 4.6) \times 10^{12}$/L. Newborn can be as high as 6×10^{12}/L. The number of the erythrocytes depends on the oxygen needs of the body and the availability of oxygen in the lung. [4] For instance, persons living at high altitudes have greater numbers of the erythrocytes.

The content of the erythrocytes consists almost entirely of the red iron–containing pigment hemoglobin [5], which binds oxygen reversibly. The average concentration of hemoglobin is 120 ~ 160 g/L in a man and 110 ~ 150 g/L in a woman. When hemoglobin is oxygen enriched (arterialized blood) it appears bright red, while it appears dark red when oxygen–poor (venous blood).

If the formation or lifespan of the red cells is insufficient as a result of pathological processes, the result is anemia [6].

---

[1] 双凹圆盘形。

[2] 无核的。

[3] 表面积与体积比值。

[4] 红细胞数量受机体需氧量和肺内氧气的利用率影响。

[5] 血红蛋白。

[6] 贫血。

1.2 Physiological characteristics of red blood cells

1.2.1 Plastic deformation.

When the erythrocytes pass through capillaries or the pores of the sinusoids, their shape changes remarkably and can be rehabilitated after passing. This phenomenon is named plastic deformation [1] of the erythrocytes. The plastic deformation ability is directly proportional to the elasticity, fluidity and surface area of the erythrocyte membrane, and is inversely proportional to the viscosity of the erythrocytes (such as hemoglobin concentration or degeneration).

1.2.2 Osmotic fragility. The phenomenon of swelling, rupture and hemolysis [2] of erythrocytes in a hypotonic solution, known as osmotic fragility [3] of erythrocytes, indicates the ability of erythrocytes to resist the hypotonic solution. Degenerated erythrocytes have greater osmotic fragility.

If erythrocytes are suspended in an isotonic solution, their shape and size remain unchanged. When erythrocytes are suspended in the hypotonic fluids of different concentrations, the erythrocytes gradually expanded and deformed with the decrease of osmotic pressure. Normal erythrocytes begin to hemolysis in 0.42% NaCl solution, complete hemolysis in 0.35% NaCl solution.

Conversely, erythrocytes shrink in hypertonic solutions.

1.2.3 Suspension stability and erythrocyte sedimentation rate. The erythrocytes are stably suspended in the blood. The phenomenon is called the suspension stability [4] due to the repelling force by the same charge of the red cells. Since erythrocytes have a slightly higher density than the suspending plasma, they normally settle out of whole blood very slowly. When a blood sample to which an anticoagulant has been added stands in a narrow tube, the red cells form aggregates which gradually sediment leaving a clear zone of plasma above. The erythrocytes sedimentation rate (ESR) [5] is measured as the length of column of clear plasma after one hour. Erythrocytes in the blood of healthy men sediment at a rate of 0 ~ 15mm per hour; those in the blood of healthy women sediment slightly faster (0 ~ 20mm per hour). The ESR can be an important diagnostic index, as values are often significantly elevated during infection, in patients with arthritis, and in patients with inflammatory diseases. ESR fast is mainly due to the rouleaux formation of erythrocytes. The rouleaux refers to the phenomenon

[1] 可塑变形性。

[2] 溶血。

[3] 渗透脆性。

[4] 悬浮稳定性。

[5] 红细胞沉降率，简称血沉。

of multiple erythrocytes stacking or aggregating with each other. [1] After the occurrence of rouleaux, surface to volume ratio of erythrocytes decrease, plasma friction is also reduced, and then erythrocyte sedimentation rate is faster. The reasons for alterations in the ESR in disease states are the concentration of plasma proteins increasing, for example, fibrinogen, immunoglobulins, etc.

1.3 Physiological function of red blood cells

The major function of erythrocytes is to carry O_2 and CO_2. For more information, see Chapter 5.

The hemoglobin in the cells is an excellent acid–base buffer (as is true of most proteins), so that the red cells are responsible for most of the acid–base buffering power of the whole blood. [2]

1.4 The hematopoietic process in bone marrow

Hematopoiesis [3], the process of blood cell generation, occurs in healthy adults in the bone marrow and lymphatic tissues, such as the spleen, thymus, and lymph nodes. During fetal development, hematopoietic cells are present in high levels in the liver, spleen, and blood. Shortly before birth, blood cell production gradually begins to shit to the bone marrow. By age 20 years, the marrow in the cavities of many long bones becomes inactive, and blood cell production mainly occurs in the bones of the chest, the base of the skull, and the upper portions of the limbs. Within the bones, hematopoietic cells germinate in extravascular sinuses called marrow stroma. Active cellular marrow is called red marrow; inactive marrow that is infiltrated with fat is called yellow marrow.

Blood cell production begins with the proliferation of multipotent stem cells [4]. Depending on the stimulating factors, the progeny of multipotent stem cells may be other uncommitted stem cells or stem cells committed to development along a certain lineage. The committed stem cells include myeloblasts, which form cells of the myeloid series (neutrophils, basophils, and eosinophils), erythroblasts, lymphoblasts, and monoblasts. Promoted by hematopoietins [5] and other cytokines, each of these blast cells differentiates further, a process that ultimately results in the formation of mature blood cells. This is a highly dynamic process, also influenced by factors from capillary endothelial cells, stromal fibroblasts, and mature blood cells.

[1] 叠连是指红细胞互相堆积或聚集在一起。

[2] 红细胞能缓冲血液酸碱度。

[3] 造血。

[4] 多能干细胞。

[5] 促红细胞生成素。

The first cell that can be identified as belonging to the red blood cell series is the pro-erythroblast[1] (also called pronormoblast), formed from the erythroid progenitor cells under appropriate stimulation(Figure 3-2). Once the proerythroblast has been formed, it divides multiple times, eventually forming many mature red blood cells.

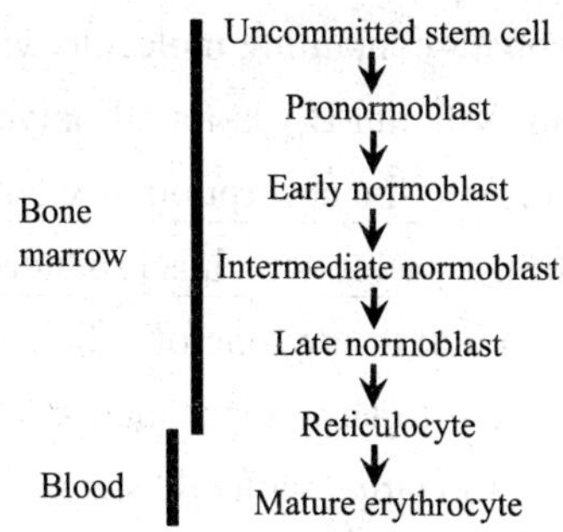

Figure 3-2 Erythropoiesis
Erythrocytes are the result of a process that begins with uncommitted stem cells and involves a series of differentiations in the bone marrow sinusoids until the final erythrocytes enter the bloodstream by diapedesis.

1.5 Erythropoiesis necessary material

The production and maturation of red blood cells requires many nutrients. Protein and iron are necessary for the synthesis of hemoglobin and become part of hemoglobin molecules. The folic acid and vitamin B_{12} are required for deoxyribonucleic acid (DNA) synthesis in the stem cells of the red bone marrow.

1.5.1 Iron

Iron is essential to the synthesis of hemoglobin.The total quantity of iron in the body averages 4 to 5 grams, about 65 per cent of which is in the form of hemoglobin. 15 to 30 per cent is stored for later use, mainly in the reticuloendothelial system[2] and liver parenchymal cells[3], principally in the form of ferritin[4].

As old erythrocytes are destroyed in the spleen (and liver), their iron is released into the plasma and bound to transferrin. Almost all of this iron is delivered by transferrin[5] to the bone marrow to be incorporated into new erythrocytes. In people who do not have adequate quantities of transferrin in their blood, failure to transport iron to the erythroblasts in this manner can cause severe hypochromic anemia (also called iron-deficiency anemia)—that is, red cells that contain much less hemoglobin than normal.

1.5.2 Folic acid and vitamin B_{12}

Folic acid is required for synthesis of the nucleotide base thymine[6]. It is, therefore, essential for the formation of DNA and thus for normal cell division. Folic acid is founded in large amounts in leafy plants, yeast, and liver.

The production of normal erythrocyte numbers also requires extremely small quantities of

---

[1] 原红细胞。

[2] 网状内皮系统。

[3] 肝细胞。

[4] 铁蛋白。

[5] 转铁蛋白。

[6] 胸腺嘧啶核苷酸。

a cobalt-containing molecule, vitamin B_{12}, since this vitamin is required for the action of folic acid. Vitamin B_{12} is found only in animal products, and strictly vegetarian diets are deficient in it. Also the absorption of vitamin B_{12} from the gastrointestinal tract requires a protein called intrinsic factor, which is produced by parietal cells of the stomach lining.[1]

Lack of any one of folic acid, vitamin B_{12} and intrinsic factor from the stomach mucosa can lead to slow reproduction of erythroblasts in the bone marrow. As a result, the red cells grow too large, with odd shapes, and are called megaloblasts[2], which have fragile membranes and rupture easily. Patients who have loss of the entire stomach after surgical total gastrectomy[3] or have intestinal sprue[4], in which folic acid and vitamin B_{12} are poorly absorbed, often develop megaloblastic anemia[5].

1.6 Regulation of erythropoiesis

The direct control of erythrocyte production is exerted primarily by a circulating hormone called erythropoietin[6], which is a glycoprotein with a molecular weight of about 34,000 and secreted mainly by a particular group of hormone-secreting connective tissue cells in the kidneys. The liver also secretes a much lesser of this hormone. Erythropoietin acts on the bone marrow to stimulate the proliferation of erythrocyte progenitor cells and their differentiation into mature erythrocytes.

Erythropoietin is normally secreted in relatively small amounts, which stimulate the bone marrow to produce erythrocytes at a rate adequate to replace the usual loss. The erythropoietin secretion rate is increased markedly above basal values when there is a decreased oxygen delivery to the kidneys. As a result of the increase in erythropoietin secretion, plasma erythropoietin concentration, erythrocyte production, and the oxygen-carrying capacity of the blood all increase. Therefore, oxygen delivery to the tissues returns toward normal.

Testosterone[7], the male sex hormone, also stimulates the release of erythropoietin. This accounts in part for the higher hematocrit in men than in women.

[1] 小肠对维生素 B_{12} 的吸收需依赖胃黏膜壁细胞分泌的内因子的帮助。

[2] 巨幼红细胞。

[3] 全胃切除术。

[4] 肠道性腹泻。

[5] 巨幼红细胞性贫血。

[6] 促红细胞生成素：英文缩写 EPO，同 hematopoietin。促红细胞生成素合成部位主要在肾，其次在肝细胞。它的生理作用是：促使造血干细胞向原红细胞转化；促进红细胞发育和血红蛋白合成；能促使成熟的红细胞释放入血。

[7] 睾酮，属雄激素。

1.7 Red blood cell destruction

The average life span of an erythrocyte is approximately 120 days, which means that almost 1 percent of the body's erythrocytes is destroyed and must be replaced every day. Erythrocyte destruction normally occurs in the spleen and the liver. Most of the iron released in the process is conserved. The major breakdown product of hemoglobin is bilirubin [1], which is returned to the circulation and gives plasma its characteristic yellowish color.

2 White blood cell

2.1 The number and classification of white blood cells count

The adult human being has about (4.0 ~ 10.0) $\times 10^9$ leukocytes per liter of blood. The number of white cells changes physiologically in a wide range: newborns are higher than adults; eating, pain, excited and strenuous exercise can increase it; during menstruation, pregnancy and childbirth, leukocytes of woman are increased too.

The various classes of leukocytes are classified according to their structure and affinity for the various dyes. According to whether there are special particles in the cytoplasm, the white blood cells can be divided into granulocytes [2] (mainly including neutrophils, eosinophils, basophils) and agranulocytes [3] (mainly including lymphocytes and monocytes) .

Of the total white blood cells, the normal percentages of the different types are approximately the following:

- Leukocytes
  - Granulocytes
    - Polymorphonuclear neutrophils 50%~70%
    - Polymorphonuclear eosinophils 0%~7%
    - Polymorphonuclear basophils 0%~1%
  - Agranulocytes
    - Monocytes 2%~8%
    - Lymphocytes 20%~40%

2.2 Physiological characteristics and functions of leukocytes

In addition to lymphocytes, leukocytes can squeeze through the pores of the blood capillaries by diapedesis [4]. Many different chemical substances in the tissues are released by the

---

[1] 胆红素：红棕色，主要在脾、骨髓及肝脏中由衰老红细胞中血红蛋白的辅基衍变而成，在血浆中以蛋白质复合物的形式运输，并以与葡萄糖醛酸结合的形式排泄至胆汁。

[2] 颗粒细胞主要包括中性粒细胞、嗜酸粒细胞、嗜碱粒细胞。

[3] 无颗粒细胞主要包括淋巴细胞和单核细胞。

[4] 渗出。

stimulation of bacteria, foreign bodies, etc, then leukocytes are attracted to the inflamed tissue areas by chemotaxis[1] and phagocytize these harmful substances.

2.2.1 Neutrophil The neutrophils are usually the most prevalent leukocyte in peripheral blood. In blood, one half of neutrophils is in circulation, the other half is adhesive to the capillary wall. Large amount of neutrophils is stored in the bone marrow. If it is needed, it can be immediately transferred from the bone marrow storage pool into the circulatory blood. They are the first defensive cell type to be recruited to a site of inflammation[2]. Defects in neutrophil function quickly lead to massive infection and, quite often, death. These cells respond instantly to microbial invasion by detecting foreign proteins or changes in host defense network proteins. Neutrophils provide an efficient defense against pathogens that have gotten past physical barriers such as the skin. Invading bacteria induce neutrophil migration to the site of infection by the release of chemotactic factors from the bacteria. And then they engulf the invading pathogen by the process of phagocytosis. A burst of metabolic events occurs in the neutrophil after phagocytosis. In the phagosome[3], the bacterium is exposed to enzymes that were originally positioned on the cell surface. Membrane–bound enzymes, activated when the phagocytic vacuole closes, work in conjunction with enzymes secreted from intracellular granules into the phagocytic vacuole[4] to destroy the invading pathogen efficiently.

2.2.2 Eosinophil[5]

Eosinophils are weak phagocytes, and they exhibit chemotaxis, but in comparison with the neutrophils, it is doubtful that the eosinophils are significant in protecting against the usual types of infection. Eosinophils, however, are often produced in large numbers in people with parasitic infections, and they migrate in large numbers into tissues diseased by parasites. Although most parasites are too large to be phagocytized by eosinophils or any other phagocytic cells, eosinophils attach themselves to the parasites by way of special surface molecules and release substances that kill many of the parasites.

Eosinophils also have a special propensity to collect in tissues in which allergic reactions occur, such as in the peribronchial tissues of the lungs in people with asthma and in the skin after allergic skin reactions. This is caused at least partly by the fact that many mast cells and basophils participate in allergic reactions. The mast cells and basophils release an eosinophil chemotactic factor that causes eosinophils to migrate toward the inflamed allergic tissue. The

---

[1] 趋化性是指白细胞具有趋向某些化学物质游走的特性。

[2] 中性粒细胞处在机体抵御微生物病原体的第一线，它可吞噬、水解细菌及坏死细胞，是炎症时的主要反应细胞。

[3] 吞噬小体。

[4] 吞噬泡。

[5] 嗜酸粒细胞的主要功能有：参与对蠕虫的免疫反应；限制嗜碱粒细胞和肥大细胞的致敏作用。

eosinophils are believed to detoxify some of the inflammation–inducing substances released by the mast cells and basophils and probably also to phagocytize and destroy allergen–antibody complexes, thus preventing excess spread of the local inflammatory process.

2.2.3 Basophil

The basophils in the circulating blood are similar to the large tissue mast cells located immediately outside many of the capillaries in the body. Both mast cells and basophils liberate heparin[1] into the blood, a substance that can prevent blood coagulation. The mast cells and basophils also release histamine, as well as smaller quantities of bradykinin[2] and serotonin[3]. Indeed, it is mainly the mast cells in inflamed tissues that release these substances during inflammation. The mast cells and basophils play an exceedingly important role in some types of allergic reactions because the type of antibody, the immunoglobulin E (IgE) type, that causes allergic reactions has a special propensity to become attached to mast cells and basophils. Then, when the specific antigen for the specific IgE antibody subsequently reacts with the antibody, the resulting attachment of antigen to antibody causes the mast cell or basophil to rupture and release exceedingly large quantities of histamine[4], bradykinin, serotonin, heparin, slow–reacting substance of anaphylaxis[5], and a number of lysosomal enzymes. These cause local vascular and tissue reactions that cause many, if not most, of the allergic manifestations.

2.2.4 Monocyte–macrophage

The monocytes are the largest of the leukocytes. Monocytes circulate in the bloodstream for about one to three days and then typically move into tissues throughout the body where many of them differentiate into macrophages, which are several times as phagocytic as neutrophils[6]. After entering the tissues, another large portion of monocytes becomes attached to the tissues and remains attached for months or even years until they are called on to perform specific local protective functions. When appropriately stimulated, they can break away from

---

[1] 肝素：由 D– 葡糖醛酸和 D– 氨基葡糖胺组成的一种酸性黏多糖，存在于许多组织内，尤以肝和肺为多，有很强的抗凝特性。

[2] 缓激肽：一种能引起多数平滑肌收缩但使小动脉和静脉扩张的 9 肽，可提高毛细血管通透性。

[3] 5– 羟色胺：是一种具有药理活性的速发型过敏性介质，由色氨酸转变而成，能引起血管扩张，毛细管渗透性增加和平滑肌收缩。

[4] 组胺：由组氨酸脱羧基形成，能引起血管舒张、毛细血管通透性增加及平滑肌收缩。

[5] 过敏性慢反应物质：可使支气管平滑肌痉挛收缩，血管通透性增加。其作用缓慢且持续时间较长，不被抗组胺药物所抑制。在过敏反应中，参与速发型超敏反应。

[6] 血液中的单核细胞尚未成熟。在血液中 1 ~ 3 天后，迁入组织转变为巨噬细胞。巨噬细胞进一步增大，吞噬能力大为增强。单核细胞和巨噬细胞二者相同但在部位不同名称不一样，共同构成单核巨噬细胞系统。

their attachments and once again become mobile macrophages that respond to chemotaxis and all the other stimuli related to the inflammatory process. Monocytes and macrophages have multiple tasks in the immune system and take part especially in nonspecific (Innate) immunity. Their function includes phagocytosis and intracellular destruction of bacteria, fungi, viruses, autologous damaged cells and other foreign particles in the tissue. If the particle is not digestible, the macrophages often form a "giant cell" capsule around the particle until such time—if ever—that it can be slowly dissolved. Such capsules are frequently formed around tuberculosis bacilli, silica dust particles, and even carbon particles. This walling–off process delays the spread of bacteria or toxic products. Beyond that they also take part in specific immunity, in that they pass information about foreign antigens to the lymphocytes. Thus, the body has a widespread "monocyte–macrophage system" in virtually all tissue areas. Monocytes and macrophages also produce a number of soluble factors (cytokines) that lead to the infiltration and activation of other cells of the nonspecific immune system.

2.2.5 Lymphocyte

Two basic but closely allied types of acquired immunity (adaptive immunity) occur in the body. In one of these, the body develops circulating antibodies, which are globulin molecules in the blood plasma that are capable of attacking the invading agent. This type of immunity is called humoral immunity[1] or B–cell immunity (because B lymphocytes produce the antibodies). The second type of acquired immunity is achieved through the formation of large numbers of activated T lymphocytes that are specifically crafted in the lymph nodes to destroy the foreign agent. This type of immunity is called cell–mediated immunity[2] or T–cell immunity (because the activated lymphocytes are T lymphocytes). T cells and B cells comprise 40 to 60% and 20 to 30% of the total circulating pool of lymphocytes respectively, and a less numerous third kind called natural killer cells. While B cells mediate immune responses by releasing antibody, T cells often exert their effects by synthesizing and releasing cytokines, hormone–like proteins that act by binding specific receptors on their target cells. Both T cells and B cells provide memory for immunity. Natural killer cells[3] destroy foreign cells by chemically rupturing their membranes.

[1] 体液免疫：由血液循环中的抗体所致的免疫，是以B淋巴细胞产生抗体来达到保护目的的免疫机制。

[2] 细胞免疫：T淋巴细胞受到抗原刺激后，增殖、分化、转化为致敏T细胞（也叫效应T细胞），当相同抗原再次进入机体的细胞中时，致敏T细胞对抗原的直接杀伤作用及致敏T细胞所释放的细胞因子的协同杀伤作用，统称为细胞免疫。

[3] 自然杀伤细胞：血液中存在一种小的类淋巴细胞。这种细胞能自然地杀死多种肿瘤细胞和病毒感染细胞，并受干扰素的作用而增强其活性。因其溶解细胞不依赖抗体，所以称为自然杀伤细胞。

2.3 Regulation of leukocyte production

All blood cells are descended from a single population of bone marrow cells called pluripotent hematopoietic stem cells, which are undifferentiated cells capable of giving rise to precursors[1] (progenitors) of any of the different blood cells. When a pluripotent stem cell divides, its two daughter cells either remain pluripotent stem cells or become committed to a particular developmental pathway. The first branching yields either lymphoid stem cells, which give rise to the lymphocytes, or so–called myeloid stem cells[2], the progenitors of all the other varieties. At some point, the proliferating offspring of the myeloid stem cells become committed to differentiate along only one path.

Proliferation and differentiation of the various progenitor cells is stimulated, at multiple points, by a large number of protein hormones and paracrine agents collectively termed hematopoietic growth factors[3] (HGFs). One example is the use of granulocyte colony stimulating factor[4] (G–CSF) to stimulate granulocyte production in individuals whose bone marrow has been damaged by anticancer drugs.

2.4 White blood cell life

The life of the granulocytes after being released from the bone marrow is normally 4 to 8 hours circulating in the blood and another 4 to 5 days in tissues where they are needed. In times of serious tissue infection, this total life span is often shortened to only a few hours because the granulocytes proceed even more rapidly to the infected area, perform their functions, and, in the process, are themselves destroyed. The monocytes also have a short transit time, 10 to 20 hours in the blood, before wandering through the capillary membranes into the tissues. Once in the tissues, they swell to much larger sizes to become tissue macrophages, and, in this form, can live for months unless destroyed while performing phagocytic functions. There is continual circulation of lymphocytes through the body. The lymphocytes have life spans of weeks or months; this life span depends on the body's need for these cells.

---

[1] 祖细胞。

[2] 骨髓干细胞。

[3] 造血生长因子：能使造血前体细胞分化增殖的生物分子，主要作用是调节机体的造血功能。

[4] 粒细胞集落刺激因子：一种主要由单核吞噬细胞在受到 γ－干扰素、α－肿瘤坏死因子或脂多糖刺激后产生的细胞因子。主要作用于粒细胞系造血细胞的增殖、分化和活化。临床主要用于预防和治疗肿瘤放疗或化疗后引起的白细胞减少症等。

3 Blood platelet

3.1 Platelet morphology and number

Platelets, also called thrombocytes, are minute discs 1 to 4 micrometers in diameter. The circulating platelets are not complete cells but colorless cell fragments from megakaryocytes[1].

A normal platelet count is normally about (100 ~ 300) $\times 10^9$ in each liter of blood. Their number may change significantly. For example, after the hard physical work the number of platelets is increased 3 ~ 5 times. It is increased also after the meal or under the influence of emotions. The platelets number is more in the day–time than at night. These changes may be connected with the rhythm of work and rest. Thrombocytopenia[2] is the term for a low platelet count.

3.2 Physiological characteristics

Platelet activation results in the sequential responses of adherence, aggregation (sticking together), and secretion[3].

Platelet adherence can be initiated by a variety of substances. For instance, factors released by platelets cause the upregulation of adherence proteins (integrins[4]) on endothelial cells. Ruptured cells at the site of tissue injury release adenosine diphosphate[5] (ADP), causing the aggregation of more platelets, which are, in turn, stabilized by fibrinogen.

Binding of platelets to collagen triggers the platelets to release the contents of their secretory vesicles, which contain a variety of chemical agents. Many of these agents, including ADP and serotonin, then act locally to induce multiple changes in the metabolism, shape, and surface proteins of the platelets, a process termed platelet activation, which introduces positive feedback. Some of these changes cause platelet aggregation, which rapidly creates a platelet plug inside the vessel. Chemical agents in the platelets' secretory vesicles are not the only stimulators of platelet activation and aggregation. Adhesion of the platelets rapidly induces them to synthesize thromboxane A_2[6]. Thromboxane A_2 is released into the extracellular fluid

---

[1] 血小板不是完整的细胞，是从骨髓中成熟的巨核细胞胞浆裂解、脱落下来的具有生物活性的小块胞质，呈梭形或椭圆形。

[2] 血小板减少症。

[3] 血小板的的生理特性：黏附、聚集和释放反应。

[4] 整合素：是一种细胞表面受体，对细胞和细胞外基质的黏附起介导作用。

[5] 二磷酸腺苷：是引起血小板聚集最重要的物质。

[6] 血栓烷 A_2：可使血管平滑肌收缩，可以激活血小板并能使其聚集。

and acts locally to further stimulate platelet aggregation and release of their secretory vesicle contents.

The platelet plug can completely seal small breaks in blood vessel walls. Its effectiveness is further enhanced by another property of platelets—contraction. Platelets contain a very high concentration of actin and myosin, which are stimulated to contract in aggregated platelets. This results in a compression and strengthening of the platelet plug.

3.3 Function of platelets

3.3.1 Participating in physiological hemostasis[1]

When a vessel is severed or ruptured, the bleeding occurs and leads to blood loss. Prevention of blood loss is called hemostasis. Platelets involved in the whole process of hemostasis.

3.3.1.1 Vascular constriction (vasoconstriction)

When a blood vessel is severed or otherwise injured, its immediate inherent response is to constrict by contraction of the smooth muscle in the vessel wall. This short–lived response slows the flow of blood in the affected area. In addition, this constriction presses the opposed endothelial surfaces of the vessel together, and this contact induces stickiness capable of keeping them "glued" together. The vascular smooth muscle contraction results from: local myogenic spasm; local autacoid factors[2] from the traumatized tissues and blood platelets; and nervous reflexes.

3.3.1.2 Formation of a platelet plug

When platelets come in contact with a damaged vascular surface, especially with collagen fibers in the vascular wall, the platelets themselves immediately change their own characteristics drastically. Therefore, at the site of any opening in a blood vessel wall, the damaged vascular wall activates successively increasing numbers of platelets that themselves attract more and more additional platelets, thus forming a platelet plug. This is at first a loose plug, but it is usually successful in blocking blood loss if the vascular opening is small. At this stage the activated platelets change their shape, liberate substances from vesicles in which they were stored, including a vasoconstrictor serotonin, and initiate the formation of the actual clot (thrombus)[3] by aggregation.

3.3.1.3 Formation of a blood clot as a result of blood coagulation

The clot begins to develop in 15 to 20 seconds if the trauma to the vascular wall has been severe. Activator substances from the traumatized vascular wall, from platelets, and from

[1] 止血。

[2] 自体有效物质：体内自然存在的一类物质。对细胞有激素或类似激素的活性，作用于体内的限定部位。如组胺、5-羟色胺、血管紧张肽及前列腺素等。

[3] 血栓。

blood proteins adhering to the traumatized vascular wall initiate the clotting process. Within 3 to 6 minutes after rupture of a vessel, if the vessel opening is not too large, the entire opening or broken end of the vessel is filled with clot.

3.3.2 Promoting coagulation

The cell membrane of the platelets is a coat of glycoproteins that repulses adherence to normal endothelium and yet causes adherence to injured areas of the vessel wall. The platelet membrane contains large amounts of phospholipids[1] that activate multiple stages in the blood-clotting process. In addition, platelets secret many procoagulant factors[2], such as factor I, to promote coagulation.

3.3.3 Repairing of vascular wall

Platelets can be integrated into vascular endothelial cells, thereby maintaining vascular barrier.

Section 3 Blood coagulation and fibrinolysis

1 Blood coagulation

Blood coagulation[3], or clotting, is the transformation of blood into a solid gel termed a clot or thrombus and consisting mainly of a protein polymer known as fibrin.

Within a few minutes after a clot is formed, it begins to contract and usually expresses most of the fluid from the clot within 20 to 60 minutes. The fluid expressed is called serum[4] because all its fibrinogen and most of the other clotting factors have been removed as a result of clotting; in this way, serum differs from plasma. Serum cannot clot because it lacks these factors.

1.1 Coagulation factors

Substances participating in the blood coagulation are called coagulation factors[5] (Table 3-1). They are referred to by number (designated by a Roman numeral) in a sequence based

[1] 血小板磷脂：可促使凝血的发生。

[2] 促凝因子，如凝血因子Ⅰ、血小板因子。

[3] 血液凝固：指血液由流动状态变成不能流动的胶冻状凝块的过程，简称为凝血。

[4] 血清：为血液凝血后血凝块收缩析出的清澈淡黄色液体。与血浆的主要区别是不含纤维蛋白原，但增加了少量在凝血过程中血小板释放出来的物质和激活了的凝血因子。

[5] 凝血因子：指血液和组织中直接参与凝血的物质。由国际凝血因子命名委员会根据其被发现的先后次序，用罗马数字编号为 12 种（Ⅰ~ⅩⅢ，其中Ⅵ是已活化的Ⅴ，不再视为单独的因子）凝血因子。此外还有前激肽释放酶、高分子量激肽原及血小板磷脂等。

on the order of the discovery of each factor. Coagulation factors but III released from injured tissue, exist in the blood. Many coagulation factors except IV and platelet phospholipid, are proteins mostly produced by the liver. Factor II, VII, IX and X are vitamin–K dependent factors. In normal state, Factor II, VII, IX, X, XI, XII and XIII are inactive in the blood, but they can be activated into active forms and can be expressed by adding ‘a’ in the right foot of these factors.

Table 3–1 Clotting factors in blood and their synonyms

Clotting Factor	Synonyms
Factor I	Fibrinogen
Factor II	Prothrombin[1]
Factor III	Tissue factor[2]; tissue thromboplastin
Factor IV	Calcium
Factor V	Proaccelerin; labile factor; accelerator globulin
Factor VII	Serum prothrombin conversion accelerator (SPCA); proconvertin; stable factor
Factor VIII	Antihemophilic factor (AHF); antihemophilic globulin (AHG); antihemophilic factor A
Factor IX	Plasma thromboplastin component (PTC); christmas factor; antihemophilic factor B
Factor X	Stuart factor; stuart–Prower factor
Factor XI	Plasma thromboplastin antecedent (PTA); antihemophilic factor C
Factor XII	Hageman factor; glass factor
Factor XIII	Fibrin–stabilizing factor; Laki–Lorand factor
PK	Prekallikrein; fletcher factor
HMWK	Fitzgerald factor; high–molecular–weight kininogen
PL	Platelet phospholipid; platelet factor (PF)

1.2 Blood coagulation process

Blood coagulation is mediated by the sequential activation of a series of coagulation factors, proteins synthesized in the liver that circulate in the plasma in an inactive state. The sequential activation of a series of inactive molecules resulting in a biological response is called a metabolic cascade. The sequential activation of coagulation factors resulting in the conversion of fibrinogen to fibrin (and, hence, clotting) is called the coagulation cascade[3].

[1] 凝血酶原。

[2] 组织因子。

[3] 瀑布学说：凝血是一系列循序发生的酶促反应过程，只要始动因子被激活，凝血过程将依次发生，最终使血浆中可溶性的纤维蛋白原转变为不溶性的纤维蛋白多聚体，交织网罗血细胞而形成血凝块。

Blood coagulation takes place in three essential steps[1] (Figure 3–3): ① In response to rupture of the vessel or damage to the blood itself, a complex cascade of chemical reactions occurs in the blood involving more than a dozen blood coagulation factors. The net result is formation of a complex of activated substances collectively called prothrombin activator[2]. ② The prothrombin activator catalyzes conversion of prothrombin into thrombin. ③ The thrombin acts as an enzyme to convert fibrinogen into fibrin fibers that enmesh platelets, blood cells, and plasma to form the clot.

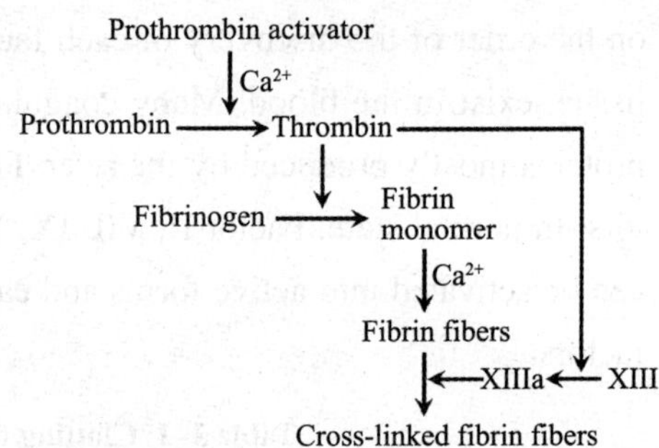

Figure 3–3 Schema for conversion of prothrombin to thrombin and polymerization of fibrinogen to form fibrin fibers

Clot retraction[3] is a phenomenon that may occur within minutes or hours after clot formation. Platelets are necessary for clot retraction to occur.

Prothrombin activator is generally considered to be formed in two ways,[4] although, in reality, the two ways interact constantly with each other: ① by the endogenous or intrinsic pathway that begins in the blood itself and ② by the extrinsic pathway that begins with trauma to the vascular wall and surrounding tissues.

1.2.1 Endogenous coagulation pathway

Trauma to the blood or exposure of the blood to vascular wall collagen alters two important clotting factors in the blood: Factor XII and the platelets. When Factor XII is disturbed, such as by coming into contact with collagen or with a wettable surface such as glass, it takes on a new molecular configuration that converts it into a proteolytic enzyme called “activated Factor XII”. Simultaneously, the blood trauma also damages the platelets because of adherence to either collagen or a wettable surface (or by damage in other ways), and this releases platelet phospholipids that contain the lipoprotein called platelet factor 3, which also plays a role in subsequent clotting reactions.

The activated Factor XII acts enzymatically on Factor XI to activate this factor as well, which is the second step in the intrinsic pathway. This reaction also requires HMW (high-molecular-weight) kininogen[5] and is accelerated by prekallikrein[6].

[1] 凝血过程分为三个基本步骤：凝血酶原激活物形成；凝血酶原转变成凝血酶；纤维蛋白原转变成纤维蛋白。

[2] 凝血酶原激活物：是由激活的因子 X、V，血小板磷脂和钙离子等形成的复合物。

[3] 血凝块回缩：此过程必须依赖血小板收缩蛋白的收缩反应，同时加固了血凝块。

[4] 根据凝血酶原激活物形成途径的不同，凝血过程可分为内源性凝血和外源性凝血。

[5] 高分子量激肽原。

[6] 前激肽释放酶。

The activated Factor XI then acts enzymatically on Factor IX to activate this factor also.

The activated Factor IX, acting in concert with activated Factor VIII and with the platelet phospholipids and factor 3 from the traumatized platelets, activates Factor X. It is clear that when either Factor VIII or platelets are in short supply, this step is deficient. Factor VIII is the factor that is missing in a person who has classic hemophilia [1], for which reason it is called antihemophilic factor. Platelets are the clotting factor that is lacking in the bleeding disease called thrombocytopenia.

The activated Factor X (Xa) combines immediately with platelet phospholipids as well as with Factor V to form the complex called prothrombin activator. Note especially the positive feedback effect of thrombin, acting through Factor V, to accelerate the entire process once it begins (Figure 3–4). Because the clotting factors in this pathway are all derived from plasma, they are called endogenous clotting pathways.

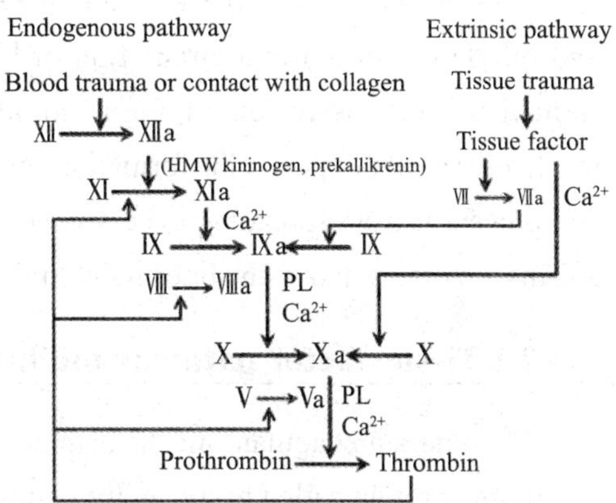

Figure 3–4 Two clotting pathways–called endogenous and extrinsic–merge and can lead to the generation of thrombin PL:platelet phospholipid

1.2.2 Extrinsic coagulation pathway

The extrinsic pathway for initiating the formation of prothrombin activator begins with a traumatized vascular wall or traumatized extravascular tissues that come in contact with the blood (Upper right of Figure 3–4). This pathway begins with a protein called tissue factor or tissue thromboplastin [2], which is a complex of several factors released by traumatized tissue. This factor is composed especially of phospholipids from the membranes of the tissue plus a lipoprotein complex that functions mainly as a proteolytic enzyme.

The lipoprotein complex of tissue factor further complexes with blood coagulation Factor VII and, in the presence of Ca^{2+}, acts enzymatically on Factor X to form Xa. In addition, it catalyzes the activation of factor IX, which can then help activate even more factor X by plugging into the intrinsic pathway.

An especially important difference between the extrinsic and endogenous pathways is that the extrinsic pathway can be explosive; [3] once initiated, its speed of completion to the final clot is limited only by the amount of tissue factor released from the traumatized tissues and

[1] 血友病：为一组遗传性凝血功能障碍的出血性疾病，其共同特征是活性凝血活酶生成障碍，凝血时间延长，终身具有轻微创伤后出血倾向，重症患者没有明显外伤也可发生自发性出血。

[2] 组织凝血活酶。

[3] 相对于内源性凝血，外源性凝血过程非常迅速。

by the quantities of Factors X, VII, and V in the blood. With severe tissue trauma, clotting can occur in as little as 15 seconds. The endogenous pathway is much slower to proceed, usually requiring 1 to 6 minutes to cause clotting.

2 Anticoagulation

Clotting should take place to stop bleeding, but too much clotting would obstruct vessels and interfere with normal circulation of blood. The body has mechanisms for limiting clot formation itself and for dissolving a clot after it has formed. There are at least four different mechanisms that oppose clot formation, once underway, thereby helping to limit this process and prevent it from spreading excessively. Defects in any of these natural anticoagulant mechanisms are associated with abnormally high risk of clotting (hypercoagulability [1]).

2.1 Tissue factor pathway inhibitor

The first anticoagulant mechanism acts during the initiation phase of clotting and utilizes the plasma protein called tissue factor pathway inhibitor (TFPI)[2], which is secreted mainly by endothelial cells. This substance binds to tissue factor–factor VIIa complexes and inhibits the ability of these complexes to generate factor Xa. This anticoagulant mechanism is the reason that the extrinsic pathway by itself can generate only small amounts of thrombin.

2.2 Thrombin

The second anticoagulant mechanism is triggered by thrombin. Thrombin can bind to an endothelial cell receptor known as thrombomodulin. This binding eliminates all of thrombin's clot–producing effects and causes the bound thrombin to bind a particular plasma protein, protein C [3]. The binding to thrombin activates protein C, which, in combination with yet another plasma protein, then inactivates factors VIIIa and Va. Thus, we saw earlier that thrombin directly activates factors VIII and V, and now we see that it indirectly inactivates them via protein C.

---

[1] 高凝状态。

[2] 组织因子途径抑制物：是体内主要的生理性抗凝物质，主要来自小血管内皮细胞的一种糖蛋白，其凝血机制一是与X a结合，直接抑制X a的活性，二是在 Ca^{2+} 存在的前提下，TEPI- X a复合物与TF- Ⅶ a复合物结合，从而灭活TF- Ⅶ a的活性，发挥抑制凝血作用。

[3] 蛋白质C：是一种维生素K依赖因子，主要由肝脏合成。以酶原的形式存在于血浆中，在凝血过程中被激活。主要作用是：通过灭活因子Ⅴ a、Ⅷ a，阻碍因子X a与血小板磷脂膜的结合；刺激纤溶酶原激活物的释放，增强纤溶酶活性，促进纤维蛋白溶解。

2.3 Antithrombin III

A third naturally occurring anticoagulant mechanism is an alpha–globulin called antithrombin III[1] or antithrombin–heparin cofactor[2], which inactivates thrombin and several other clotting factors. To do so, circulating antithrombin III must itself be activated, and this occurs when it binds to heparin, a substance that is present on the surface of endothelial cells. Antithrombin III prevents the spread of a clot by rapidly inactivating clotting factors that are carried away from the immediate site of the clot by the flowing blood.

2.4 Heparin

The fourth anticoagulant is heparin[3], but its concentration in the blood is normally low, so that only under special physiologic conditions does it have significant anticoagulant effects. However, heparin is used widely as a pharmacological agent in medical practice in much higher concentrations to prevent intravascular clotting.

The coagulability of blood can be reduced by medications such as oxalates[4] and dicumarol[5] (e. g., dicumarin, warfarin[6]). Clotting can be prevented if Ca^{2+} is removed from the blood by the addition of substances such as oxalates, which form insoluble salts with Ca^{2+}, or chelating agents binding Ca^{2+}.

3 Fibrinolysis and anti – fibrinolysis

3.1 Fibrinolysis

3.1.1 Process of fibrinolysis

Fibrinolysis[7] is the process of breaking down the product of coagulation, a fibrin clot.

---

[1] 抗凝血酶Ⅲ：是肝脏和血管内皮细胞合成的脂蛋白。能与凝血酶结合形成复合物，使凝血酶失去活性；能使激活的因子Ⅶa、Ⅸa、Ⅹa、Ⅺa、Ⅻa失活。

[2] 抗凝血酶肝素辅助因子。

[3] 肝素：是由肥大细胞和嗜碱粒细胞产生的一种酸性黏多糖。其主要作用是：与抗凝血酶Ⅲ结合，能显著增强抗凝血酶Ⅲ与凝血酶的亲合力，并使二者的结合更稳定，从而促使凝血酶失活；能抑制凝血酶原被激活，阻止血小板的黏着、聚集、释放反应，促使血管内皮细胞释放凝血抑制物和纤溶酶原激活物。

[4] 草酸盐。

[5] 双香豆素。

[6] 华法林：是香豆素类抗凝剂的一种，在体内有对抗维生素 K 的作用。

[7] 纤维蛋白溶解：简称纤溶，指纤维蛋白或纤维蛋白原在纤维蛋白溶解酶的作用下，被降解液化的过程。其生理意义是：使血液经常保持液态，血流通畅，防血栓形成。

The fibrinolytic (or thrombolytic) system is the principal effector of clot removal. The physiology of this system is analogous to that of the clotting system. The plasma proteins contain a euglobulin [1] called plasminogen [2] (or profibrinolysin) that, when activated becomes a substance called plasmin [3] (or fibrinolysin). Plasmin is a proteolytic enzyme that resembles trypsin [4] the most important proteolytic digestive enzyme of pancreatic secretion. Plasmin digests fibrin fibers and some other protein coagulants such as fibrinogen Factor V, Factor VIII, prothrombin, and Factor XII Therefore, whenever plasmin is formed, it can cause lysis of a clot by destroying many of the clotting factors, thereby sometimes even causing hypocoagulability of the blood (Figure 3–5).

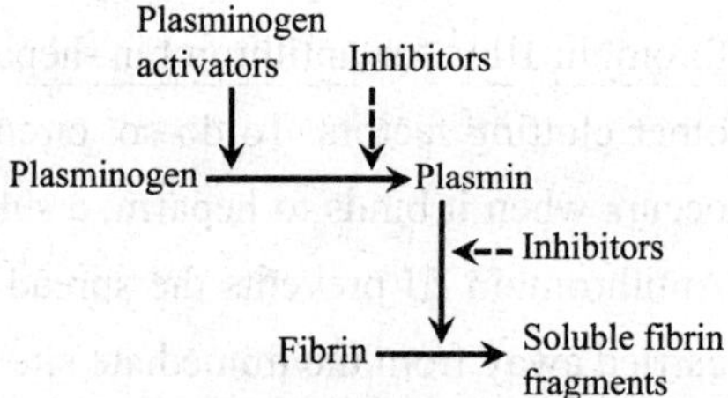

Figure 3–5 Basic fibrinolytic system. There are many different plasminogen activators and many different pathways for bringing them into play.

3.1.2 Plasminogen activators

Plasminogen activators or tissue kinase are widely distributed and of various sorts. Mainly there are three types. The first type is depending on the activity of XII, which can activate the tissue prokinase into kinase. The second type is a tissue activator contained in many tissues. It is released mainly during tissue repairing and wound healing. The urokinase [5], also known as urokinase–type plasminogen activator (u-PA), released by kidney is a representative. The third type is a vessel activator which is synthesized and released in the endothelium of the vessel. It is released whenever there is a clot formation in the vessel canal. The injured vascular endothelium very slowly release a powerful activator called tissue plasminogen activator (t–PA) [6] that a few days later, after the clot has stopped the bleeding, eventually converts plasminogen to plasmin, which in turn removes the remaining unnecessary blood clot. In fact, many small blood vessels in which blood flow has been blocked by clots are reopened by this mechanism. Thus, an especially important function of the plasmin system is to remove minute clots from millions of tiny peripheral vessels that eventually would become occluded were there no way to clear them.

---

[1] 优球蛋白。

[2] 纤维蛋白溶解酶原，简称纤溶酶原。

[3] 纤维蛋白溶解酶，简称纤溶酶。

[4] 胰蛋白酶。

[5] 尿激酶。

[6] 组织型纤溶酶原激活物。

3.2 Inhibitors of fibrinolysis

Plasminogen activators can be inhibited by plasminogen activator inhibitor–1 (PAI–1), plasminogen activator inhibitor–2 (PAI–2), protein C inhibitor, alpha–2–antiplasmin (or α_2–antiplasmin or plasmin inhibitor) and alpha–2–macroglobulin (or α_2– macroglobulin).

PAI–1, also known as endothelial plasminogen activator inhibitor[1] or serpin[2] E1, is mainly produced by the endothelium, but is also secreted by other tissue types, such as adipose tissue. PAI–1 is a serine protease inhibitor (serpin) that functions as the principal inhibitor of u–PA and t–PA. PAI–1 inhibits u–PA via active site binding, preventing the formation and mediating the degradation of plasmin.

PAI–2 (placental PAI), a serine protease inhibitor of the serpin superfamily, is a coagulation factor that inactivates t–PA and u–PA. It is present only at detectable quantities in blood during pregnancy, as it is produced by the placenta, and may explain partially the increased rate of thrombosis during pregnancy.

Protein C inhibitor, which limits the activity of protein C, is also a serine protease inhibitor inactivating t–PA.

Alpha–2–antiplasmin[3], which is produced mainly by the liver, is also a serine protease inhibitor responsible for inactivating plasmin.

Alpha–2–macroglobulin[4] is a large plasma protein found in the blood. It is produced mainly by the liver. Alpha–2–macroglobulin acts as an antiprotease and is able to inactivate an enormous variety of proteinases. It functions as an inhibitor of fibrinolysis by inhibiting plasmin and kallikrein.

Section 4 Blood types and blood transfusion

1 Blood type

Blood type[5] (also called a blood group) is a classification of blood based on the presence or absence of inherited antigenic substances on the surface of the red blood cells. The surface

[1] 纤溶酶原激活物抑制物。

[2] 丝氨酸蛋白酶抑制剂。

[3] α_2– 抗纤溶酶：由肝脏合成，平时储存于血小板的 α 颗粒中，是循环血液中纤溶酶的主要抑制物。

[4] α_2– 巨球蛋白：由肝细胞与单核吞噬细胞系统中合成，是血浆中分子量最大的蛋白质。它能与多种蛋白水解酶结合而影响这些酶的活性。

[5] 血型：指血细胞膜上特异凝集原的类型。一般是指红细胞血型。

membrane of erythrocytes contains a large number of various saccharides (glycolipids, glycoproteins), the so-called blood group antigens. They are called antigens because in foreign organisms they induce the formation of antibodies. Antibodies in the plasma of one blood type will react with antigens on the surfaces of the red cells of another blood type. At this point, red blood cells condense into clusters. This phenomenon is called red cell agglutination[1]. Human blood contains more than 100 such antigens, of which especially the ABO and Rh systems are of clinical importance.

1.1 ABO blood group system

1.1.1 Classification of ABO blood group system

Two antigens—type A and type B—occur on the surfaces of the red blood cells in a large proportion of human beings. The ABO (O = none) system[2] consists of four blood groups: erythrocytes with the A antigen (blood group A), the B antigen (blood group B), antigens A and B (blood group AB), or neither antigen (blood group O) (Table 3–2). Additionally, plasma contains antibodies against whichever antigen is missing, i.e., persons with blood group A have antibodies against B (anti–B). Correspondingly, the plasma of blood of group B contains antigens against A (anti–A). In the case of blood group AB, the plasma contains neither antibody; and blood group O plasma contains both anti–A and anti–B.

Table 3–2 Human ABO blood groups

Blood group	Antigen on RBC	Genetic possibilities	Antibody in blood
A	A	AA、AO	Anti–B
B	B	BB、BO	Anti–A
AB	A and B	AB	Neither anti–A nor anti–B
O	Neither A nor B	OO	Both anti–A and anti–B

Unlike normal antibody formation, the formation of antibodies of the ABO system does not require contact with foreign antigens. They develop in the first months of life. Because of their agglutinating effect they are also called agglutinins[3], while the erythrocyte antigens are called agglutinogens[4].

[1] 凝集反应：指某一血型的红细胞和与其对应的凝集素相遇时，红细胞彼此聚集黏合在一起，成为一簇簇不规则的细胞团的现象。凝集的红细胞可以堵塞毛细血管，产生的大量血红蛋白将损害肾小管，同时伴有过敏反应，严重者危及生命。

[2] ABO 血型系统分型依据是红细胞膜上是否存在 A 凝集原和（或）B 凝集原。

[3] 凝集素：指能与凝集原结合的特异抗体。

[4] 凝集原：指红细胞膜上的抗原物质（糖蛋白或糖脂上的寡糖链）。

1.1.2 ABO blood group inheritance

Two genes, one on each of two paired chromosomes, determine the O–A–B blood type. These genes can be any one of three types but only one type on each of the two chromosomes: type O, type A, or type B. The type O gene is either functionless or almost functionless, so that it causes no significant type O agglutinogen on the cells. Conversely, the type A and type B genes do cause strong agglutinogens on the cells. The six possible combinations of genes, as shown in Table 3–2, are OO, AO, BO, AA, BB, and AB. These combinations of genes are known as the genotypes, and each person is one of the six genotypes. One can also observe from Table 3–2 that a person with genotype OO produces no agglutinogens, and therefore the blood type is O. A person with genotype AO or AA produces type A agglutinogens and therefore has blood type A. Genotypes BO and BB give type B blood, and genotype AB gives type AB blood.

The ABO blood group system is inherited according to Mendelian laws [1], and therefore the possible blood groups of children can be predicted if the blood groups of the parents are known (Table 3–3).

Table 3–3 Genetic relationship of ABO blood group

One of parents	Another of parents	Child's possible blood group	Child's impossible blood group
A	A	A、O	B、AB
B	B	B、O	A、AB
A	B	A、B、O、AB	
AB	A	A、B、AB	O
AB	B	A、B、AB	O
O	A	O、A	B、AB
O	B	O、B	A、AB
O	AB	A、B	O、AB
AB	AB	A、B、AB	O
O	O	O	A、B、AB

1.2 Rh blood group system

There are six common types of Rh antigens[2], called an Rh factors, among which the type D antigen is widely prevalent in the population and considerably more antigenic than the other

[1] 孟德尔定律：由奥地利遗传学家格里哥·孟德尔在 1865 年发表并催生了遗传学诞生的著名定律。他揭示出遗传学的两个基本定律——分离定律和自由组合定律，统称为孟德尔遗传规律。

[2] Rh 血型抗原：与临床关系密切有 C、c、D、d、E、e 六种抗原，以 D 抗原的抗原性最强。有 D 抗原为 Rh 阳性 (Rh^+)，无 D 抗原为 Rh 阴性 (Rh^-)。

Rh antigens. Anyone who has this type of antigen is said to be Rh positive (Rh+), whereas a person who does not have type D antigen is said to be Rh negative(Rh–). Rh positive in Han nationality and most other ethnic groups in China accounted for about 99%, Rh negative only 1%.

If an Rh–negative person has never before been exposed to Rh–positive blood, transfusion of Rh–positive blood into that person will likely cause no immediate reaction.[1] However, anti–Rh antibodies can develop in sufficient quantities during the next 2 to 4 weeks to cause agglutination of those transfused cells that are still circulating in the blood. These cells are then hemolyzed by the tissue macrophage system. Thus, a delayed transfusion reaction occurs, although it is usually mild. On subsequent transfusion of Rh–positive blood into the same person, who is now already immunized against the Rh factor, the transfusion reaction is greatly enhanced and can be immediate and as severe as a transfusion reaction with hemolysis and possible kidney damage caused by mismatched type A or B blood.

Rh disease of the newborn may also be called erythroblastosis fetalis[2] and is the result of an Rh incompatibility between mother and fetus. During a normal pregnancy, maternal blood and fetal lood do not mix in the placenta. However, during delivery of the placenta, some fetal blood may enter maternal circulation.

If the woman is Rh negative and her baby is Rh positive, this exposes the woman to Rh–positive erythrocytes. In response, her immune system will now produce anti–Rh antibodies following this first delivery. In a subsequent pregnancy, these maternal antibodies will cross the placenta and enter fetal circulation. If this next fetus is also Rh positive, the maternal antibodies will cause destruction (hemolysis) of the fetal erythrocytes.

1.3 White blood cells and platelet blood group

White blood cells and platelets also have antigens same as those in red cells. Human leukocyte antigens (HLA)[3] are antigens on leukocytes that are representative of the antigens present on all the cells of an individual. The HLA system antigens are widely distributed in the cells of skin, kidney, liver, and heart. Its importance in organ transplantation should receive special attention.[4] The HLA system also shows race speciality and therefore, it is also very

[1] 第一次将 Rh 阳性血液输给 Rh 阴性患者，不会引起输血反应。

[2] 胎儿成红细胞增多症。

[3] 人类白细胞抗原：编码基因是人类的主要组织相容性复合体，位于 6 号染色体上（6p21.31），与人类的免疫系统功能密切相关。

[4] 人类白细胞抗原又称移植抗原，其研究是在器官移植研究推动下开展起来的，同时其在器官移植中起重要作用。

important in anthropology research.

Furthermore, the platelet also has its own specific antigen systems such as Zw, Ko, and PI system which are important not only in platelet infusion therapy, but also in pregnancy with mother–fetus incompatible groupings.

2 Blood transfusion and cross–match test

Before blood transfusion, the blood type must be identified first, and the blood types of the donor and the recipient can be ensured to be compatible [1]. During the transfusion of incompatible blood, the red cells clump together (agglutinate) as a result of the interaction of the blood group antigens with their corresponding antibodies. This damages the red cells, which hemolyze. Such a transfusion reaction is especially severe when the plasma of the recipient contains antibodies against the red cells of the donor. In the reverse case, where the donor blood contains antibodies against the red cells of the recipient, the reaction is less marked, because the antibodies are diluted in the recipient's bloodstream.

With this information as background, we can predict what happens if a type A person were given type B blood. There are two incompatibilities: ① The recipient's anti–B antibodies cause the transfused cells to be attacked, and ② the anti–A antibodies in the transfused plasma cause the recipient's cells to be attacked. However, the transfused antibodies become so diluted in the recipient's plasma that the latter is generally ineffective in inducing a response. It is the destruction of the transfused cells by the recipient's antibodies that produces the problems.

Similar analyses show that the following situations would result in an attack on the transfused erythrocytes: a type B person given either A or AB blood; a type A person given either type B or AB blood; a type O person given A, B, or AB blood.

There is a saying that type O people are sometimes called universal donors, whereas type AB people are universal recipients (Figure 3–6). This kind of different blood type transfusion can only be used in emergencies with a small amount of slow blood transfusion, preventing from agglutination of the recipient's red blood cell by the donor's antibody.

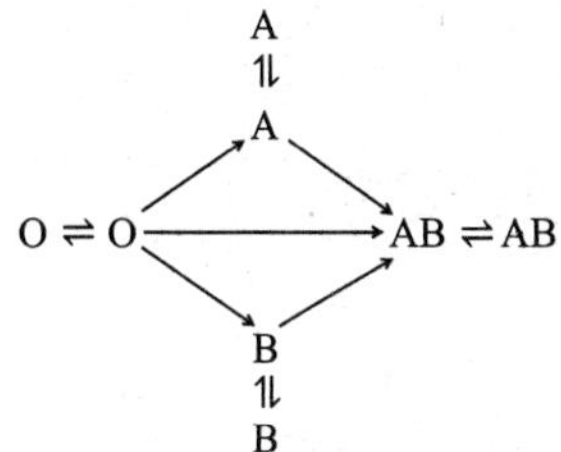

Figure 3–6 Transfusion between different blood types

However, since besides antigens of the ABO system, there are a host of other erythrocyte antigens and plasma antibodies against them. Therefore, except in a dire emergency, the blood

[1] 在输血前，首先必须鉴定血型，保证供血者与受血者的血型相合。输血原则是：同型血互输，异型血慎输，输血前要进行交叉配血试验。

of donor and recipient must be tested for incompatibilities directly by the procedure called cross-match test[1] (Figure 3-7). The recipient's serum is combined on a glass slide with the prospective donor's erythrocytes (a 'major' cross-match), and the mixture is observed for rupture (hemolysis) or clumping (agglutination) of the erythrocytes; this indicates a mismatch. In addition, the recipient's erythrocytes can be combined with the prospective donor's serum (a 'minor' cross-match), looking again for mismatches.

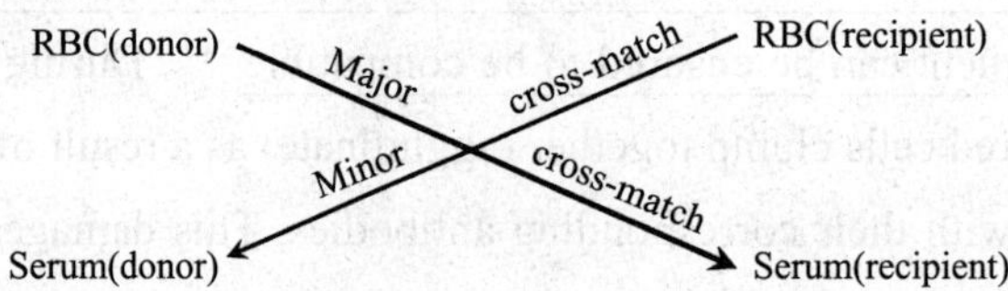

Figure 3-7 Cross-match test of blood

[1] 交叉配血试验：主侧指供血者的红细胞与受血者的血清配合，次侧指受血者的红细胞与供血者的血清配合，观察它们是否发生凝集。如果主次侧都没有发生凝集现象，即为配血相合，可以进行输血；如果主侧不凝集而次侧凝集，则只能在紧急情况下输血（如将O型血输给其他血型的受血者），且输血速度要缓慢，数量一般不超过200mL，并须密切观察，如有输血反应，立即停止。

Chapter 4 BlOOD CIRCULATION

A cardiovascular system,a closed loop, consists of the heart (a pump), blood vessels (a set of interconnected tubes), and blood (a mixture of extracellular fluid and cells). Blood circulation is a physiological phenomenon that the heart, as power organs, pumps blood through a closed system of vessels continuously along a specific route. Since the valves keep blood from reversing its direction of flow, and the blood flows in one direction only. Arteries take blood away from the heart, and veins carry blood back to the heart. The primary function of the cardiovascular system is the transport of materials, including nutrients, water, and gases that enter the body from the external environment, and metabolic wastes that the cells eliminate, and other materials (hormones and agents, etc.) that move from cell to cell within the body. In addition, the cardiovascular system plays an important role in defending the body against foreign invaders by white blood cells and antibodies. In general, cardiovascular system maintains an appropriate environment in all the tissue fluids of the body for optimal survival and function of the cells.

Section 1 Bioelectrical phenomena and physiological properties of the cardiac muscle

The heart, as a pump, is a muscular organ that contracts and relaxes continually without any external stimulus. Cardiac muscle is composed of cardiac muscle cells, or myocardial cells[1]. Cardiac muscle cells, like skeletal muscle cells and neurons, is an excitable cells with the ability to generate action potentials. Most cardiac muscle is contractile, but about 1% of the myocardial cells are specialized to generate action potentials spontaneously.

1 Bioelectrical phenomena of the cardiac muscle

The excitation or stimulus for the heart arises from the cardiac muscle itself. The cardiac muscle cells are divided into two types by their properties: the first is the cardiac working

[1] 心肌细胞。

cells[1], or myocardial contractile cell, including atrial muscle (AM)[2] and ventricular muscle (VM)[3] for the contractility. The second is the cardiac autorhythmiccells[4], includingsino–atrial node (SA node)[5], atrioventricularnode (AV node)[6], bundle of His (BH)[7], Purkinje fibers (PF)[8] and terminal of Purkinje fiber (TPF)[9]. From a functional point of view, the AV nodal region can be divided into atrio–nodal (AN)[10], nodal (N)[11], and nodal–His (NH)[12] zones. Each of the two types of cardiac muscle cells has a distinctive action potential (Figure 4–1).

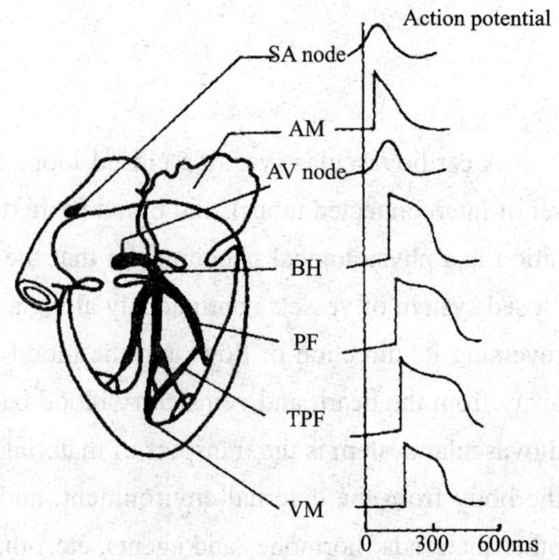

Figure 4–1 The action potential of myocardial cells in each part of the heart

The myocardial cells can be divided into fastresponse cells[13] and slow response cells[14] according to the speed and mechanism of depolarization during action potentials are obtained. The fast response cells include AM, VM and PF, while slow response cells include SA node and AV node, etc. The action potentials of fast response cells are characterized by the larger amplitude and faster velocity of depolarization and faster excitation conduction speed than that of slow response cells.

---

[1] 心肌工作细胞。
[2] 心房肌。
[3] 心室肌。
[4] 心肌自律细胞。
[5] 窦房结。
[6] 房室结。
[7] 希氏束或房室束。
[8] 浦肯野纤维。
[9] 末梢浦肯野纤维。
[10] 房结区。
[11] 结区。
[12] 结希区。
[13] 快反应细胞。
[14] 慢反应细胞。

1.1 The membrane potentials of cardiac working cells

The ventricular cells, one of cardiac working cells, play an important role in cardiac ejection blood. Generally ventricular membrane potential is divided into 5 phases, and the details are shown as follows.

1.1.1 Resting membrane potential

Ventricular cells have a stable resting potential of about –90 mV. The ionic basis of the ventricular cell is similar to that of the neurons and skeletal muscle cells due to K^+ leaving the cell.

1.1.2 Action potential

Ventricular action potential includes depolarization phase and replarization phase. (Figure 4–2)

(1)Phase 0 Depolarization. When a wave of depolarization from SA nodes moves into a ventricular cell through gap junctions, the membrane potential becomes more positive and rapidly reaches the overshoot [1] about +20 mV. The potential change in phase 0 is caused by Na^+ rapid influx through the voltage–gated Na^+ channels, called fast channels,which can be activated and open in a fraction of a millisecond and are inactivated after several milliseconds. Na^+ channel has two gates,similar to the voltage–gated Na^+ channels of the neuron.

(2) Phase 1 Initial repolarization. When the Na^+ channels close, the cell begins to rapidly repolarize as K^+ leaves through open K^+ channels, which produces a transient, early outward current (I_{to}), and leads to the incomplete repolarization.

(3) Phase 2 The plateau [2]. After initial repolarization, the action potential flattens into a plateau that lasts for as long as 0.2 ~ 0.3 second.The plateau is due to the combination of increased Ca^{2+} influx and decreased K^+ efflux. Voltage–gated Ca^{2+} channels activated by depolarization are slow to open and therefore are called slow channels. When they finally open, prolonged Ca^{2+} current(I_{ca-L}) enters the cell. At the same time, some "fast" K^+ channels close, however, the other "slow" voltage–gated K^+ channels often not open much until the end of the plateau.

(4) Phase 3 Rapid repolarization. When Ca^{2+} channels close and K^+ efflux increases once more. The "slow" K^+ channels are activated by depolarization and open slowly, K^+ exits rapidly, returning the cell to its resting potential (phase 4). The time taken from phase 0 to phase 3 is the action potential duration.

(5) Phase 4 Resting membrane potential. The membrane potential roaches the resting levels, however, the ionic distribution is not recover. Na^+–Ca^{2+} exchanger can be activated

---

[1] 超射。

[2] 平台期。

in phase 4 to move three Na^+ ions inside the cell and one Ca^{2+} ion outside the cell, which can transport Ca^{2+} entering into the cell in phase 2 outwardly. Meanwhile, Na^+–K^+ pump can work on moving three Na^+ ions outside the cell and two K^+ ions inside the cell, leading to Na^+ ions entering into the cell during phase 0 outward and K^+ ions leaving the cell during phase 1, 2, 3 inward. By the interaction of Na^+–Ca^{2+} exchanger and Na^+–K^+ pump, the ionic distribution can return to the original state.

Table 4–1 Ventricular action potential and ion flow

Phase	Membrane channels
0	Na^+ channels open
1	Na^+ channels close
2	Ca^{2+} channels open; fast K^+ channels close
3	Ca^{2+} channels close; slow K^+ channels open
4	Resting potential

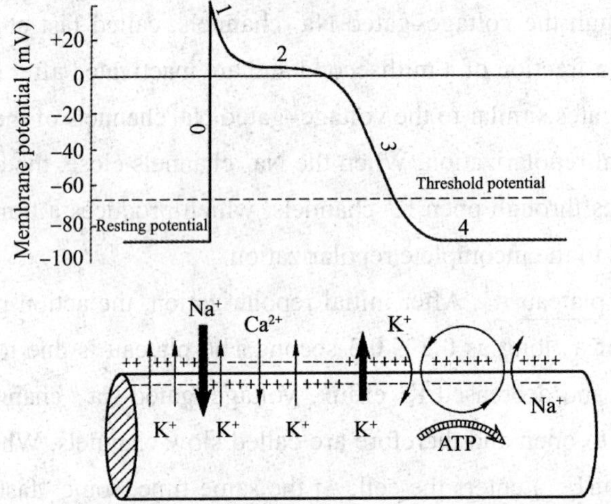

Figure 4–2 Ventricular action potential and ion flow

1.2 The membrane potentials of cardiacautorhythmic cells

Autorhythmic cells possess unique ability to generate action potentials spontaneously without input from the nervous system. Phase 4 demonstrates a slow, continuous diastolic depolarization, so that during diastole, the membrane potential of SA node and Purkinje fibers progressively becomes less negative. This unstable membrane potential reaches maximum polarization state, which is called maximal repolarization potential[1] rather than a resting mem-

[1] 最大复极电位。

brane potential.

1.2.1 The membrane potentials of SA node

Figure 4–3 shows that the action potentials are obtained from SA node. The maximal repolarization potential is about –60 mV. When the threshold potential reaches about –40 mV, a set of voltage–gated Ca^{2+} (I_{Ca-L}) channels open. Ca^{2+} rushes into the cell, creating the slower depolarization process of the action potential in phase 0. This phase is different from that in cardiac working cells, in which the opening of voltage–gated Na^+ channels leads to the depolarization phase. At the peak of the action potential, the Ca^{2+} (I_{Ca-L}) channels close and slow K^+ channels have opened. The entire process of repolarization is slow and results from efflux of K^+ in phase 3 without phase 1 and 2.

Following the repolarization, there is a progressive decline and unstable membrane potential in phase 4.SA node has three types of membrane ion channels that play important roles in causing the voltage changes of the action potential in phase 4. ① A separate K^+ channel, usually labeled I_k, shows inactivation which results in a decreased permeability to K^+. ② When the membrane potential is about –60 mV, I_f channels open and allow Na^+ to flow into cells. When Na^+ influx exceeds K^+ efflux, the membrane potential becomes more positive, the I_f channels gradually close. ③ Meanwhile, a different set of transient Ca^{2+} (I_{Ca-T}) channels open and influx of Ca^{2+} results in depolarization toward threshold steadily. After reaching the threshold potential, the slowly opening Ca^{2+}(I_{Ca-L}) channels are activated and result in depolarization in phase 0.

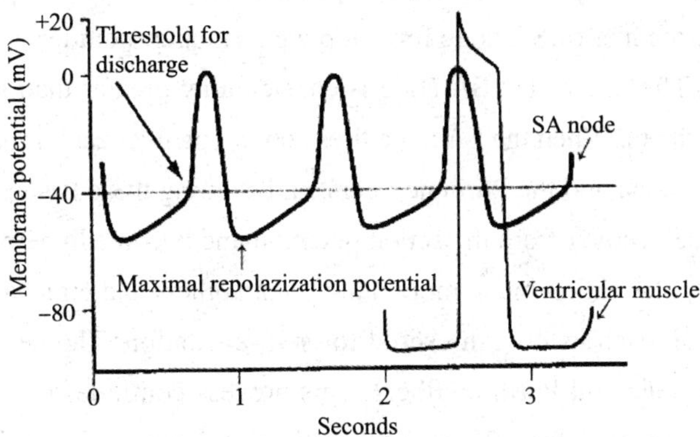

Figure 4–3 Rhythmic discharge of a SA nodal fiber compared with that of a ventricular muscle fiber

1.2.2 The membrane potentials of Purkinjefibers

When Purkinje fibers excite and generate action potentials with faster response, the shape of their action potentials are similar to that of ventricular cells.Theiraction potentials also are divided into five phase including 0, 1, 2, 3 and 4, whose bioelectrical mechanism in phase 0 ~ 3 are also basically the same as that of ventricular cells. However, the significant difference of action potentials between Purkinje fibers and ventricular cells is the membrane potential of

Purkinje fibers is unstableinphase 4. The generation mechanism of the automatic depolarization obtained in Purkinje fibers is similar to that of SA node in phase 4.

2 Physiological properties of cardiac muscle cell

The physiological properties of cardiac muscle cell include autorhythmicity, conductivity, excitability and contractility. The latter is the mechanical property of cardiac muscle. The others are the electrophysiological properties of cardiac muscle.

2.1 Autorhythmicity

Autorhythmicity, also called automaticity, means the capacity of certain specialized "pacemaker" cells to initiate an action potential by spontaneous depolarization, in the absence of an external stimulus. The autorhythmicity of different cells can be evaluated by their autorhythmic excitation frequencies.

2.1.1 Heart pacemaker

In the heart, the normal pacemaker cell of the SA node is the fastest pacemaker and thus sets the normal heart rate. The intrinsic rate of SA node generating impulse is approximately 100 per minute. The rate of the AV node is 50 per minute, and the rate of the Purkinje cell is 25 per minute, so they are called the latent pacemaker.If their rhythm controls the heart, they would be called the ectopic pacemaker.

2.1.2 The control of SA node for ectopic pacemaker

The controlling manner of SA node for ectopic pacemaker include:

(1) Capture [1] The rate of the SA node is considerably greater than that of either the AV node or the Purkinje fibers. When the SA node fires action potential each time, its impulse is conducted to both the AV node and the Purkinje fibers, and exciting these tissues. Then these tissues, as well as the SA node, recover from the action potential and become hyperpolarized. But the SA node loses this hyperpolarization much more rapidly than others and emits a new impulse before either one of them can reach its own threshold for self-excitation. The new impulse again discharges both the AV node and Purkinje fibers. This process continues on and on, the SA node always excites other potentially self-excitatory tissues before self-excitation can actually occur. The SA node controls the pace of the heartbeat, because its rhythm is faster than that of any other part of the heart. The refore, the SA node is the normal pacemaker of the heart.

(2) Overdrive suppression [2] The cause of the prolonged delay before establishing the new rhythm is the phenomenon called overdrive suppression. When the SA node drives the Purkinje system at a rhythmical frequency far above its natural frequency, normally, the Pur-

---

[1] 抢先占领或夺获。

[2] 超速驱动压抑。

kinje system is found to be overdriven, and the excitabilities of the Purkinje fibers are temporarily suppressed.Therefore, an extra period of time is required before they can become self-excitatory. This is a very valuable effect on keeping the other parts of the heart besides the SA node suppressed enough so that it is difficult for them to take over a pacemaker function.

2.1.3 Influence factorsforautorhythmicity

There are three factors that influence the cardiac autorhythmicity separately, including the velocity of spontaneous depolarization in phase 4, maximal repolarization potential, and threshold potential (Figure 4–4). In Figure 4–4 A, the slopes can imply the depolarization velocities of two cells. The reduction in the slope of the pacemaker potential (from a to b) will diminish the frequency, so the autorhymicity is reduced. In Figure 4–4 B, a rise in the threshold potential (from TP–2 to TP–1) or an increase in the magnitude of the maximal repolarization potential (from c to d) will also diminish the frequency, and the autorhymicity will decrease.

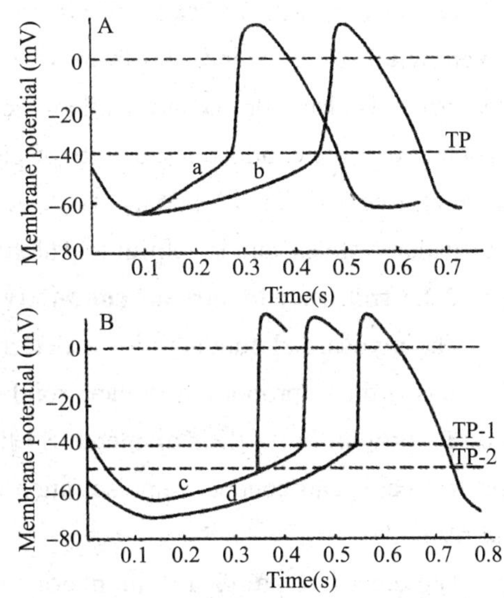

Figure 4–4 Changes of firing frequency in pacemaker. TP: threshold potential

2.2 Conductivity

Conductivity indicates the ability or characteristics of cardiac cells and tissues for transmitting excitation (action potential). The cardiac muscles can be regarded as a functional syncytium [1], and there are intercalated disks [2] between cardiac cells.Thus, the action potential transported so rapidly to adjacent cells through gap junctions [3] in the intercalated disks by local current. In the same way, individual myocardial cell can depolarize and contract in a coordinated fashion so that the heart is to create enough force to eject and circulate the blood.

2.2.1 Conduction pathway and feature

The electrical signals from the SA node activates the atrial myocardial cells to contract, and then reaches the main conduction system at the level of the AV node. The impulse is delayed in the AV node, and this delay allows the atrial systole to squeeze extra blood into the ventricles just before the ventricular systole occurs. The bundle of His is a rapid conduction

[1] 合胞体。

[2] 闰盘。

[3] 缝隙连接。

pathway that the electrical signals from the AV node is transmitted down.The bundle of His is composed of the right and left bundle branches, by which electrical signals can reach and stimulate the right and the left ventricle to contract. Purkinje fibers are large diameter cells and transmit impulses very rapidly, with speeds up to 4 m/sec, so that all contractile cells in the apex [1] contract nearly simultaneously.

For an adult with 75 beats per minute, time needed for electrical signals from the SA node to ventricle is 0.22 second, and from SA node to AV node is 0.06 second, and from AV node to ventricle is also 0.06 second, while the conducting time in AV node is 0.1 second. The phenomenon that the conduction velocity of electrical signal through the AV node is very slow is called atrioventricular (AV) delay [2], which can insure the atrial systoles always occur before ventricular systoles, and is helpful for the filling and ejecting blood of ventricles.

2.2.2 Influence factors for conductivity

The myocardial conductivity is determined by their structure. The diameter of myocardial cells is direct proportion to their conducting velocity, because their myocardial resistance is direct proportion to their diameter. So the thick myocaridac cells, such as ventricular and Purkinje cells, can conduct impulse much more quickly than the thin myocardial cells of SA and AV node.

The electric features are the major factors affecting conductivity. If the depolarization velocity increases in phase 0, the adjacent myocardial excitation can be easily produced, so the conduction is more easily. And the depolarization amplitude is much greater, the potential differences between myocardial cells are greater, so the conduction velocity will increase. Another factor is the ionic channel state of adjacent myocardial cells. If the ionic channels are at resting state, impulse can be conducted easily, while the ionic channels are at inactivated state, the conductivity will decrease.

2.3 Excitability

2.3.1 Cycling change of cardiac cell excitability

Figure 4–5 shows the cycling change of cardiac cell excitability during action potential. The excitable cycle of myocardial cell is divided into three periods:

(1) Effective refractory period[3] (ERP) From phase 0 to –60mV in Phase 3. There are two periods, absolute refractory period (phase 0 to –55mV in Phase 3) and local response period (–55mV to –60mV in Phase 3). During the absolute refractory period, Na^+ channels are inactivated and cannot activated to fire new action potential by any stimuli, which means the excit-

[1] 心尖。

[2] 房 – 室延搁。

[3] 有效不应期。

ability of myocardial cells is zero. During the local response period, only a few Na^+ channels can be activated. When one hyper threshold stimulus is applied to the myocardial cell, there is not enough Na^+ influx. Though the local potential appears, action potential will not occur. Thus, the myocardial excitability in local response period is also zero.

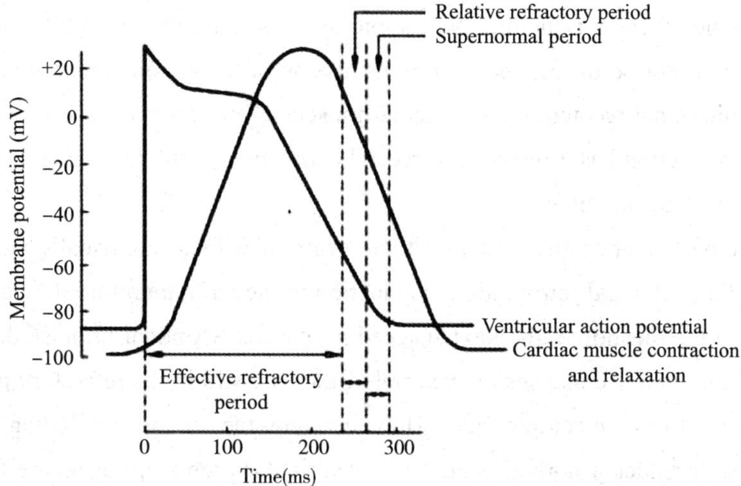

Figure 4–5 The ventricular action potential, myocardial systolic curve and the change in excitability

(2) Relative refractory period [1] (RRP) From –60 mV to –80 mV in Phase 3. In this period, much more Na^+ channels are reactivation. So one hyperthreshold stimulus is applied, more Na^+ flow into the myocardial cell, which may make the membrane potential reach threshold potential and cause excitation. But in this period, the quantity of Na^+ channels that can be activated is less than that in the normal state, so the hyperthreshold stimulus is needed.

(3) Supranormalperiod [2] (SNP) From –80mV in Phase 3 to –90mV in Phase 4. In this period, the membrane potential is close to the resting potential, that is, the distance between the membrane potential and threshold potential is smaller than that in normal state. Moreover, the quantity of Na^+ channels that can be activated is nearly the same to that in the normal state. So one subthreshold stimulus can excite the myocardial cell. The excitability in supranormal period is great.

2.3.2 Premature contraction and compensatory pause

Often, a small area of the heart becomes much more excitable than normal and causes an abnormal impulse to be generated during the time interval between the normal impulses. This can occur in either the atria or the ventricles. A depolarization wave spreads outward from the

[1] 相对不应期。

[2] 超常期。

irritable area and initiates a premature contraction [1], also called premature beats or premature systole (Figure 4–6). The point at which the abnormal impulse is generated is called an ectopic focus. Frequently, an ectopic focus is an irritable area in cardiac muscle that becomes self–excitable. This can result from a local area of muscle ischemia, overuse of stimulants such as caffeine or nicotine, lack of sleep, anxiety, or other debilitating states. However, in many instances, especially when there is ischemia, the ectopic focus is caused by a re–entrant signal that is delayed for a short period of time by slow transmission of the action potential in the ischemic muscle; then this signal reenters the ventricular muscle a few tenths of a second later after the normal heart contraction has already occurred. This obviously will cause a second contraction of the heart at an abnormal time.

Premature beats that originate in an ectopic ventricular focus are usually incapable of exciting the bundle of His and retrograding conduction to the atria, therefore they does not occur continuously. In the meantime, the next succeeding normal SA nodal impulse depolarizes the atria. If the normal impulse reaches the ventricles, they are still in the refractory period following depolarization from the ectopic focus. However, only the second succeeding impulse from the SA node can produce a normal beat. Thus, ventricular premature beats are followed by a compensatory pause [2] that is often longer than the pause after an atrial extrasystole.

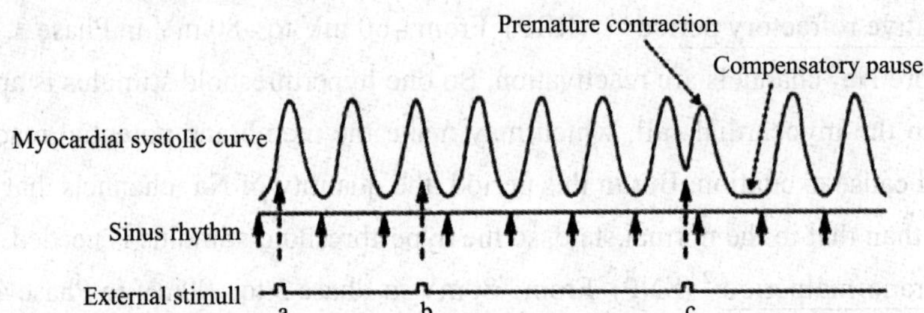

Figure 4–6 Premature contraction and compensatory pause

a ~ c: External stimuli

Stimuli "a" and "b" fall within ERP, no reaction induced; Stimulus "c"falls within RRP, premature contraction and compensatory pause are induced.

2.3.3 Influence factors for excitability

(1) Distance between the membrane potential and threshold potential To the working cells or autorhythmic cells, the distance between the membrane potential or maximal potential and threshold potential is direct proportion to the excitability. The distance is smaller, the cost time reaching threshold potential is less, and so the excitability is greater.

[1] 期前收缩。

[2] 代偿间歇。

(2) States of channel Take quick response cell as an example, the states of Na^+ channel can be divided into 3 states: resting state, activation and inactivation. When the membrane potential is –90 mV, the Na^+ channel is at rest, which can be activated to allow enough Na^+ influx, then action potential is produced. But Na^+ channels will be inactivated quickly after activation, and cannot be activated soon after that, so the myocardial excitability will be zero.

2.4 Contractility

The molecular mechanism of myocardial contraction is very similar to that of skeletal muscular contraction, here the characteristics of myocardial contraction are introduced.

2.4.1 Characteristics of contractility

(1) All–or–none contraction [1] Because the resistance of the intercalated disks between cardiac muscles is very low, sinus impulse conduction between the atria or ventricle is so rapid that cardiac muscles can contract synchronously. Thus, the heart can be looked as a functional syncytium, that is, when sinus impulse reaches the atria or ventricle, atrial or ventricular muscles can contract synchronously.

(2) No tetanus [2] The effective refractory period of myocardial cells is very long,any stimuli cannot cause the heart to excitation in this period. So myocardial cells cannot contract as the way of skeletal muscle with tetanus when a serial of stimuli is given.

(3) Extracellular Ca^{2+} dependence [3] For lack of Ca^{2+}in the myocardial cells, more $Ca^{2+}$are needed to enter into the myocardial cells for causing contraction. So the extracellular Ca^{2+} concentration is very important for the normal contraction function of myocardial cells.

2.4.2 Influence factorsforcontractility

The factors that affect stroke volume can affect contractility, such as preload, afterload, myocardial contractility, and extracellular Ca^{2+}. See below for details (Section 2 Pumping function of heart: 5 Factors controlling cardiac output).

3 Body surface electrocardiogram

The human body can be seen as a volume conductor, because our NaCl–based extracellular fluid are good conductors of electricity.When the electrical impulse from all parts of the heart can spread from the heart to the surface through the surrounding conductive tissues and fluids. If electrodes are placed on the skin's surface, electrical activity of the heart can be recorded, and the recording is known as an electrocardiogram (ECG) [4]. An ECG is different

[1] “全或无” 式收缩。

[2] 不发生强直收缩。

[3] 对细胞外 Ca^{2+} 依赖性。

[4] 心电图。

from a single action potential. The action potential represents a electrical event in a single cell, recorded using an intracellular electrode. The ECG shows the sum of multiple action potentials generated by all cells of the heart, recorded using an extracellular electrode. The first electrocardiogram was recorded in 1887, and Dutch physiologist Walter Einthoven was known as the father of the modern ECG.

3.1 The recording of ECG

The ECG can be recorded by using an active or exploratory electrode connected to an indifferent electrode at zero potential, or by using two active electrodes. Depolarization moving toward an active electrode in a volume conductor produces a positive deflection, whereas depolarization moving in the opposite direction produces a negative deflection.As action potentials spread from the atria to the ventricles, the voltage measured between these two electrodes will vary in a way that provides a curve graph of the electrical activity of the heart.

There are three types of ECG recording electrodes, or "leads[1]", including bipolar leads, unipolar limb leads and unipolar chest leads. The bipolar limb leads record the voltage between electrodes placed on the wrists and legs. These bipolar leads include lead Ⅰ (right arm to left arm), lead Ⅱ (right arm to left leg), and lead Ⅲ (left arm to left leg). The right leg is used as a ground lead. In the unipolar leads, voltage is recorded between a single exploratory electrode-placed on the body and an electrode that is built into the electrocardiograph and maintained at zero potential (ground).The unipolar limb leads are placed on the right arm, left arm, and left leg, and are abbreviated aVR, aVL, and aVF, respectively. The unipolar chest leads are labeled V_1 ~ V_6, starting from the midline position. A standard 12–lead ECG is now the standard for clinical use.

3.2 Characteristics of the normal ECG

An ECG is divided into waves (P, Q, R, S, T), segments (PR and ST segments) between the waves, and intervals (PR and QT intervals) consisting of a combination of waves and segments. The various waves and segments of the ECG can be recorded from lead Ⅱ for one cardiac cycle (Figure 4–7). The normal ECG includes a P wave, a QRS complex, and a T wave. Occasionally, U wave appears after

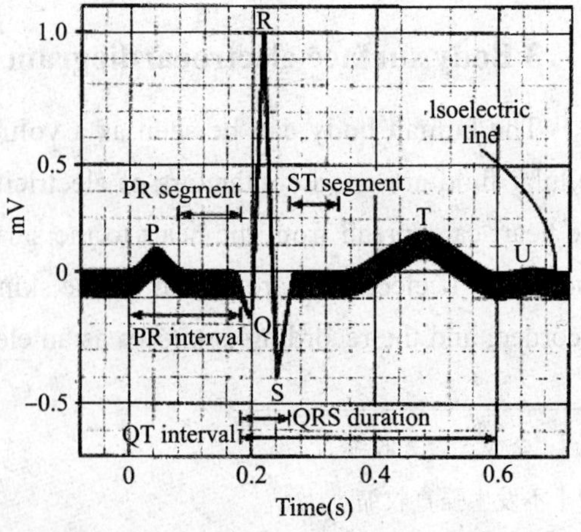

Figure 4–7 Waves of the ECG recorded by Lead Ⅱ

[1] 导联。

T wave. The different waves reflect depolarization or repolarization of the atria and ventricles. Both the P wave and QRS complex are depolarization waves. However, T wave is repolarizaton wave.

(1) P wave For each cardiac cycle, the ECG begins with atrial depolarization and P wave appears at first. P wave represents atrial depolarization and occurs at the beginning of contraction of the atria. The normal duration of P wave is about 0.08 ~ 0.11 second, and amplitude is less than 0.25 mV.

(2) QRS complex The QRS complex consists of three separate waves: Q wave, R wave, and S wave. The three waves are not always appear simultaneously in different lead records. The QRS complex represents ventricular depolarization and occurs at the beginning of ventricular contraction. Ventricular contraction begins just after the Q wave and continues until after the end of the T wave. The normal QRS complex lasts about 0.06 ~ 0.10 second.When the left or right bundle branch is blocked by disease,the QRS complex is prolonged more than 0.12 second.

(3) T wave The T wave is positive in most leads, represents ventricular repolarization and has the same direction as the QRS complex. The process of ventricular repolarization extends over a long period, about 0.05 ~ 0.25 second. When the QRS complex is positive and the T wave is negative, it indicates that the repolarization proceeds in a wrong direction. Abnormal T waves are due to cardiac hypertrophy, myocardial damage or electrical disturbances.

(4) U wave The U wave is an inconstant finding, believed to be due to slow repolarization of the papillary muscles.

(5) PR interval and PR segment The PR interval, normally 0.12 ~ 0.2 second, from the beginning of the P wave to the beginning of the QRS complex, measures the impulse speed through the supraventricular tissue from the SA node to the bifurcation of the His bundle. Prolonged PR interval is caused by disturbances of AV conduction.

The PR segment, from the end of the P wave to the beginning of the QRS complex, indicates conduction through AV node and AV bundle. During the PR segment, the electrical signal is slowing down as it passes through the AV node and AV bundle (AV delay).

(6) QRS duration QRS duration is the time taken by ventricular depolarization and atrial repolarization.

(7) ST segment The ST segment, from the beginning of the QRS complex to the beginning of the T wave, represents the period, where the entire ventricular myocardium is depolarized. Therefore it is isoelectric. Any deviation, up or down from the isoelectric level, indicates anoxic damage of the myocardium.

(8) QT interval The QT interval, from the beginning of the QRS complex to the end of the T wave, represents the time of ventricular depolarization plus ventricular repolarization.

Section 2 Pumping function of heart

The function of the circulatory system is to maintain an optimum environment for cellular function. The optimum environment requires control of concentrations of nutritive, hormonal, and waste materials, tensions of respiratory gases, and temperature. Because of continuous cellular activity, an optimum environment may be maintained only by an uninterrupted flow of blood to the tissues to renew nutrients and remove wastes. To maintain this continuous flow, the heart pumps the blood via succession of heart contractions, which plays a important role in the cardiovascular system.

1 Heart rate and cardiac circle

1.1 Heart rate

Heart rate[1] (HR) is the heartbeats per minute. For the adult, the normal heart rate at rest ranges between 60 and l00 beats per minute and averages about 70. For the newborn, the heart rate is about 135 beats per minute and for the elderly, about 80 beats per minute. The heart of the trained athlete at rest often beats less than 50 times per minute. The heart rate has relationship with the age, size of body, body position, physical training and gender.

1.2 Cardiac cycle

One cardiac cycle[2] has two phases: systole[3] (contraction) and diastole[4] (relaxation). The atria and ventricles do not contract and relax at the same time. Each cardiac cycle includes atrial systole and diastole, ventricular systole and diastole. After atrial systole, atrial diastole occurs, then ventricular systole and ventricular diastole. Note that there is overlap of atrial diastole and ventricular systole. The common period of atrial and ventricular diastole is half a cardiac cycle. If the heart rate is 75 beats per minute, each cardiac cycle is 0.8 second, and atrial systole is 0.1 second, ventricular systole is 0.3 second, atrial diastole is 0.7 second, ventricular diastole is 0.5 second. Thus, the atria act as primer pumps in cardiac cycle, and the ventricles in turn play the major role in moving blood through the body's vascular system.

---

[1] 心率。

[2] 心动周期。

[3] 收缩。

[4] 舒张。

2 Cardiac pumping – ejection and filling process

One cardiac cycle is divided into seven phases, and the relative events are also shown in Figure 4–8. We will discuss left atrial and left ventricular events separately.

2.1 Isovolumetric contraction phase [1]

In response to the ventricularcontraction, the pressure in the ventricle increases very rapidly, but normally there is no change in intraventricular volume because the AV (atrioventricular) valves and semilunar (aortic and pulmonary)valves are closed. Vibrations following closure of the AV valves create the first heart sound [2] (S_1). Therefore, during this phase, ventricular contraction is occurring, but the volume of blood in the ventricle is not changing.

2.2 Rapid ejection phase [3]

As the ventricles contract continually, and the pressure in the ventricles exceed the pressure in the aorta and pulmonary artery. Thus, the ventricularpressures push the semilunar valves open and about 70 % of blood into artery during this first third of ejection phase. Therefore, the first third is called the rapid ejection phase. At the onset of ventricular contraction, the “c” wave of atrial pressure is caused mainly by bulging of the AV valves backward to the atria because of increasing pressure in the ventricles.Soon the atrial pressure comes a decrease in pressure. The ventricular and atrial pressure can approach their maximum and ventricular is greater than the aortic pressure in this phase.

2.3 Slow ejection phase [4]

The remaining 30% of blood emptying occurs during the last two thirds of ejection phase, called the slow ejection phase. During this phase, the contractile forces of the heart are decreasing and the ventricular pressures are lower by a few millimeters of mercury than the aortic pressures. Because of the momentum of the rapidly ejecting of blood, the semilunar valves are opened continuously and the blood in ventricles are pushed to outflow slowly into artery. At the end of this phase, the end–systolic volume [5] (ESV) can be decreased to minimum. Simultaneously, the “v” wave of atrial pressure occurs, results from slow flow of blood into the

---

[1] 等容收缩期。

[2] 第一心音。

[3] 快速射血期。

[4] 减慢射血期。

[5] 收缩末期容积。

atria from the veins while the AV valves are closed during ventricular contraction.

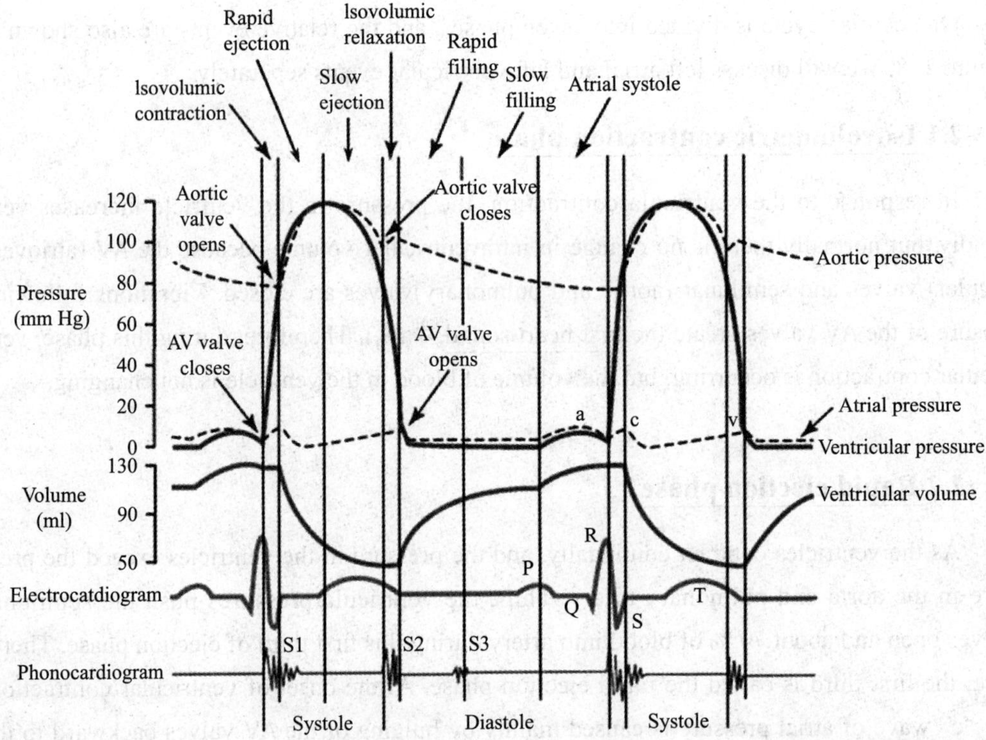

Figure 4–8 Events of the cardiac cycle

2.4 Isovolumic relaxation phase [1]

When ventricular contraction is over, the ventricles begin to relax suddenly. In this phase, the ventricular pressure decreasesrapidly. Once ventricular pressure falls below aorticpressures, blood starts to flow backward into the heart, which forces semilunar valves to be closed. The vibrations following closure of semilunar valves create the second heart sound [2] (S_2). Because ventricular pressures are still higher than atrial pressure, the AV valves remain closed. Thus, there is no change in ventricular volume in this period, called isovolumic relaxation phase.

2.5 Rapid filling phase [3]

During ventricular contraction, large amounts of blood accumulate in the atria with the closed AV valves. Once systole is over, ventricular relaxation causes the pressure in the ven-

[1] 等容舒张期。

[2] 第二心音。

[3] 快速充盈期。

tricle to become less than in the atria.The increased atrial pressure immediately pushes the AV valves open, and blood rushes into the ventricles and ventricular volume starts to increase again. Filling of the ventricles occurs quickly because ventricular pressure is at its minimum value and the AV pressure gradient is relatively high. The rapid filling phase lasts for about the first third of diastole.

2.6 Slow filling phase [1]

During this phase, only a small amount of blood flows slowly into the ventricles. The filling of blood from the veins can pass through the atria directly into the ventricles. The slow filling phase lasts for about the middle third of diastole.

During the last third of diastole, the atria contract and give an additional squeeze to the filling of blood into the ventricles, which accounts for about 20% of the ventricular filling. Consequently, the volume of the ventricle increases to maximum at the end of ventricular diastole, this volume is called the end–diastolic volume [2] (EDV).

2.7 Atrial systole

Atrial systole [3] is the beginning of the sequence of events. A pacemaker cell in the SA node depolarizes, and there is a spread of excitation across the atria. Atrial contraction follows, causing a development of pressure in the right atrium. This gives "a" wave in the atrial pressure. The increased pressure causes additional ventricular filling, of which accounts for about 25% . Finally, as a result of the filling due to contraction, the ventricular pressure is slightly increased to the value called the end–diastolic ventricular pressure [4] .The atrial systole can be used as a primary pump.

3 Evaluation of pumping function of heart

3.1 Stroke volume

Stroke volume [5] (SV) is the amount of blood ejected by one ventricle during a systole. It can be calculated as follows:

Stroke volume = end–diastolic volume (EDV) –end–systolic volume (ESV)

For a person at rest, the normal SV: 135 mL – 65 mL = 70 mL. Stroke volume can in-

[1] 减慢充盈期。

[2] 舒张末期容积。

[3] 房缩期。

[4] 舒张末期心室内压。

[5] 每搏输出量，简称搏出量。

crease to more than double normal during exercise.

3.2 Ejection fraction

Ejection fraction [1] is the proportion of the end-diastolic volume that is ejected.

Ejection fraction =stroke volume/end diastolic volume

This is a useful index of contractility. The stroke volume is 70mL. The EDV is about 135 mL. Thus, about 65 ml of blood remains in each ventricle at the end of systole. The ejection fraction is usually about 50% ~ 60%.

3.3 Cardiac output

Cardiac output [2] (CO) is the volume of blood ejected by one ventricle per minute.

Cardiac output = stroke volume × heart rate

For an average resting heart rate (75 beats per minute)and a stroke volume (70 mL/ beat):
CO = 75 beats/min ×70 mL/ beat= 5250 mL / min (or approx. 5 L/ min)

Cardiac output is used to assess the effectiveness of the heart as a pump.

3.4 Cardiac index

The Cardiac output per square meter of body surface is the cardiac index [3].

Cardiac index = cardiac output/ square meter of body surface

For a resting person, the average square meter of body surface is about 1.6 ~ 1.7 m^2, the cardiac index averages about 3.0 ~ 3.5L/min·m^2.It can be used as a measure of the heart function for different individuals. At the age of 10, the cardiac index of resting heart rate is highest 4 L/min·m^2. The cardiac index decreases with age, and by the age of 80 is close to 2 L/min·m^2.

3.5 Work output of the heart

Stroke work [4] is the amount of energy that the heart converts to work during a ventricular systole while pumping blood into the arteries. Minute work [5] is the total amount of energy converted to work per minute.

Minute work = stroke work × heart rate

[1] 射血分数。

[2] 每分输出量或心输出量。

[3] 心指数。

[4] 每搏功，简称搏功。

[5] 每分功。

Stroke work includes two forms. Firstly, the major proportion of the energy is called external work or pressure–volume work [1], which is used to pump the blood from the low–pressure veins to the high–pressure arteries. Secondly, a minor proportion is internal work or kinetic energy of blood flow component, which is used to accelerate the blood to its velocity of ejection through the aortic and pulmonary valves. Ordinarily, kinetic energy of blood flow is ignored in the calculation of the total stroke work output because of only about 1 per cent of the total work output of the ventricle. Therefore,

Stroke work = pressure–volume work + kinetic energy
≈pressure–volume work
= stroke volume× increment of ventricular pressure in each systole

Under normal condition, the stroke volume of left and right ventricle are same, but the pulmonary artery pressure is only about 1/6 of the average arterial pressure. So the stroke work of right ventricle is only about 1/6 of the left ventricle.

4 Cardiac reserve

The maximum percentage that the cardiac output can increase above normal is called the cardiac reserve[2]. Thus, in the normal young adult the cardiac reserve is 300% to 400%. In the athletically trained person it is occasionally as high as 500% to 600%, whereas in the asthenic person it may be as low as 200%. As an example, during severe exercise the cardiac output of the normal healthy young adult can rise to about five times normal; this is an increase above normal of 400% – that is, a cardiac reserve of 400%.

Any factor that prevents the heart from pumping blood decreases the cardiac reserve. This can result from ischemic heart disease, primary myocardial disease, vitamin deficiency, damage to the myocardium, valvular heart disease, and many other factors.

5 Factors controlling cardiac output

Variations in cardiac output can be produced by changes in heart rate or stroke volume. The heart rate is controlled primarily by the cardiac innervation, sympathetic stimulation increasing the rate and parasympathetic stimulation decreasing it. Stroke volume can be affected by preload [3], afterload [4], myocardial contractility [5].

---

[1] 压力－容积功。

[2] 心力储备。

[3] 前负荷。

[4] 后负荷。

[5] 心肌收缩能力。

5.1 Preload

For the heart, the preload is the degree to which the myocardium is stretched before it contracts. The relation of length and tension in cardiac muscle can indicate the length of the muscle fibers is proportionate to the end–diastolic volume. Stroke volume is based on end–diastolic volume. Frank–Starling law states “energy of contraction is proportional to the initial length of the cardiac muscle fiber”. Thus, the greater the heart muscle is stretched during filling, the greater is the energy of contraction and the greater the volume of blood pumped into the aorta. So stroke volume can change with end–diastolic volume, but stroke volume will not increase after preload (end–diastolic volume) gets an optimal degree and the ventricle is full of blood. The relation between ventricular stroke volume and end–diastolic volume is called the Frank–Starling curve (Figure 4–9).Regulation of cardiac output as a result of changes in cardiac muscle fiber length is called heterometric regulation.

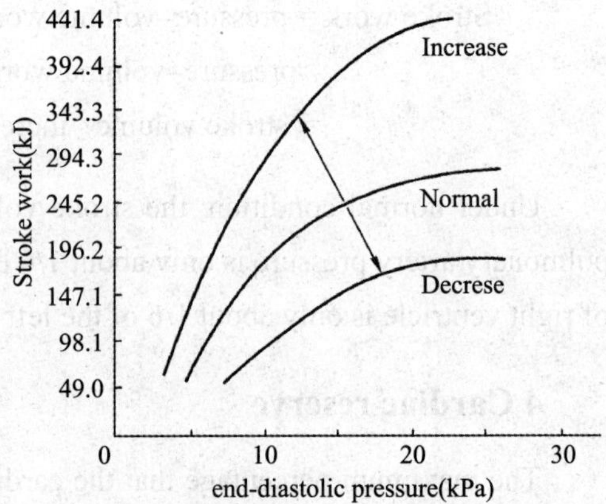

Figure 4–9 The Frank–Starling curve

5.2 Afterload

Afterload is the combined load of end–diastolic volume and the arterial pressure, which is the resistance against blood ejection from ventricles. When the peripheral resistance is increased, the heart pumps less blood than it receives for several beats, leading to the decrease in stroke volume. Blood accumulates in the ventricles, and the size of the heart increases, so that the accumulated blood in the ventricles becomes the preload of the ventricle in the following cardiac cycles. The amplified heart beats more forcefully, and stroke output returns to its previous level. So, increasing the arterial pressure load (up to a limit) does not decrease the stroke volume. Mean arterial pressure is a clinical indicator of afterload.

5.3 Myocardial contractility

Myocardial contractility is the intrinsic ability of a cardiac muscle fiber to contract at any given fiber length and is a function of Ca^{2+} interaction with the contractile filaments. It exerts a major influence on stroke volume, and is proportional to stroke volume. Myocardial contractility is regulated by the nervous and endocrine systems. The chemical and drugs, such as catecholamines epinephrine and norepinephrine and digitalis, enhance myocardial contractility. So they are considered to have a positive inotropic effects. Chemicals and drugs with negative inotropic effects can decrease myocardial contractility. Figure 4–9 shows that the whole Frank–Starling curve shifts upward and to the left due to norepinephrine. The mechanism of norepinephrine is that they bind to β_1–adrenergic receptors and increase Ca^{2+} entry and storage and exert their positive inotropic effects. There is a positively inotropic effects of sympathetic nerve due to the norepinephrine released at nerve endings. However, there is a negatively inotropic effects of vagal stimulation on the atrial muscle and a small negatively inotropic effects on the ventricular muscle.

Regulation of cardiac output due to changes in contractility independent of length is sometimes called homometric regulation.

5.4 Heart rate

Normally the heart rate at the range of 40 ~ 180 beats per minute is proportional to the cardiac output. However, when the heart rate is more than 180 beats per minute, the ventricular filling phases will shorten markedly, causing end–diastolic volume decrease. The result is that stroke volume reduces obviously, and the decline of cardiac volume is followed. On the contrary, the heart rate less than 40 beats per minute can prolong ventricular filling time, causing more blood entering into the ventricle, but the ventricular volume is limit and the actual ventricular volume will not increase after reaching the peak, so the cardiac output decreases.

6 Heart sounds [1] and Echocardiography [2]

Although the opening of the valves is a slower, essentially silent process, the valves close rather suddenly with pressure changes, along with vibrations of the valves and adjacent walls and major vessels around the heart.The sevibrations result in the noises called heart sound, 'lub–dup', that is heard by using the stethoscope and phonocardiogram on chest.

6.1 First heart sound

At the onset of isovolumetric contraction phase, vibrations following closure of the AV valves create the first heart sound (S_1), the 'lub'. S_1 is a low, slightly long–lasting and associated with the following dynamic phenomena: the beginning of cardiac muscle contraction, closing of the AV valves, rapid development of pressure,thenopening of the semilunar valves, and outflow.

6.2 Second heart sound

The second heart sound (S_2), a shorter, high–pitched 'dup', appears at the beginning of isovolumetric relaxation phase. Meantime,blood in the roots of the aorta and pulmonary artery

[1] 心音。

[2] 超声心动图。

rushes back toward the ventricular chambers, but this movement is abruptly arrested by closure of the semilunar valves. So S_2 is caused mainly by the closure of the semilunar valves and the resulting vibrations of the valves, heart, and large arteries. S_2 is associated with the following dynamic phenomena: the beginning of cardiac muscle relation, closing of the semilunar valves,drop of pressure,thenopening of the AV valves, and backflow of blood.

6.3 Third heart sound

The third heart sound (S_3)occurs at the time of transition between rapid filling and reduced filling, when filling slows abruptly, giving a transient soft thud. The mechanism is not clearly understood. The sound is occasionally heard in adults, but may be heard in many people under age 30; it is of low pitch and intensity. When S_3 is of pathological significance, it is associated with a dilated ventricle and high atrial pressure.

6.4 Fourth heart sound

The fourth sound (S_4),also called atrial heart sound, is almost always inaudible in normal adults and occurs at the time of the peak of atrial contraction. When heard, it is associated with a high atrial pressure, vigorous atrial contraction, and filling of the ventricle. Clinically it occurs when the ventricle is stiff, as in ventricular hypertrophy or ischemia.

6.5 Echocardiography

Wall movement[1] and other aspects of cardiac function can be evaluated by echocardiography, a noninvasive technique that does not involve injections or insertion of a catheter. In echocardiography, pulses of ultrasonic waves, commonly at a frequency of 2.25 MHz, are emitted from a transducer that also functions as a receiver to detect waves reflected back from various parts of the heart. Reflections occur wherever acoustic impedance changes, and a recording of the echoes displayed against time on an oscilloscope provides a record of the movements of the ventricular wall, septum, and valves during the cardiac cycle. When combined with Doppler techniques, echocardiography can be used to measure velocity and volume of flow through valves. It has considerable clinical usefulness, particularly in evaluating and planning therapy in patients with valvular lesions.

Section 3 Physiology of vessel

Blood vessels[2] form a tubular network throughout the body permit blood to flow from

[1] 室壁运动。

[2] 血管。

heart to all the living body cells and then back to heart. The rate of blood flow through most tissues is controlled in response to the tissue need for nutrients. What are the mechanisms for controlling blood volume, blood pressure, blood flow and the exchange between blood and tissues? There are some of the topics and questions that we discuss in this chapter.

1 Functional organization of the vessel

The vascular system in each separate tissue has its own special characteristics,however, some general principles of vascular function apply in all parts of the systemic circulation[1]. Before attempting to discuss details of function in the systemic circulation, it is important to understand the overall role of its various parts. This section mainly describes the physiological function of blood vessels, and also introduces the features of lymphatic circulation[2].

1.1 Windkessel vessels

The large arteries, such as aorta[3] and arteriapulmonalis[4], are elastic, because of their vessel walls are rich in elastic fibers. The elastin and smooth muscles in vessel wall enable arteries to distend during ventricular systole and recoil during diastole. Commonly, there is only 1/3 of stroke volume flow to the peripheral during systolic, the remaining 2/3 stored temporarily in aorta and large arteries, which will flow to peripheral during diastole. As the blood flow into capillaries and veins, volume of arterial system declines and blood pressure falls, and diastolic pressure is supported by the energy of elastic recoil. And forward the blood flow is continuous because of the recoil during diastole of vessel walls which have been stretched during systole. At the same time, effect of elastic reservoir can significantly reduce the fluctuation of blood pressure in each cardiac cycle. This recoil effect is called the windkessel effect, and these vessels are called windkessel vessels[5]. Windkessel is a general word for an elastic reservoir.

1.2 Resistance vessels

For fluid flowing through a pipe, there is a resistance to flow is present in all blood vessels, precapillary as well as postcapillary. The elements of precapillary resistance[6] are the

[1] 体循环。

[2] 淋巴循环。

[3] 主动脉。

[4] 肺动脉。

[5] 这种回缩作用称为弹性储器作用，这种血管被称为弹性储器血管。

[6] 毛细血管前阻力。

small arteries, arterioles[1], and precapillary sphincters[2]. The small arteries and arterioles walls are rich in smooth muscles, and their diameter is small, so they represent the major variable elements of resistance that determine the extent of total tissue blood flow[3]. On the other hand,precapillary sphincters determine the extent of capillary flow velocity, capillary surface area, the mean extravascular diffusion distance, and the distribution of capillary blood flow, by adjusting the number of opened capillaries.In short, precapillary sphincter activity exerts a great influence on the nature of transcapillary exchange. Postcapillary resistance vessels include the small veins and venules[4]. Although they show only small changes in resistance, their strategic position enables them to influence capillary pressure markedly. The ratio of precapillary to postcapillary resistance primarily determines capillary hydrostatic pressure[5].

1.3 Exchange vessels

Effective exchange between vascular and extravascular tissues occurs across parts of preferential channels, true capillaries and venules. These vessels are uniquely suited for exchange by virtue of their high ratio of surface area/volume and their thin walls. Moreover, the true capillary[6] is composed of a single layer of endothelial cells[7], only a thin basement membrane outside, so exchange vessels[8] are usually located within 20 to 50 μm of tissue cells, diffusion distances are minimal. In different tissues the capillary walls possess varying relative permeability.Greater exchange occurs across the venous end of exchange vasculatures, because it is more permeable to water and solutes than arterial end. Where macromolecules can pass by filtration in a pressure determined fluid transport. Passage as a whole plasma portion through fenestrations is also possible by pores of 40 ~ 60 nm.

1.4 Shunt vessels

The shunt vessels[9] serve as elements that bypass the effective exchange circulation of

---

[1] 微动脉。

[2] 毛细血管前括约肌。

[3] 小动脉和微动脉管壁富含平滑肌，且口径较小，所以它们是总外周阻力的主要影响因素。

[4] 毛细血管后阻力血管包括小静脉和微静脉。

[5] 毛细血前后阻力的比率决定了毛细血管的流体静压。

[6] 真毛细血管。

[7] 内皮细胞。

[8] 交换血管。

[9] 短路血管。

a tissue. They include arteriovenous anastomoses [1] and preferential (or thoroughfare) channels [2]. Their precise functional significance is unclear, except for those in the skin that subserve temperature regulation. There are many shunt vessels in the skin of auricle [3], finger and toe. A fraction of total flow to an organ or tissue will not participate in exchange,when effective shunts are present.

1.5 Capacitance vessels

In vivo, the venous system is an important blood reservoir. Normally the veins are partially collapsed and oval in cross section. A small change in the diameter of vein, the blood volume of vein can be greatly changed. When a segment of vena cava or another large distensible vein is filled with blood, the pressure does not rise rapidly until a large volume of fluid are injected. So a large amount of blood can be added to venous system before the volume produce a large rise in venous pressure. When quiet, the venous system contains 60% ~ 70% of total circulating blood volume, therefore, the veins are called capacitance vessels [4].

2 Hemodynamics [5]

Hemodynamics is a series of physical problems in the flow of blood in the cardiovascular system. It is a branch of hydrodynamics[6], which focuses on blood flow, blood flow resistance, blood pressure and their relationships.

2.1 Blood flow

Blood always flows from the areas of high pressure to low pressure, except in certain situations when momentum [7] transiently sustains flow. There must be a pressure gradient [8] between the two ends of the vessel. There is a general relationship between blood flow (Q), blood pressure gradient (ΔP), and resistance (R) in the vessels is analogous for fluid flow through a pipe.

$$Q=\Delta P/R$$

[1] 动－静脉吻合支。

[2] 优先（或直捷）通路。

[3] 耳郭。

[4] 安静状态时，静脉系统容纳了全身循环血量的 60% ~ 70%，因此静脉被称为容量血管。

[5] 血流动力学。

[6] 流体力学。

[7] 动量。

[8] 压力梯度。

In any portion of the vascular system, the rate of blood flow (Q) is equal to the size of pressure gradient (ΔP) divided by resistance(R)[1].ΔP is the mean pressure at arterial end minus the mean pressure at venous end. Applying this to the systemic circulation, ΔP is the pressure gradient between aorta and atrium. Since atrial pressure is negligible in comparison with arterial pressure, ΔP effectively equals to arterial blood pressure. The cardiac output is the total blood flow through the systemic circulation, i.e. Q. Thus:

Arterial pressure (ΔP) = Cardiac output (Q) × Resistance (R)

Where, the total resistance to blood flow through systemic circulation is R. This equation indicates that blood pressure may be regulated through changes in either peripheral resistance or cardiac output.

2.2 Blood resistance

The resistance to blood flow through a blood vessel is known as blood resistance[2]. Within the blood vessels, an infinitely thin layer of blood in contact with the wall of vessel does not move. The next layer has a low velocity, the next a higher velocity, and so forth, velocity being greatest in the center of the stream. A feature of laminar flow is the direction of each particle in the liquid are consistent[3].When turbulence occurs, all the particles in the blood are constantly changing the direction of the flow, so the energy consumption is more than laminar flow, the flow resistance is also large. Blood flow resistance generally needs to be calculated.Mainly due to blood flow in the process, the friction between blood and vessel wall or internal components of energy consumption, and transformed into heat, so the blood pressure is gradually reduced. When the laminar flow occurs, the blood resistance can be expressed as follows:

$$R = \frac{8\eta L}{\pi r^4}$$

Since resistance varies inversely with the fourth power of the radius, resistance and blood flow in vivo are markedly affected by small changes in the caliber of the vessels. Thus, for example, flow through a vessel is doubled by a decrease of only 19% in its radius, and when the radius is doubled, resistance is reduced to 1/16 of its previous value. This is why organ blood flow is so effectively regulated by changing the caliber of the arterioles and why small variations in arteriolar diameter have such a pronounced effect on systemic arterial blood pressure.

[1] 在血管的任何部分，血流量 Q 都与压力梯度 ΔP 成正比，与血流阻力 R 成反比。

[2] 血液流经血管时所遇到的阻力，称为血流阻力。

[3] 层流的特征是流体中的每个质点的方向是一致的。

3 Arterial blood pressure and arterial pulse

There is a lateral pressure exerted by blood flow against any unit area of vessel wall, which is blood pressure [1], and always is measured in millimeters of mercury (mmHg). Blood pressure is initially derived from cardiac contraction, but the measurements can be made at different sites around systemic circulation, which can be grossly divided into three types, arterial blood pressure, capillary blood pressure and venous blood pressure[2]. Clinically, arterial blood pressures are routine measurements,andthat reflects the status of cardiovascular system. Capillary blood pressure is important to keep fluid balance between the capillary and tissue. Venous blood pressure reflects the balance between myocardial contractility [3] and venous return.

3.1 Definition

Blood pressure refers to the pressure of blood flowing through blood vessel to the side wall of unit area [4].The pressure in aorta is high, because the heart pumps blood continually into aorta, averaging about 100 mmHg.The blood pressure refers to blood flow in the large arteries per unit area of the vessel wall, namely arterial blood pressure[5].There is only a small drop along their length from large to medium-sized arteries, because their resistance to flow is small. Also, because the pumping is pulsatile, the arterial blood pressure is pulsatile too (Figure 4–10).

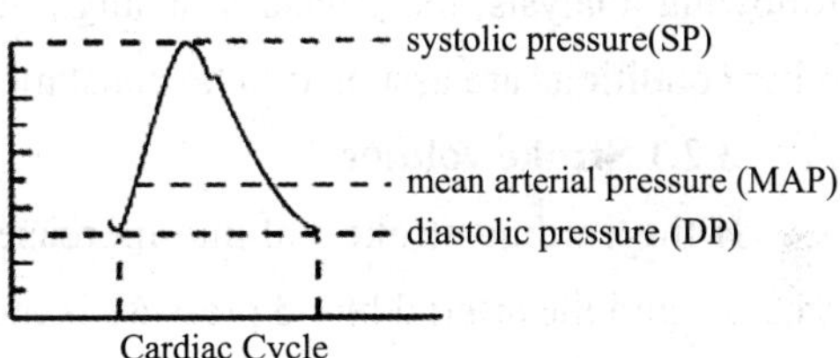

Figure 4–10 Blood pressure of the aorta

The arterial blood pressure rises to a peak value during each cardiac cycle, which is systolic pressure (SP) [6], when the arterial blood pressure falls to a minimum value, which is diastolic pressure (DP) [7]. The arterial blood pressure is written as systolic pressure over diastolic pressure conventionally, e.g. 120/70 mmHg. The difference between SP and DP, about 40mmHg, is called the pulse pressure (PP)[8]. The average pressure throughout cardiac cycle is

---

[1] 血管中流淌的血液对于单位面积血管壁的侧压力称为血压。

[2] 血压被大体分为三种类型：动脉血压、毛细血管血压和静脉血压。

[3] 心肌收缩能力。

[4] 血压是指血管内流动的血液对单位面积血管壁的侧压力。

[5] 血管内流动的血液对单位面积动脉管壁的侧压力，即动脉血压。

[6] 在一个心动周期中，动脉血压升高达到的最高值称为收缩压。

[7] 在一个心动周期中，动脉血压降低达到的最低值称为收缩压。

[8] 收缩压和舒张压的差值称为脉压，大约 40 mmHg。

mean arterial pressure (MAP) [1] , which approximately equals the DP plus 1/3 of the PP:

$$MAP=DP+\frac{PP}{3}$$

The normal ranges of blood pressure in the Chinese adult are shown in Table 4–2.

Table 4–2 The normal value of arterial blood pressure of the Chinese adult

	mmHg	kPa
Systolic pressure	90 ~ 140	12.00 ~ 18.70
Diastolic pressure	60 ~ 90	8.00 ~ 12.00
Pulse pressure	30 ~ 40	4.00 ~ 5.33
Mean arterial pressure	70 ~ 103	9.33 ~ 13.78

3.2 Factors affecting arterial blood pressure

Any factors that affect the formation of arterial blood pressure can affect it too. In the following analysis, the effects of a single factor on arterial blood pressure are analyzed when other conditions are assumed to be constant.

3.2.1 Stroke volume

If the cardiac stroke volume increases, the amount of blood flow into the aorta is increased, and the arterial blood pressure is more obviously increased in systole. Due to increased blood pressure, elastic expansion of arterial wall is more obvious, more energy reserves, diastolic wall elastic recoil effect increased. Compared with normal, blood velocity increased significantly, and the blood volume flows into peripheral arteries from heart increased too, ultimately the blood volume remained in the aorta at the end of diastole increased is not many. Therefore, when the volume of cardiac stroke is increased, the increase of arterial blood pressure is mainly manifested in the increase of SP, and the increase of DP is relatively small. On the contrary, when the volume of stroke decreased, the SP and PP decreased. Therefore, under normal circumstances, the level of SP mainly reflects the amount of cardiac stroke [2] .

3.2.2 Heart rate

The heart rate increases, the cardiac cycle becomes shorter, diastole shortened more significantly, the blood volume flow into peripheral decreased in diastole, the volume remnant in aorta at the end of diastole is increased, therefore, DP increased. The SP increased too, due to the increase of aortic blood volume in systole, and elevated blood pressure makes the blood flow faster, there will be more blood flow to peripheral, so SP increased less than DP, and PP

[1] 一个心动周期中每一瞬间动脉血压的平均值称为平均动脉压。

[2] 所以，在一般情况下，收缩压的高低主要反映心脏搏出量的多少。

decreased. On the contrary, when the HR slows down, the droped amplitude of DP is lower than that of SP.

3.2.3 Peripheral resistance

When the peripheral resistance increases, the resistance to diastole blood flow from heart to periphery increased, and the blood velocity slow down, so that the blood volume remaining in aorta at the end of diastole is higher than normal, and DP increased obviously. SP also increased, but because of elevated blood pressure, blood flow speed up, there will be more blood flow to the peripheral, the volume of blood remaining in aorta at the end of systole increase not too much, so when the peripheral resistance increased, SP increased not as much as DP, and PP decreases. On the contrary, when the peripheral resistance decreased, DP decreased more than SP significantly, so the PP will increase. Therefore, the DP is usually used to reflect the size of the peripheral resistance[1].

3.2.4 Ratio of circulating blood volume to vascular system capacity[2]

Normally, the circulatory blood volume and the vascular system capacity is appropriate, the filling degree of vascular system is steady, the mean circulatory filling pressure[3] changes is little, so the blood pressure maintains normal. When the blood loss, circulatory blood volume reduced, if the volume of vascular system is not changed, then the mean circulatory filling pressure will be reduced and the arterial blood pressure is also reduced. In other cases, arterial blood pressure may be reduced if circulating blood volume remains unchanged and the vascular system capacity increases.

3.2.5 The elastic reservoir effect of aorta

As mentioned earlier, the windkessel vessels have a role in buffering the fluctuation of blood pressure. With the increase of age, the elastic fibers of arterial wall decreased gradually, the arterial compliance decreased gradually. Arterial compliance is the inverse of elasticity and determined by physical properties of arterial wall.As the arteries become hardened with arteriosclerosis[4], SP rises to a greater extent, and DP falls, so that PP increases markedly, because of less energy is absorbed by arterial wall during systole then less energy is restored to the blood by elastic recoil during diastole.

Conditions that varied SV, HR, TPR (totevl peripheral resistance), and/or arterial compliance change SP and DP[5]. Frequently, these varieties occur in combination as a result of the cardiovascular regulatory adjustment to stress.

---

[1] 所以，通常用舒张压的高低来反映外周阻力的大小。

[2] 循环血量和血管系统容量的比值。

[3] 平均充盈压。

[4] 动脉硬化。

[5] 每搏输出量、心率、外周阻力和（或）动脉顺应性改变都会影响收缩压和舒张压。

3.3 Mean arterial blood pressure

As blood flow through the systemic circulation, blood pressure falls progressively to about 0 mmHg when it reaches the termination of venae cave where vessels empty into the right atrium. Both the mean pressure and amplitude of PP falls rapidly in the small arteries, but the largest drop of blood pressure occurs within arterioles. At the end of arterioles, mean pressure is 30 ~ 38 mmHg, PP also decreases rapidly to about 5 mmHg. All of these indicate that the largest contribution to the peripheral resistance comes from arterioles, which produce about 55% of total resistance (Figure 4–11). Arterioles have a amount of smooth muscles in their walls, both the blood pressure and peripheral resistance considerably depending upon whether they are constricted or dilated.

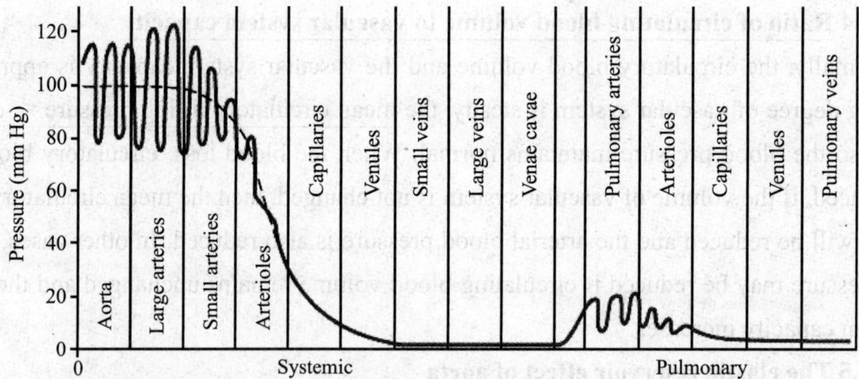

Figure 4–11 Blood pressure in different portions of the body

Factors that determine the mean arterial blood pressure can be defined easily by an application of Ohm's law [1] to the cardiovascular system, which provides the relationship between these factors.

$$MAP = CO \times TPR$$

MAP is mean arterial blood pressure (mmHg); CO is cardiac output (L/min); TPR is total peripheral resistance [2] (mmHg/L·min). Thus, MAP can be modified by changes in either CO or TPR or both of them.

3.4 Pulse pressure

PP that occurs during each cardiac ejection (dP/dt) depends on the change in arterial vol-

[1] 欧姆定律。

[2] 总外周阻力。

ume (dV) relative to the change in arterial compliance (dC). Thus:

$$dP/dt=dV/dC$$

The dV is determined by temporal relationship between inflow (Qi) and outflow (Q_o) through arterial system in turn.The dP/dtis also determined by the changes in inflow and outflow during cardiac cycle. The pressure and volume increase while inflow exceeds outflow, and reach maxima when inflow equals to outflow, and decrease as outflow exceeds inflow. Therefore, systolic pressure depends primarily on the stroke volume of the heart(cardiac contractility[1]), peak of cardiac ejection rate, residual arterial volume[2], and arterial compliance. Diastolic pressure depends on residual arterial volume, TPR, and elastic recoil ability of arterial[3]. In general, the greater stroke volume output, the greater amount of blood that must be accommodated in arterial duct, therefore, the greater pressure rise and fall during cardiac cycle, thus causing a greater PP. Conversely, the less compliance of arterial system, the greater rise in pressure for a given volume of blood pumped into arteries. In effect, PP is determined approximately by the ratio of stroke volume to arteries compliance.

3.5 Arterial pulse

During each cardiac cycle, the pressure and volume of arteries will fluctuate periodically. Whenblood is forced into aorta during systole, it sets up a pressure wave that travels along arteries.The pressure wave expanding along arterial walls is arterial pulse[4]. The velocity of pulse wave is faster than the velocity of blood flow. The greater the distensibility of arterial wall, the slower the propagation[5] of pulse wave.The pulse wave velocity is the slowest in aorta, about 3 ~ 5 m/s, because of aortic distensibility is the greatest. It accelerated to 15 ~ 35 m/s in arterioles. Consequently, the pulse is felt in radial artery[6] about 0.1 s after the peak of systolic. In old people, arteries become more inflexible, and the pulse wave moves faster. The strength of pulse is determined by pulse pressure and has little relation to mean pressure.

---

[1] 心肌收缩力。

[2] 残余动脉容积。

[3] 动脉弹性回缩能力。

[4] 沿动脉管壁扩展的压力波即为脉搏。

[5] 传播。

[6] 桡动脉。

4 Venous pressure and venous return

4.1 Venous pressure

The venous system is situated between capillary and right atrium. In this location, venous pressure [1] can be influenced by both capillary and cardiac function. Venous pressure depends on the volume relative to compliance, as anywhere else.Venous pressure is quite low compared with arterial pressure,and cm H_2O is used to express venous pressure besides mmHg.

Blood from systemic veins flows into right atrium, therefore, the pressure in right atrium is called the central venous pressure [2], which is normally low, about range in 4 ~ 12 cmH_2O, and almost equal to the atmospheric pressure. Central venous pressure is regulated by a balance between the cardiac function to pump blood out of right atrium and the blood flow from peripheral veins into right atrium. Central venous pressure can be increased to about 20 ~ 30 mmHg under very abnormal conditions, such as heart failure [3] or massive transfusion [4], which greatly increases the total blood volume and causes quantities of blood to flow into heart from peripheral vessels. The low limit to central venous pressure is usually about –3 ~ –5mmHg, which is the pressure in chest cavity. It approaches this lowest value when blood flow into the heart is greatly depressed, such as severing hemorrhage [5].

According to the central venous pressure as zero reference point [6], the pressure in veins above this point is negative. So the cerebral vein pressure [7] would be as low as –28 mmHg, that leads to a negative transmural pressure [8], and then veins in the head and neck are collapse. As blood volume build up behind the collapsed vessels, they open to allow blood to flow through after that collapse again as pressure falls. Veins in the cranium [9] do not collapse because hydrostatic influence is balanced by equal extravascular influence. The hydrostatic pressure at foot is about 90 mmHg in erect position. In reclining position [10], the mean blood

---

[1] 静脉压。

[2] 右心房内的压力称为中心静脉压。

[3] 心力衰竭。

[4] 大量输液。

[5] 大失血。

[6] 参考零点。

[7] 脑静脉压。

[8] 跨壁压。

[9] 头盖骨。

[10] 卧位。

pressure in arteriaedorsalispedis[1] is about 90 mmHg. This pressure rise to about 180 mmHg in erect position, that is the sum of reclining pressure and hydrostatic pressure.

4.2 Venous return

Venous return is depended on the pressure gradient between peripheral venous pressure and central venous pressure and the resistance to blood flow imposed by the large venous system. Therefore, the factors that can affect central venous pressure, peripheral venous pressure and venous resistance can affect the amount of venous return. In venous system[2], the resistance to blood flow is small, results in blood pressure from micro vein to right atrium drops only about 15mmHg. The resistance in veins accounts for 15% of TPR, which is compatible with the function of vein.

4.2.1 Mean circulatory filling pressure

Peripheral venous pressure[3] is the pressure generated by blood volume flow from capillaries into peripheral veins relative to compliance of veins. The venous resistance and compliance, primarily of the small veins and venules, is revealed in the mean circulatory filling pressure[4] which generated by the total blood volume in vascular system. If tissue blood flow is zero then the mean systemic pressure throughout system is equal. When mean systemic pressure is high, peripheral venous pressure will be high, and then the pressure head for venous return is high.

4.2.2 Myocardial contractility

Since cardiovascular system is a closed–tube network[5], and the system is, in a steady state, venous return and cardiac output are equal. Actually, in a short term, cardiac output is substantially determined by venous return in normal subjects. When the central venous pressure is increased due to instances of reduce cardiac function, results in reduction of venous return.

4.2.3 Gravity and position

Assumption of the standing position increases peripheral venous transmuralpressure,becausea shift of blood from the central of circulatory system to the peripheral veins of the lower extremities.This shift causes cardiac output and venous return to decline, and results in syncope when compensation is absent.

---

[1] 足背动脉。

[2] 静脉系统。

[3] 外周静脉压。

[4] 循环系统平均充盈压。

[5] 闭管网络。

4.2.4 Thoracoabdominal pump

The intrapleural pressure[1] below atmospheric pressure, in general, thus large veins in thoracic cavity[2] are dilated. Respiration is a factor that contributes to maintain venous return by changing the pressure gradient between thoracic and abdominal cavity[3]. During inspiration, intrathoracic pressure[4] decreases, so that expansion of large veins and the right atrium was more obvious. Increased intraabdominal pressure[5] causes peripheral venous pressure to increase, augments the pressure gradient for venous return. During expiration the opposite effects occur.

4.2.5 Skeletal muscle pump

In upright position, there is a great difference, with or without muscle contraction, in the amount of venous return. On quiet standing, venous pressure of foot may rise to as high as 90 mmHg. While walking, repeated muscle contraction can discharge enough blood from leg veins toward heart to maintain foot venous pressure below 25 mmHg. The skeletal muscle pump is composed of muscles and venous valves[6]. Contraction of skeletal muscles squeezes the underlying and adjacent veins. On the other hand, every venous valve is oriented toward heart, they ensure blood flow in the direction of heart, thereby increasing venous return with muscle contraction together. The muscle pump makes significant contribution to maintain venous return and to reduce peripheral venous blood retention during walking. Under these circumstances, the work of skeletal muscle pump accelerates systemic circulation to a great extent.

5 Microcirculation

The circulation between arterioles and venules is namedasmicrocirculation, where is materials exchange place between blood and tissue fluid[7]. The exchange in microcirculation is responsible for transport of nutrients and O_2 to tissues, and for removal of CO_2 and cell excreta[8]. So that physical and chemical factors of internal environment are maintained relatively stable, so as to ensure normal metabolism of tissue cells. Each tissue, in most instances, controls its blood flow in relation to the individual needs by change the diameters of arterioles.

[1] 胸膜腔内压。

[2] 胸腔。

[3] 腹腔。

[4] 胸内压。

[5] 腹内压。

[6] 静脉瓣。

[7] 微动脉与微静脉之间的血液循环称为微循环，是血液和组织液进行物质交换的场所。

[8] 排泄物。

5.1 The compositions of a microcirculation unit

In general, each nutrient artery[1] entering an organ branches 6 ~ 8 times before the arteries become small enough to be called arterioles that characterized by well-developed smooth musculature[2] in its wall, and their internal diameters only 10 ~ 15 micrometers. A unit of microcirculation is a collection of vessels that originate from an arteriole, thereof, the role of arteriole is to shrink or expand vessel diameter through contraction or relaxation of smooth muscle, thereby to control the blood flow as a "total gate" of the microcirculation. And then, arterioles branch 2 ~ 3 times, at their ends, reaching diameters of 5 ~ 9 micrometers which are named metarterioles[3], where they supply blood to the capillaries. Either several true capillaries supplied blood from one metarteriole, or one to one. Usually, there are 1 ~ 2 smooth muscle cells in the initial parts of capillaries, forming as a ring, are called precapillary sphincter[4], which plays a role of "parted gate" to regulate blood flow into capillary. Also, There are smooth muscle cells in venule, which determines postcapillary resistance to control capillary pressure, then plays a role as "post gate".

The typical microcirculation consists of 7 parts following: arteriole, metarteriole, precapillary sphincter, true capillary (circuitous channel) , thoroughfare channel, arterio-venous anastomosis[5] and venule(Figure 4-12). There are three different types of structure and function in microcirculation.

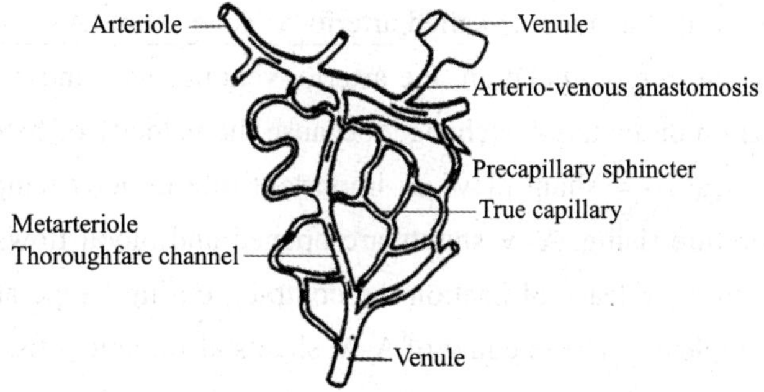

Figure 4-12 A microcirculatory unit

[1] 营养动脉。

[2] 肌肉组织。

[3] 后微动脉。

[4] 毛细血管前括约肌。

[5] 动静脉吻合支。

5.1.1 Circuitous channel

Circuitous channel [1] is the most important function of microcirculation blood flow, where the blood flow pass through arteriole, metarteriole, precapillarysphincter,true capillary network[2], and finally into venule. Circuitous channel is characterized by true capillary, which is composed of a unicellular layer by endothelial cells and is surrounded by a thin basement membrane outside of the wall. The total thickness of capillary wall is only about 0.5μm. The internal diameter of capillary is 4 ~ 9μm, barely large enough for all blood cells to squeeze through. All of these factors are conducive to exchange quickly and easily, so it is called "nutritional channel [3] " too.

5.1.2 Thoroughfare channel

In certain tissues, the arteriole branches into metarterioles, without nervous supply, often in open state, and continue into large capillaries and then shunt blood to venules directly. Thoroughfare channels [4] are bypasses of true capillaries, so they are also called preferential channels [5]. Thoroughfare channels relatively more express in skeletal muscle, where material exchange is weak, because the diameter is wide, so that blood flow is fast and not conducive to exchange. The main function of thoroughfare channel is to make blood flow through microcirculation and back into vein quickly.

5.1.3 Arterio–venous shunt

Arterioles of the human skin, especially in the face, ear, fingers and toes, often branch into arterio–venous anastomoses [6], which have function as shunt vessels leading blood back into venous directly, so that channel is called arterio–venous shunt (A–V shunt) [7]. Different from other pathways of microcirculation, the arterio–venous anastomoses branched from arteriole have no function on material exchange, because the velocity of blood flow is high and vessel wall is thick. But A–V shunt plays an important role in body temperature regulation. During body temperature rising, A–V shunts are opened and blood flows to skin increased, which is conducive to the release of heat;on the contrary, during temperature reducing, A–V shunts are closed completely. The opening of A–V shunts also reduces tissue oxygen supplied from blood.

---

[1] 迂回通路。

[2] 真毛细血管网。

[3] 营养通路。

[4] 直捷通路。

[5] 优先通路。

[6] 动 – 静脉吻合支。

[7] 动 – 静脉短路。

5.2 Regulation of microcirculation

In general, blood does not flow continuously through the capillaries. Instead, the blood flows intermittently, because the vessels turning on and off every few seconds or minutes. This phenomenon is called vasomotion[1], which means intermittent contraction of metarterioles and precapillary sphincters, and sometimes even the very small arterioles contract as well.

5.2.1 Local product of metabolism

The most important factor found to affect blood flow of microcirculation is the rate of metabolism of local tissues.When metarterioles and precapillary sphincters contract, true capillaries are closed, then the rate of oxygen decreased, and metabolites[2] (such as CO_2, histamine, lactic acid, adenosine[3]) around vascular tissues accumulated. Hypoxia and metabolic products[4] cause local metarterioles and precapillary sphincters relaxation, followed by true capillary network open again.Whenthe local accumulation of metabolites in blood is removed and local oxygen is increased, true capillary network closed again. Thus, the blood flow of microcirculation is proportionate to the level of metabolic activity. In quiet, the level of tissue metabolism is low, at the same time, only 20% ~ 35% of true capillaries in the skeletal muscle is open.

5.2.2 Resistance of microcirculation

Generally, blood flow in microcirculation is laminar, which is proportional to the pressure gradient from arteriole tovenule,anddivided by the total resistance of microcirculation. Capillary blood pressure depends on the ratio of precapillary resistance and postcapillary resistance, when the ratio is increased, capillary pressure is reduced by reduction of blood; in contrast, when the ratio is decreased, the opposite effects occur.

5.2.3 Neural and humoralregulation

The smooth muscle in the walls of the arterioles and venules are controled by sympathetic vasoconstrictor fibers[5],in addition, there are vasoactive substances[6] such as angiotensin II, vasopressin, epinephrine and norepinephrine in blood.When the sympathetic vasoconstrictor nerve fibers were excited, arterioles and venules contracted both, but the degrees of their contraction were different. Because the nerve density of arteriole greater than venule's, therefore, when sympathetic nervous activity increased, the contraction of arterioles is stronger than ve-

[1] 血管运动。

[2] 代谢产物。

[3] 腺苷。

[4] 代谢产物。

[5] 交感缩血管纤维。

[6] 血管活性物质。

nule's, so that blood flow into microcirculation and capillary pressure will be reduced. In the contrary condition, the result is contrary too. The volume and distribution of blood flow are mainly affected by local metabolites, and a relatively small regulating effect bynervaland humoral factors.

6 Tissue fluid and lymph

6.1 Tissue fluid

About one sixth of the total volume of body consists of spaces between cells, and the fluid in these spaces is called interstitial fluid[1] or tissue fluid[2]. The interstitial fluid is exchange media of blood and cell. Substances in blood can pass through the junctions between endothelial cells and through fenestrations[3]. In the case of lipid-soluble substances[4], they also pass through cells by vesicular transport[5] .Quantitatively,diffusion is the most important factor in terms of exchange for nutrients and waste materials between blood and tissue. Glucose and O_2 are in higher concentration in bloodstream than interstitial fluid and diffuse into interstitial fluid, whereas CO_2 diffuses in the opposite direction.

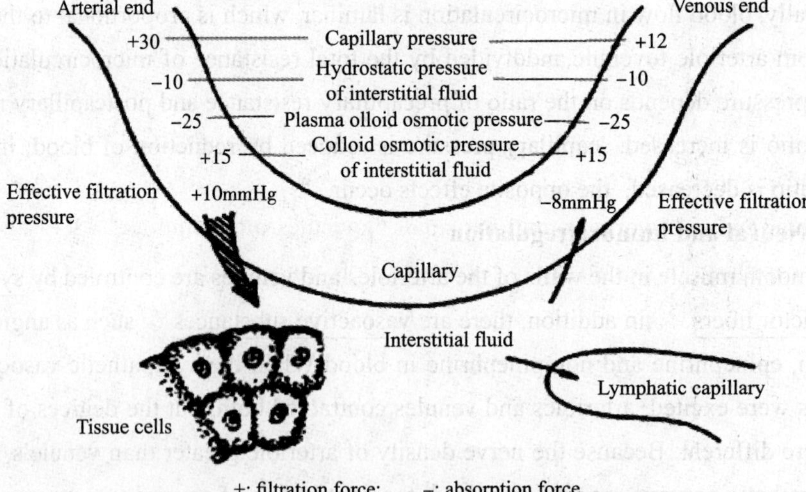

Figure 4-13 Formation and return of interstitial fluid

[1] 间质液。
[2] 组织液。
[3] 窗孔。
[4] 脂溶性物质。
[5] 囊泡运输。

The rate of filtration at any point along capillaries depends upon a force named effective filtration pressure[1],which is a balance of filtration force and absorption force which sometimes called the Starling forces[2], and which determines whether fluid will move out of blood vessel into interstitial fluid or in the opposite direction (Figure 4–13). One of these forces is the hydrostatic pressure gradient[3](hydrostatic pressure in capillary minus hydrostatic pressure of interstitial fluid). The other force is the osmotic pressure gradient[4] across capillary wall (colloid osmotic pressure of plasma minus colloid osmotic pressure of interstitial fluid). Thus:

$$Fluid\ movement = k[(P_c + \pi_i) - (P_i + \pi_c)]$$

Where, k = capillary filtration coefficient, Pc = capillary pressure, Pi = hydrostatic pressure of interstitial fluid, πi = colloid osmotic pressure of interstitial fluid, πc = capillary colloid osmotic pressure.

Pc tends to force fluid and dissolved substances through capillary pores into interstitial spaces. Pi varies from one organ to another, and there is considerable evidence that it is subatmospheric[5] about –2 mmHg in subcutaneous tissue[6] and positive in liver and kidneys and brain.π_i is usually negligible, so osmotic pressure gradient (π_c –π_i) usually equals the osmotic pressure caused by plasma proteins, and which normally prevents significant loss of fluid volume from blood into interstitial spaces. Takes the capillary filtration coefficient[7] into account, and is proportionate to, the permeability and area of capillary wall available for filtration.If the sum of these forces–the net filtration pressure[8], is positive, there will be a net fluid filtration[9] into interstitial spaces across capillaries. On the contrary, there will be a net fluid absorption[10] from interstitial spaces into capillaries. Therefore,fluid moves into interstitial space at the arteriolar end of capillary, where filtration pressure exceeds oncotic pressure, and moves into capillary at venular end.It is worth noting that small molecules often equilibrate with the tissues nearby each capillary. In this situation, total diffusion can be increased by increasing blood

[1] 有效滤过压。

[2] 斯塔林力。

[3] 静水压差。

[4] 渗透压差。

[5] 负压。

[6] 皮下组织。

[7] 滤过系数。

[8] 净滤过压。

[9] 液体净滤出量。

[10] 液体净吸收量。

flow, i.e., exchange is blood flow-limited [1].

The effective filtration pressure is slightly positive under normal conditions, resulting in a net fluid filtration into interstitial space across capillaries in most organs. It has been estimated that about 24 L of fluid are filtered through capillaries per day. This is about 0.3% of cardiac output. About 90% of filtered fluid is reabsorbed into capillaries, and the remainder returns to circulation via lymphatics [2].

6.2 Lymph

Fluid that returns to circulation from tissue space by the way of lymphatic system [3] is defined as lymph [4]. The rate of lymph flow is very low under normal circumstances in mammals [5]. But lymphatic drainage is important for transporting chylomicrons [6] absorbed from intestine, and to return proteins from tissue spaces, neither of which can be replaced by absorption directly into capillaries.

Lymphatics are composed of endothelium-lined vessels similar to capillaries. They are equipped with one-way valves, so rhythmic activity in skeletal muscles returns lymph to circulation via thoracic duct [7]. Lymph vessels originate as blind-ended sacs close to capillaries, those are permeable to proteins, macromolecules and even to cells from interstitial fluid. such as bacteria, can push their way between endothelial cells of lymphatic vessels and enter the lymph. As lymph passes through lymph nodes [8], these particles are almost entirely removed and destroyed.

Section 4 Cardiovascular regulatory mechanism

Cardiovascular activity is regulated by multiple mechanisms. These mechanisms increase blood supply to active tissues,and maintain homeostasis of blood pressure, and increase or decrease heat loss from body by redistributing blood. In the face of challenges such as hemorrhage [9], the blood flow to heart and brain must be ensured. When the hemorrhage is severe,

[1] 血流量限制性。

[2] 淋巴管。

[3] 淋巴系统。

[4] 淋巴。

[5] 哺乳动物。

[6] 乳糜微粒。

[7] 胸导管。

[8] 淋巴结。

[9] 出血。

blood flow to these vital organs is maintained at the decrease of blood supply to the rest of body. The homeostatic control of blood pressure involves the integrated activity of cardiovascular system acting over short term, in conjunction with the systems concerned with body fluid and electrolyte balance acting over long term[1].

1 Neuroregulation

Nervous regulation of circulation that such as increasing or decreasing cardiac activity, especially, redistributing blood flow to different areas of body, providing very rapid control of systemic arterial pressure by minutes. The nervous system controls circulation almost entirely through autonomic nervous system[2], and the most important part of autonomic nervous system for regulating circulation is sympathetic nervous system[3]. The innervation[4] of heart and blood vessels, such as cardiac sympathetic, cardiac vagal[5], sympathetic vasoconstrictor, vasodilator, has unitary effects on cardiovascular activity, comparatively, adjustment of tissue blood flow is mainly by the function of local control mechanisms.

1.1 Cardiac innervations

The myocardiac cells[6] are innervated by sympathetic and vagal nerves both. Impulses in noradrenergic[7] sympathetic cardiac nerves increase the heart rate (positive chronotropic effect[8]) and the force of cardiac contraction (positive inotropic effect[9]). These effects caused by norepinephrine (NE) that combines with β_1 adrenergic receptor[10] on myocardiac cell membrane. They also inhibit the effects of vagal stimulation, probably by release of neuropeptide Y[11], which is a cotransmitter[12] in the sympathetic endings. Impulses in cholinergic[13] vagal

[1] 在维持动脉血压稳定方面，心血管活动的调节发挥短期作用，体液和电解质平衡的维持发挥长期作用。

[2] 自主神经系统。

[3] 交感神经系统。

[4] 神经支配。

[5] 心迷走神经。

[6] 心肌细胞。

[7] 去甲肾上腺素能。

[8] 变时作用。

[9] 正性肌力作用。

[10] β_1 肾上腺素能受体。

[11] 神经肽 Y。

[12] 共同递质。

[13] 胆碱能。

cardiac fibers decrease heart rate.

Although parasympathetic nervous system[1] is exceedingly important for many other autonomic functions, it plays only a minor role in regulation of circulation. Its most important circulatory effect is to control heart rate by the way of vagal cardiac nerves. Principally, vagal stimulation causes a marked decrease in heart rate and a slight decrease in heart muscle contractility by releasing acetylcholine[2], which can combine with muscarinic cholinergic receptor[3] on myocardiac cell membrane. The functions are known as negative chronotropic effect and negative inotropic effect.

There is a moderate amount of tonic discharge[4] in cardiac sympathetic nerves at rest, but there is a good deal of tonic vagal discharge, named as vagal tone[5], in humans and other large animals. When vagus is cut in experimental animals, heart rate rises, and after administration of parasympatholytic drugs[6] such as atropine[7], heart rate in humans increases from its normal value of 70 to 150 ~ 180 beats/min because sympathetic tone[8] is unopposed. In humans heart rate is approximately 100, in whom both noradrenergic and cholinergic systems are blocked.

1.2 Innervations of blood vessels

Sympathetic vasomotor nerve fibers innervate mainly the vasculature of internal viscera[9] and heart, almost immediately, they distribute to the vasculature of peripheral areas. They leave spinal cord[10] through all thoracic spinal nerves[11] to the first one or two lumbar spinal nerves[12]. Sympathetic vasomotor nerve fibers end on vessels in all parts of body, most of them are noradrenergic and vasoconstrictor in function. In addition to their vasoconstrictor innervation, resistance vessels of skeletal muscles are innervated by vasodilator fibers, which, although travel with sympathetic nerves, are cholinergic named as sympathetic vasodilator sys-

---

[1] 副交感神经系统。

[2] 乙酰胆碱。

[3] 毒蕈碱胆碱能受体。

[4] 紧张性放电。

[5] 迷走神经紧张。

[6] 副交感神经阻断药。

[7] 阿托品。

[8] 交感神经紧张。

[9] 内脏。

[10] 脊髓。

[11] 脊髓胸段。

[12] 脊髓腰段。

tem[1]. Bundles of noradrenergic and cholinergic fibers form a plexus[2] on adventitia of arterioles[3]. Fibers with multiple varicosities[4] extend from this plexus to media and end, primarily on outer surface of smooth muscle of media without penetrating it. Transmitters reach inner portions of the media by diffusion, and current spreads from one smooth muscle cell to another via gap junctions[5].

There is no tonic discharge in vasodilator fibers, but vasoconstrictor fibers to most vascular beds have tonic activity. When sympathetic nerves are cut, blood vessels dilate. In most tissues, vasodilation is produced by decreasing the rate of tonic discharge in vasoconstrictor nerves, although in skeletal muscles it can also be produced by activating sympathetic vasodilator system.

Nerves containing polypeptides[6] are found on many blood vessels. The cholinergic nerves also contain vasoactive intestinal peptide (VIP)[7], which produces vasodilation. The noradrenergic postganglionic sympathetic nerves[8] also contain neuropeptide Y, which is a vasoconstrictor. Substance P[9] and calcitonin gene–related peptide α[10], which produce vasodilation, are found in sensory nerves near blood vessels. Afferent impulse[11] in sensory nerves from skin are relayed antidromically[12] down branches of sensory nerves that innervate blood vessels, and these impulses cause release of substance P which causes vasodilation and increased capillary permeability. This local neural mechanism is called axon reflex[13].

1.3 Cardiovascular center

Vasomotor and blood pressure are adjusted by variations in the rate of tonic discharge of nervous system. The sympathetic nervous system constricts arterioles and veins, and increases heart rate and stroke volume, discharge in a tonic fashion. Spinal reflex activity affects blood

---

[1] 交感舒血管系统。
[2] 丛。
[3] 动脉外膜。
[4] 曲张体。
[5] 缝隙连接。
[6] 多肽。
[7] 血管活性肠肽。
[8] 去甲肾上腺素能交感节后纤维。
[9] P 物质。
[10] 降钙素基因相关肽 α。
[11] 传入冲动。
[12] 逆向。
[13] 轴突反射。

pressure. But the main control of blood pressure is exerted by groups of neurons in the medulla oblongata [1] that are called the cardiovascular enter [2].

Neurons that mediate increased sympathetic discharge to blood vessels and heart project directly from sympathetic preganglionic neurons[3] in the intermediolateral (IML) gray column of spinal cord [4]. On each side, cell bodies of these neurons are located in the rostral ventrolateral medulla (RVLM) [5], where is called vasoconstrictor area [6]. The axons [7] originated from this area course dorsally and medially and then descend in the lateral column [8] of spinal cord to IML. It appears that the excitatory transmitter they secrete is glutamate [9] rather than epinephrine [10]. A vasodilator area [11] located bilaterally in the anterolateral portions of lower half of medulla[12]. Fibers from these neurons project upward to inhibit the activity of vasoconstrictor area, thus causing vasodilation. Impulses reaching the medulla also affect heart rate via vagal discharge to heart. The vagal fibers arise are in the dorsal motor nucleus [13] of vagus and nucleus ambiguus [14], where were known as cardiac inhibitory area [15].

A sensory area located bilaterally in the tractus solitaries in posterolateral portions of medulla and lower pons[16]. The neurons in this area receive sensory nerve signals from circulatory system mainly through vagus and glossopharyngeal nerves [17], then output signals to medulla and other parts of high central nervous system, such as cerebral cortex[18]. Where control activities of both the vasoconstrictor and vasodilator areas, thus providing “reflex” control of many

---

[1] 延髓。

[2] 心血管中枢。

[3] 交感节前神经元。

[4] 脊髓灰质中间外侧柱。

[5] 延髓头端腹外侧区。

[6] 缩血管区。

[7] 轴突。

[8] 侧柱。

[9] 谷氨酸。

[10] 肾上腺素。

[11] 舒血管区。

[12] 延髓尾端腹外侧部。

[13] 运动背核。

[14] 疑核。

[15] 心抑制区。

[16] 延髓与脑桥下部外侧的孤束核。

[17] 舌咽神经。

[18] 大脑皮层。

circulatory functions.

When vasoconstrictor discharge is increased, there are increased arteriolar constriction and a rise in blood pressure, and venoconstriction, and a decrease in the store of blood in venous reservoir, although changes in capacitance vessels do not always parallel changes in resistance vessels. Heart rate and stroke volume are increased because of activity in sympathetic nerves to heart. There is usually an associated decrease in tonic activity of vagal fibers. Conversely, a decrease in vasomotor discharge causes vasodilation and a fall in blood pressure, and usually a concomitant decrease in heart rate, but this is mostly due to the stimulation of cardiac vagal innervation.

1.4 Reflex regulation of cardiovascular activity

1.4.1 Baroreceptors and baroreceptor reflex

Baroreceptor reflex[1] is basically initiated by stretch receptors[2] located at specific points in the walls of heart and blood vessels, such as carotid sinus[3] and aortic arch[4] receptors that monitor arterial circulation.

Carotid sinus is a small dilation of internal carotid artery just above the bifurcation that common carotid[5] branches into external and internal carotid[6] (Figure 4–14). Baroreceptors are also found in the wall of aortic arch. They are located in the adventitia[7] of vessels, extensively branched, knobby, coiled, and intertwined the ends of myelinated nerve fibers[8]. The afferent nerve fibers from carotid sinus and carotid body form a distinct branch, named as Hering's nerve[9] or ca-

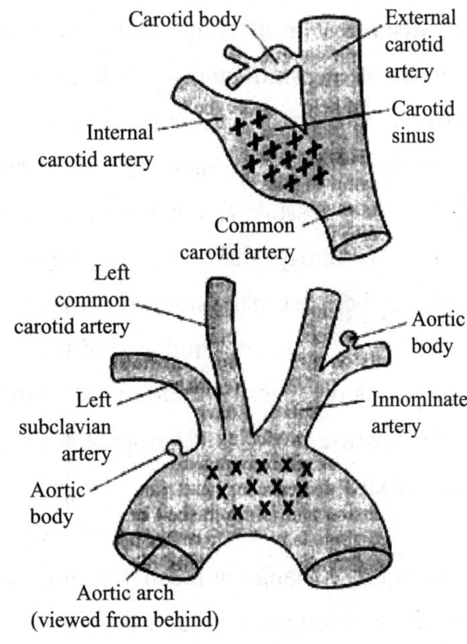

Figure 4–14 Baroreceptor areas in the carotid sinus and aortic arch. "×" sites where receptors are located.

[1] 压力感受性反射。

[2] 牵张感受器。

[3] 颈动脉窦。

[4] 主动脉弓。

[5] 颈总动脉。

[6] 颈外和颈内动脉。

[7] 外膜。

[8] 有髓神经纤维。

[9] 赫林神经。

rotid sinus nerve[1], then integrate into glossopharyngeal nerve in the high neck, and then to the NTS in medullary area of brain stem[2]. The fibers from aortic arch form a distinct branch and transmit signals through vagus nerves also to the same NTS of medulla in human. The carotid sinus nerves and vagal fibers from aortic arch are commonly called buffer nerves[3].

At normal blood pressure levels, the buffer nerves fibers discharge at a low rate (Figure 4–15). When the pressure in carotid sinus and aortic arch rises, the discharge rate increases; and when blood pressure falls, the discharge rate declines. When one carotid sinus of a monkey is isolated and perfused in vivo, and other baroreceptors are denervated[4], there is no discharge in afferent fibers from the perfused carotid sinus and no drop in monkey's arterial blood pressure or heart rate when the perfusion pressure[5] is below 30 mmHg. As perfusion pressure fluctuated in the range of 70 ~ 110 mmHg, there is an essentially linear relation between perfusion pressure and blood pressure or heart rate produced in the monkey. At perfusion pressures above 150 mmHg there is no further increase in response, presumably because the rate of baroreceptor discharge and the inhibition degree of vasomotor center are maximal.

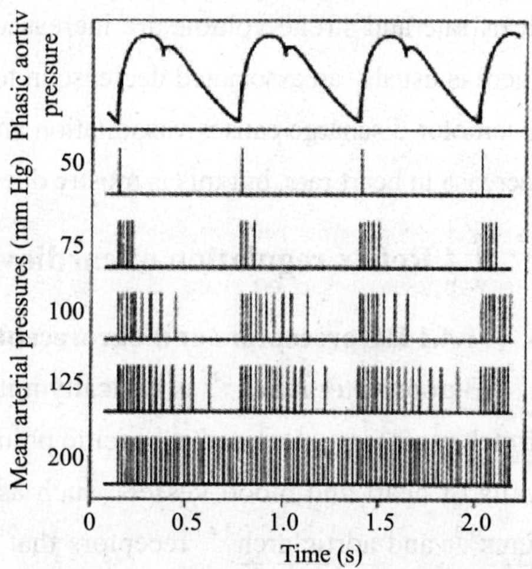

Figure 4–15 Discharges (vertical lines) in a single afferent nerve fiber from the carotid sinus at various arterial blood pressures, plotted against changes in aortic pressure with time.

The carotid receptors respond both to arterial pressure and pulse pressure. A decline in PP without any change in mean pressure decreases the rate of baroreceptor discharge and leads to a rise in blood pressure and tachycardia. The receptors also respond to changes in pressure as well as steady pressure, when the pressure is fluctuating, the rate of discharge rises with blood pressure and silent during it falls. When the pressure steads at mean pressure, has no fluctuations, there would be a steady discharge.

So it can be seen from the experiments above that when baroreceptors are excited by high pressure, discharge signals enter the NTS of medulla which produce secondary signals. These

[1] 窦神经。

[2] 脑干。

[3] 缓冲神经。

[4] 去神经。

[5] 灌注压。

secondary signals inhibit the vasoconstrictor center and excite the vagal cardiac inhibitory area of medulla. The net effects are vasodilation of arterioles and veins throughout peripheral circulatory system, and decreased heart rate and strength of heart contraction. Therefore, excitation of baroreceptors reflexly causes arterial pressure to decrease. Conversely, low pressure has opposite effects, reflexly causes the pressure to rise back toward normal, i.e. baroreceptor reflex can maintain a steady pressure.

1.4.2 Atrial stretch receptors

Stretch receptors are also located in the walls of right and left atria[1] at the entrance of superior and inferior venae cavae[2], as well as in pulmonary circulation[3]. These receptors in low–pressure part of circulation are referred to collectively as cardiopulmonary receptors[4]. There are two types of stretch receptors in atria: those discharge primarily during atrial systole[5] are type A, those discharge primarily late in diastole[6], at the time of peak atrial filling, are type B. The discharge of type B baroreceptors is increased when venous return is increased and decreased by positive–pressure breathing[7], indicating that these baroreceptors respond primarily to distention of atrial walls. The reflex circulatory adjustments initiated by increased discharge from type B receptors include vasodilation and a fall in blood pressure. However, the heart rate is increased rather than decreased.

1.4.3 Chemoreceptor reflex initiated by the carotid and aortic bodies

Chemoreceptor reflex operates in the same way as baroreceptor reflex except that chemoreceptors[8] initiate the response instead of baroreceptors. The chemoreceptors are cells that sensitive to oxygen lack, carbon dioxide[9] and hydrogen ion[10] excess. They are located in several small chemoreceptor organs about 2 mm in size, which include two carotid bodies[11] and 1 ~ 3 aortic bodies[12]. Carotid bodies lie in the bifurcation of each common carotid artery, and aortic bodies usually adjacent to aorta. Chemoreceptors excite nerve fibers that along with buf-

[1] 左右心房。

[2] 上下腔静脉。

[3] 肺循环。

[4] 心肺感受器。

[5] 心房收缩期。

[6] 舒张期。

[7] 正压呼吸。

[8] 化学性感受器。

[9] 二氧化碳。

[10] 氢离子。

[11] 颈动脉体。

[12] 主动脉体。

fer nerves into the center of medulla, and then exert their main effect on respiration. However, the afferents also converge on vasomotor area. The cardiovascular responses to chemoreceptors stimulation consist of peripheral vasoconstriction and bradycardia. Indirectly, hypoxia also produces hyperpnea and the increased catecholamine[1] secretion from adrenal medulla[2], both of which produce an increase in cardiac output and tachycardia.

Hemorrhage produces hypotension[3] leading to chemoreceptor stimulation, which is due to the decreased blood flow to chemoreceptors and consequent stagnant anoxia[4] of these organs. However, chemoreceptor reflex is not a powerful controller of arterial pressure until the pressure falls below 80 mmHg. Therefore, this reflex becomes important to help prevent still further fall in such a low pressure.

2 Humoral regulation

Humoral regulation of the circulation means control by substances secreted or absorbed into the body fluids. Many circulating hormones affect the cardiovascular system , including norepinephrine, epinephrine, angiotensin[5] and endothlin[6], and the vasodilator hormones include kinin[7], adrenomedullin[8], histamine[9], and atrial natriuretic peptide (ANP)[10]. Some of these substances are secreted by special glands and transport into blood throughout entire body, and others are formed in local tissue areas and cause only local circulatory effects.

2.1 Norepinephrine and epinephrine

Norepinephrine and epinephrine both increase the rate and force of contraction in isolated heart. These responses are mediated by β_1 receptors. They also increase myocardial excitability, causing extrasystoles[11] and, occasionally, more serious cardia arrhythmias[12]. Norepinephrine is an especially powerful vasoconstrictor hormone, and produces vasoconstriction in most

[1] 儿茶酚胺。
[2] 肾上腺髓质。
[3] 低血压。
[4] 淤血性缺氧。
[5] 血管紧张素。
[6] 内皮素。
[7] 激肽。
[8] 肾上腺髓质素。
[9] 组胺。
[10] 心房钠尿肽。
[11] 期前收缩。
[12] 心律失常。

organs via α_1 receptors. But epinephrine dilates coronary arteries[1] and blood vessels in skeletal muscle and liver via β_2 receptors, which usually overbalances the vasoconstriction produced by epinephrine elsewhere, and the total peripheral resistance drops. When norepinephrine is infused slowly in a normal animal or human, the systolic and diastolic blood pressures rise. The hypertension stimulates carotid and aortic baroreceptors, produce reflex bradycardia that overrides the direct cardioacceleratory[2] effect of norepinephrine. Consequently, the cardiac output falls. But epinephrine causes rise in both heart rate and cardiac output and a wide pulse pressure,because its effect by baroreceptor reflex is insufficient to obscure the direct effect on heart.

When the sympathetic nervous system is stimulated during stress or exercise, their nerve endings release norepinephrine which can excite heart and contracts veins and arterioles. In addition, sympathetic nerves of the adrenal medullae cause these glands to secrete both norepinephrine and epinephrine into blood. These hormones then circulate to all areas of body and cause almost the same effects on circulation as direct sympathetic stimulation, thus providing a dual system of control.

2.2 Angiotensin

The octapeptide[3] angiotensin II has a generalized vasoconstrictor action. It is a so powerful vasoconstrictor substance that as little as 1 microgram can increase the arterial pressure by 50 mmHg or more in human. The effect of angiotensin II is to constrict powerfully small arterioles, so the total peripheral resistance is increased, and arterial pressure is increased too, at the same time the blood flow to that area can be severely depressed. Angiotensin II is formed from angiotensin I that liberated by the action of renin on circulating angiotensinogen[4]. The formation of angiotensin II is increased because renin secretion is increased when blood pressure falls or the volume of ECF is reduced, which helps to maintain blood pressure. Angiotensin II also increases water intake by cause thirst, and stimulates aldosterone[5] secretion, and increased formation of angiotensin II is a part of homeostatic mechanism that operates to maintain ECF volume. Thus, angiotensin II plays an integral role in regulation of arterial pressure. In addition, there are renin–angiotensin systems[6] in many different organs, and there may be one in the walls of blood vessels. Angiotensin II produced in blood vessel walls could

[1] 冠状动脉。

[2] 心动加速。

[3] 8 肽。

[4] 血管紧张素原。

[5] 醛固酮。

[6] 肾素血管紧张素系统。

be important in some forms of clinical hypertension[1].

2.3 Vasopressin

Vasopressin[2] is even slightly more powerful than angiotensin II as a vasoconstrictor, thus making it perhaps one of the most potent vascular constrictor substance in human. It is formed in hypothalamus[3] of the brain, then transported downward by the nerve axons to posterior pituitary[4], where is finally secreted into blood. Normally, only minute amounts of vasopressin is secreted, so it plays little role in vascular control. However, experiments have shown that the concentration of circulating vasopressin after severe hemorrhage can rise high enough to increase the arterial pressure as much as 60 mmHg. In many instances, vasopressin can bring the arterial pressure almost back up to normal by itself. Also, it has a major function to increase greatly water reabsorption into blood from the renal tubules[5], which helps to control body fluid volume. That is why vasopressin is also called antidiuretic hormone (ADH)[6], which is discussed in Chapter 8.

2.4 Endothelin

Endothelin is a powerful vasoconstrictor in damaged blood vessels, which requires only nanogram[7] quantities to cause powerful vasoconstriction. It is a kind of large peptide with 21 amino acids[8], and presented in the endothelial cells of all or most blood vessels. The usual stimulus for release is damage to endothelium, such as that caused by crushing the tissues or by injecting a traumatizing[9] chemical into the blood vessel. After severe blood vessel damage, it is probably that the release of local endothelin and subsequent vasoconstriction helps to prevent extensive bleeding from arteries.

2.5 Kinin

Several substances called kinins cause powerful vasodilation when formed in the blood

[1] 高血压。
[2] 血管升压素。
[3] 下丘脑。
[4] 垂体后叶。
[5] 肾小管。
[6] 抗利尿激素。
[7] 纳克。
[8] 氨基酸。
[9] 创伤。

and tissue fluids of some organs. The most important two kinins are nonapeptide[1] bradykinin and decapeptidelysylbradykinin[2], which also known as kallidin[3]. Bradykinin and lysylbradykinin are formed from two precursor proteins[4], high-molecular-weight kininogen[5] and low-molecular-weight kininogen. Lysylbradykinin can be converted to bradykinin by aminopeptidase[6]. Both of them persist for only a few minutes then are metabolized to inactive fragments by carboxypeptidase enzyme[7] which named as kininase[8] I. In addition, one converting enzyme called kininase II inactivates bradykinin and lysylbradykinin too. The same enzyme also plays an essential role in activating angiotensin.

The biologic activities of bradykinin and lysylbradykinin[9] are generally similar, both of them cause powerful arteriolar dilation and increased capillary permeability. Kinins cause contraction of visceral smooth muscle[10], but they relax vascular smooth muscle via NO and lower blood pressure.

2.6 Atrial natriuretic peptide

ANP is synthesized and released by the myocardial cells of atrium when it is stretched. ANP has several actions which are not yet fully understood. In general, the effections of ANP are included as following: vasodilatation within kidney, inhibition of renin secretion by granular cells[11], inhibition of aldosterone secretion by the adrenal cortex[12], inhibition of ADH secretion by posterior pituitary, the actions of ADH on water transport in collecting duct[13], and an increase in sodium and water excretion. In conclusion, atrial natriuretic peptide can relax the vascular smooth muscle, decrease peripheral resistance, promote the excretion of water and sodium, and decrease blood pressure.

---

[1] 9肽。

[2] 10肽的赖氨酸缓激肽。

[3] 血管舒张素。

[4] 前体蛋白。

[5] 激肽原。

[6] 氨基肽酶。

[7] 羧基肽酶。

[8] 激肽酶。

[9] 赖氨酰舒缓激肽。

[10] 内脏平滑肌。

[11] 颗粒细胞。

[12] 肾上腺皮质。

[13] 集合管。

2.7 Adrenomedullin

Adrenomedullin (AM) is a depressor polypeptide first isolated from pheochromocytoma [1] cells. Its pro–hormone [2] is also the source of another depressor polypeptide, proadrenomedullin amino terminal 20 peptide (PAMP) [3]. AM also inhibits aldosterone secretion in salt–depleted [4] animals and appears to produce its depressor effect by increasing production of NO. PAMP appears to act by inhibiting peripheral sympathetic nerve activity. Both AM and PAMP are found in plasma and in many tissues in addition to adrenal medulla, including the kidney and brain.

2.8 Histamine

Histamine is released in essentially every tissue of body when the tissue becomes damaged or inflamed, or the subject of an allergic reaction [5]. Most of histamine is derived from mast cells in the damaged tissues and from basophils in blood. Histamine has a powerful vasodilator effect on the arterioles and, like bradykinin, has the ability to increase capillary porosity, allowing leakage of both fluid and plasma protein into tissues. In many pathological conditions, the intense arteriolar dilation and increased capillary porosity produced by histamine cause tremendous quantities of fluid to leak out of the circulation into tissues, inducing edema. The local vasodilator and edema–producing effects of histamine are especially prominent in allergic reactions.

3 Autoregulation

In addition to the mechanisms of neural and humoral regulation, the regulatory mechanisms in the local tissue also affect blood flow and pressure. It is proved that the organs and tissues still can adapt to the change of blood pressure within a certain range even after removing external nerves and humoral factors, and the blood flow can be adjusted properly through the local mechanism. The mechanism of regulation, which is present in organ tissues or blood vessels without neural and humoralregulation is called autoregulation [6]. There is also aautoregulation mechanism of the heart pumping function (Section 1 of this chapter). There are two kinds of mechanisms of local metabolism and muscle origin of autoregulation.

---

[1] 嗜铬细胞瘤。

[2] 促激素。

[3] 肾上腺髓质素前体氨基端 20 肽。

[4] 盐耗尽。

[5] 变态反应。

[6] 这种存在于器官组织或血管本身，不依赖神经和体液的调节机制，称为自身调节。

3.1 Autoregulation of local metabolites

The main substance that regulates metabolic autoregulation of local blood flow in tissue is oxygen and metabolites in tissues. The metabolism of tissue cells requires oxygen and produces various metabolites. When the metabolic activity of tissue enhances, partial pressure of oxygen [1] in the local tissue is decreases, and the accumulated metabolites increases, thereby contributing to relaxation of local arterioles. Tissue metabolites such as CO_2, H^+, adenosine, ATP, K^+ and other tissue metabolites have the effect of relaxation to local arterioles and anterior sphincter. Local blood flow increasing can provide more oxygen to the tissue, and take away metabolites, adapting to the strengthening local metabolic activities (such as muscle movement). This metabolic local vasodilator effect is sometimes quite obvious, even if accompanied with sympathetic nerve activity enhancing, the blood vessels of this local tissue are still play a relaxation role in local regulation .

As mentioned above, NO, kinins, prostaglandins, histamine, these humoral factors can also be formed in local tissues, and to regulate blood flow, but these substances are special humoral factors, so they are grouped in humoral regulation.

3.2 Myogenic autoregulation

Most vascular beds [2] have an intrinsic capacity to compensate for moderate changes in perfusion pressure by changes in vascular resistance, so that blood flow remains relatively constant. This capacity is well developed in kidneys, but it has also been observed in mesentery[3], skeletal muscle, brain, liver, and myocardium. It is probably due in part to the intrinsic contractile response of smooth muscle to stretch, myogenic theory [4] of autoregulation. As the pressure rises, blood vessels are distended and the vascular smooth muscle fibers surround vessels contract. As a result, blood flow resistance increases, buffering the increased blood flow of this organ caused by increased perfusion pressure[5], so that organ blood flow can maintain relative stability within a certain range of blood pressure fluctuations. Inhibiting the activities of vascular smooth muscle with papaverine [6], chloral hydrate and sodium cyanide [7] and other drugs, the myogenic autoregulation phenomenon will disappear.

---

[1] 氧分压。

[2] 血管床。

[3] 肠系膜。

[4] 肌原理论。

[5] 灌注压。

[6] 罂粟碱。

[7] 氰化钠

These three regulation mechanisms exist at the same time in different organs, but the interaction of their effects are different. Each mechanism is playing a regulatory role, but can not complete the whole process of complex regulation. Neural regulation mainly play a role in fast, short–term regulation; long–term regulation mainly depends on regulation of extracellular fluid volume by renal. They can cooperate in most cases, but in some cases also play a role of mutual confrontation. But all of these were integrated with the overall functional activities.

Section 5 Circulation through special regions

This section is concerned with the circulations of the heart, the lung and the brain.

1 Coronary circulation [1]

The right and left coronary arteries [2] arise at the root of the aorta behind the right and left cusps of the aortic valve, respectively. These arteries provide the entire blood supply to the myocardium. After the coronary arterial blood has passed through the capillary beds, most of it returns to the right atrium through the coronary sinus, but some of the coronary venous blood reaches the right atrium by way of the anterior coronary veins. A very small amount of coronary venous blood also flows back into the heart through small thebesian veins [3], which empty directly into all chambers of the heart.

The major coronary arteries sit on the surface of the heart and send numerous rather stout branches through the myocardium toward the endocardial surface [4]. These vessels divide frequently within the myocardium and supply a capillary network that provides an almost 1:1 ratio of capillaries to muscle fibers [5] and is among the densest found in the body.

1.1 Normal coronary blood flow

The normal coronary blood flow in the resting human being averages 225ml/min, which is about 4% to 5% of the total cardiac output. In strenuous exercise the coronary blood flow increases threefold to fourfold to supply the extra nutrients needed by the heart.

[1] 冠脉循环：心脏的血液循环。

[2] 左右冠状动脉：心肌的血液供应来自左右冠状动脉。左冠状动脉分为前降支和旋支，与右冠状动脉构成冠状动脉的三支主干。

[3] 心最小静脉。

[4] 冠状动脉主干及其大分支走行于心脏的表面，其小分支常以垂直方向穿入心肌至心内膜下。

[5] 毛细血管数和心肌纤维数的比例为 1：1。

1.2 Phasic changes in coronary blood flow

In addition to providing the pressure to drive blood through the coronary vessels, the heart also influences its blood supply by the squeezing effect of the contracting myocardium on the blood vessels that course through it. This force is so great during early ventricular systole that blood flow in the large coronary arteries that supply the left ventricle is briefly reversed[1], which is opposite to the flow in other vascular beds of the body. Maximal left coronary inflow occurs in early diastole, when the ventricles have relaxed and extravascular compression of the coronary vessels is virtually absent. This pattern is seen in the phasic coronary flow curve for the left coronary artery (Figure4–16). After an initial reversal in early systole, left coronary blood flow follows the aortic pressure until early diastole, when it rises abruptly and then declines slowly as aortic pressure falls during the remainder of diastole.

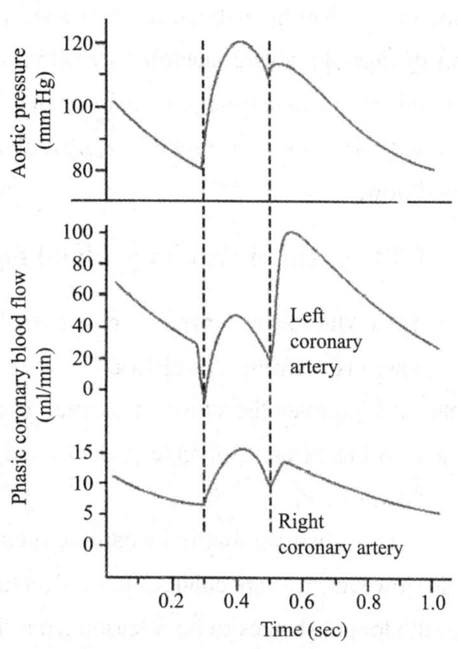

Figure 4–16 Blood flow in the left and right coronary arteries during various phases of the cardiac cycle. Systole occurs between the two vertical dashed lines.

Blood flow through the right coronary artery also undergoes phasic changes during the cardiac cycle. However, because of the lower pressure developed during systolic by the thin right ventricle, reversal of the blood flow does not occur in the right ventricle in early systole. Thus the shape of the right coronary artery blood flow curve resembles the aortic pressure curve, with the highest flow occurring during systole (Figure 4–16).

Left ventricular myocardial pressure is greatest near the endocardium[2] and least near the epicardium[3]. The importance of this pressure gradient[4] is that the intramyocardial pressure compresses the subendocardial blood vessels far more than the outer vessels. However, under normal conditions, this pressure gradient does not impair endocardial blood flow, because a

[1] 倒流、逆流。

[2] 心内膜：衬于心房和心室壁内面的一层光滑的薄膜，与血管的内膜相续。

[3] 心外膜：包在心肌外面的一层光滑的浆膜。

[4] 压力梯度：心室肌内的压力以内膜侧最高，朝向外膜侧递减。

greater blood flow to the endocardium during diastole compensates for the greater blood flow to the epicardium during systole. The cubendocardial tissue is much more vulnerable to ischemic injury than the subepicardial tissue. Subendocardial blood flow is dependent upon duration of diastole, aortic diastolic pressure, and left ventricular end–diastolic pressure. Factors that reduce diastolic time (e.g.,tachycardia[1]), lower arterial pressure (aortic insufficiency[2], coronary stenosis[3]), or raise ventricular end–diastolic pressure tend to reduce coronary blood flow.

1.3 Control of coronary blood flow

1.3.1 Metabolic control of coronary blood flow

There is a strong correlation between myocardial metabolism and coronary blood flow. That is, whenever the vigor of cardiac contraction is increased, the rate of coronary blood flow also increases. Conversely, decreased heart activity is accompanied by decreased coronary flow.

The mechanism that links cardiac metabolic rate and coronary blood flow remains unsettled. However, it is speculated that a decrease in the oxygen concentration in the heart causes vasodilator substances to be released from the muscle cells and that these substances dilate the arterioles. A substance with great vasodilator propensity is adenosine[4]. Adenosine enters the interstitial fluid space to reach the coronary resistance vessels, and induces vasodilation by activating adenosine receptors. After the adenosine causes vasodilation, much of it is reabsorbed into the cardiac cells to be reused for production of ATP, so that it cannot go elsewhere in the circulation to cause unwarranted vasodilatation.

Adenosine is not the only vasodilator product that has been identified. Others include adenosine phosphate compounds, potassium ions, hydrogen ions, carbon dioxide, prostaglandins, and nitric oxide.

1.3.2 Nervous control of coronary blood flow

The coronary vessels are innervated by both sympathetic and parasympathetic fibers. Sympathetic stimulation, which releases norepinephrine from the sympathetic nerves and epinephrine as well as norepinephrine from the adrenal medullae, increases both heart rate and heart contractility and increases the rate of metabolism of the heart. In turn, the increased metabolism of the heart sets off local blood flow regulatory mechanisms for dilating the coronary vessels, and the blood flow increases approximately in proportion to the metabolic needs of the

[1] 心动过速：心率加快时，心动周期缩短，舒张期缩短。

[2] 主动脉瓣关闭不全。

[3] 冠状动脉狭窄。

[4] 腺苷：由 AMP 在 5'－核苷酸酶的作用下分解而产生。

heart muscle. In contrast, vagal stimulation, with its release of acetylcholine, slows the heart and has a slight depressive effect on heart contractility. These effects decrease cardiac oxygen consumption and, therefore, indirectly constrict the coronary arteries.

1.3.3 Humoral regulation

Epinephrine and norepinephrine, both of which are secreted into the blood by the adrenal medulla, increase coronary blood flow by enhancing myocardial metabolism and oxygen consumption; and they can also cause coronary arterioles contraction or relaxation via directly effect on the coronary vascular alpha and beta adrenergic receptors. Thyroid hormones increase myocardial metabolic activity which in turn leads tocoronaryvasodilation. Angiotensin II and vasopressin, twopowerful vasoconstrictor substances in the blood, make coronary arterioles contraction and decrease coronary blood flow.

2 Pulmonary circulation

The lung has two circulations, a bronchial circulation[1] and a pulmonary circulation[2].

The bronchial circulation provides systemic arterial blood to the trachea, the bronchial tree, surface secretory cells, glands, nerves, visceral pleural surface, lymph nodes, pulmonary arteries and pulmonary veins. After this bronchial arterial blood has passed through these tissues, it empties into[3] the pulmonary veins and enters the left atrium.

The pulmonary circulation begins with the right ventricle. The pulmonary artery, which receives blood from the right ventricle, and its arterial branches carry blood to the alveolar capillaries for gas exchange, and the pulmonary veins then return the blood to the left atrium to be pumped by the left ventricle though the systemic circulation. The functions of the pulmonary circulatory system are ① reoxygenation of blood and to dispense of carbon dioxide[4], ② to aid in fluid balance in the lung, and ③ to distribute metabolic products of the lung.

The present discussion is concerned specifically with some features of the pulmonary circulation.

2.1 Anatomical and physiological characteristics of pulmonary circulation

2.1.1 Physiologic anatomy of the pulmonary circulation

The arteries of the pulmonary circulation are thin walled, with minimal smooth muscle.

---

[1] 支气管循环：体循环中的支气管动脉源自胸主动脉或其分支，对支气管和肺起营养性作用。肺循环与支气管动脉末梢之间有吻合支相通，部分支气管静脉的血液可经过吻合支直接进入肺静脉和左心房。

[2] 肺循环：从右心室、肺动脉经肺泡毛细血管、肺静脉到左心房的血液循环。

[3] 流注、注入。

[4] 使血液充氧和释出二氧化碳。

They are seven times more compliant[1] than systemic vessels, and they are easily distensible[2]. This highly compliant state of the pulmonary arterial vessels requires much less work for blood flow through the pulmonary circulation than do the more muscular, noncompliant arterial walls of the systemic circulation. The vessels in the pulmonary circulation, under normal circumstances, are in a dilated state and have larger diameters than do similar arteries in the systemic system. All of these factors contribute to a very compliant, low-resistance circulatory system, which aids in the flow of blood through the pulmonary circulation via the relatively weak pumping action of the right ventricle.

2.1.2 Pressures in the pulmonary circulation

The pulmonary circulation is a low-pressure, low-resistance system with a driving pressure that is almost one-sixteenth that of the systemic circulation.

The systolic pressure in the right ventricle of the normal human being averages about 22mmHg and the diastolic pressure averages about 0 to 1mmHg. During systole, the pressure in the pulmonary artery is essentially equal to the pressure in the right ventricle. The diastolic pulmonary arterial pressure averages about 8 mmHg, and the mean pulmonary arterial pressure[3] is about 15mmHg. The mean pulmonary capillary pressure has been estimated by indirect means to be about 7mmHg. The mean pressure in the left atrium and the major pulmonary veins averages about 2mmHg in the recumbent human being[4], varying from as low as 1 mmHg to as high as 5mmHg. When the left heart fails[5], the left atrial pressure is increased and the blood becomes dammed up[6] in the pulmonary system. When left atrial pressure has risen above 30mmHg, causing similar increases in capillary pressure, pulmonary edema[7] is likely to develop.

2.1.3 Negative pulmonary interstitial pressure

Because of the very low pulmonary capillary pressure, about 7 mmHg, the hydrostatic force[8] tending to push fluid out the capillary pores into the interstitial spaces is also very slight. Yet, the colloid osmotic pressure of the plasma[9], about 28 mmHg, is a large force tending to pull fluid into the capillaries. Therefore, there is continual osmotic tendency to de-

[1] 顺从，顺应。

[2] 容易扩张。

[3] 平均肺动脉压。

[4] 人在静息状态下。

[5] 左心衰竭。

[6] 阻塞。

[7] 肺水肿。

[8] 静水压：指血液在血管内因其本身的重力作用，对血管壁产生一定的压力。

[9] 血浆胶体渗透压。

hydrate[1] the interstitial spaces of the lungs. The interstitial fluid pressure in the lung, which has been measured by measuring the absorption pressure of fluid from the alveoli, giving a value of about −8 mmHg, is tending to pull the alveolar epithelial membrane toward the capillary membrane, thus squeezing the pulmonary interstitial space down to almost nothing[2]. As a result, the distance between the air in the alveoli and the blood in the capillaries is minimal, averaging about 0.4 micron in distance; this obviously allows very rapid diffusion of oxygen and carbon dioxide. Any factor that increases fluid filtration out of the pulmonary capillaries or that impedes pulmonary lymphatic function and causes the pulmonary interstitial fluid pressure to rise from the negative range into positive range will cause rapid filling of the pulmonary interstitial spaces and alveoli with large amounts of free fluid.

2.1.4 The blood volume of the lungs

The total blood volume of the lungs[3] is about 500 ml, which is about 10% of the circulating blood volume. It is estimated that 75 ml of blood is present in the alveolar–capillary network of normal adults at any one time. During exercise this blood volume can be increased by over 50% to 150 to 200 ml, due to the recruitment of new capillaries[4] secondary to an increase in pressure and flow. This recruitment of new capillaries is a unique feature of the lung, and it allows for compensation and adjustments[5] to stress, as in the case of exercise. Under various physiological and pathological conditions, the quantity of blood in the lungs can vary from as little as one–half normal up to twice normal. For instance, when a person blows out air so hard that high pressure is built up in the lungs, as much as 250 ml of blood can be expelled from the pulmonary circulatory system into the systemic circulation. Also, loss of blood from the systemic circulation by hemorrhage[6] can be partly compensated for by the automatic shift of blood from the lungs into the systemic vessels. The lungs serve as a blood reservoir[7].

2.2 Regulation of pulmonary circulation blood flow

2.2.1 Neural control of pulmonary vessels

Pulmonary vascular smooth muscle is supplied by autonomic nerves but, in contrast to their role in the systemic circulation, those nerves do not appear to participate significantly in pulmonary blood flow regulation.

---

[1] 使……脱水。

[2]（肺组织液负压）促使肺泡上皮细胞膜向毛细血管膜贴近，使得肺组织间隙非常小，几乎不存在。

[3] 肺总的血容量。

[4] 新的毛细血管募集。

[5] 补偿和调整。

[6] 出血。

[7] 储血库。

Stimulation of the vagal fibers[1] to the lungs causes a very slight decrease in pulmonary vascular resistance (PVR)[2], and stimulation of the sympathetic nerre[3] causes a slight-to-moderate increase in resistance. Sympathetic stimulation causes considerably more vasoconstriction in the presence of alveolar hypoxia[4], which suggests that the sympathetic nervous system might contribute significantly to the hypoxia mechanism to redistribute the blood flow.

2.2.2 Chemical control of pulmonary blood flow

Low and high oxygen levels have a major impact on blood flow. Hypoxia vasoconstriction occurs in small arterial vessels in response to decreased arterial PO_2. The response is local, and it may be a protective response by shifting the blood flow from the hypoxia areas to normal areas in an effort to enhance gas exchange. Low inspired oxygen levels due to exposure to high altitude will have a greater effect on PVR. High concentrations of inspired oxygen can dilate pulmonary vessels and decrease PVR.

In addition to alterations in oxygen, a wide range of other factors and mediators can influence vessel caliber, such as thromboxane A_2[5], epinephrine, norepinephrine, angiotensin[6], leukotrienes[7], neuropeptides[8], serotonin[9], endothelin[10], histamine[11], prostaglandins[12], high CO_2. These compounds can cause pulmonary vasoconstriction. Contrarily, prostacyclin[13], nitric oxide, acetylcholine[14], bradykinin[15], dopamine[16] can cause pulmonary vasodilation.

Under normal conditions, these factors play a very minor role; however, in pathological conditions their influence can be dramatic. These factors have a short half-life and their effects

---

[1] 迷走神经纤维。

[2] 肺血管阻力。

[3] 交感神经。

[4] 缺氧。

[5] 血栓烷 A_2。

[6] 血管紧张素。

[7] 白三稀。

[8] 神经肽。

[9] 5- 羟色胺。

[10] 内皮素。

[11] 组胺。

[12] 前列腺素。

[13] 前列环素。

[14] 乙酰胆碱。

[15] 缓激肽。

[16] 多巴胺。

are usually local.

3 Cerebral circulation

Blood reaches the brain through the internal carotid[1] and vertebral arteries[2]. The vertebral arteries join to form the basilar artery, which, in conjunction with branches of the internal carotid arteries, forms the *circle of Willis*[3] at the base of the brain. The arteries arising from the circle of Willis travel along the brain surface and give rise to pial arteries, which branch out into smaller vessels called penetrating arteries and arterioles. The penetrating vessels dive down into the brain tissue, giving rise to intracerebral arterioles, which eventually branch into capillaries. The cerebral capillaries are drained by veins that open into a number of wide venous spaces or sinuses on the surface of the brain.

3.1 Normal rate of cerebral blood flow

A unique feature of the cerebral circulation is that it lies within a rigid structure, the cranium. Because intracranial contents are incompressible, any increase in arterial inflow, as induced by arteriolar dilation, must be associated with a comparable increase in venous outflow. In the brain, the volume of blood and extravascular fluid is relatively constant, and the rate of total cerebral blood flow is maintained within a narrow range in contrast to most other organs. Normal blood flow through the brain of the adult person averages 50 to 65 mL /min/100 g of brain. For the entire brain, this amounts to 750 to 900 mL/min. Thus, the brain constitutes only about 2% of the body weight but receives 15% of the resting cardiac output.

3.2 Blood–cerebrospinal fluid and blood–brain barriers

Blood–cerebrospinal fluid barrier[4] and blood–brain barrier[5], exist between the blood and the cerebrospinal fluid and brain fluid, respectively. In general, these barriers are highly permeable to water, carbon dioxide, oxygen, and most lipid–soluble substances such as free forms of steroid hormones, alcohol and anesthetics; slightly permeable to electrolytes such as sodium, chloride, and potassium; and almost totally impermeable to plasma proteins and most non–lipid–soluble large organic molecules.

---

[1] 颈内动脉：供应大脑半球和间脑的各前 2/3 部。

[2] 椎动脉：供应脑干和小脑以及大脑半球和间脑的各后 1/3 部。

[3] Willis 环：两侧大脑前动脉、颈内动脉和大脑后动脉，借前交通动脉和左、右后交通动脉，在脑底吻合成一动脉环，也称大脑动脉环。此动脉环使颈内动脉与椎 – 基底动脉相互沟通，以保证大脑的血液供应。

[4] 血 – 脑脊液屏障：在毛细血管血液和脑脊液之间存在的限制某些物质交换的特殊屏障。

[5] 血 – 脑屏障。

The cause of the low permeability of the two barriers is the manner in which the endothelial cells of the brain tissue capillaries are joined to one another. That is, the membranes of the adjacent endothelial cells are tightly fused rather than having large slit pore between them, as is the case for most other capillaries of the body. In addition, the brain capillaries are surrounded by the end–feet of astrocytes[1]. These end–feet are closely applied to the basal lamina of the capillaries, but they do not cover the entire capillary wall, and gaps of about 20 nm occur between end–feet. However, the end–feet induce the tight junctions in the capillaries.

The blood–cerebrospinal fluid and blood–brain barriers probably maintain the constancy of the environment of the neurons in the central nervous system. These neurons are so dependent upon the concentrations of K^+, Ca^{2+}, Mg^{2+}, H^+, and other ions in the fluid bathing them that even minor variations have far–reaching consequences. The constancy of the composition of the extracellular fluid in all parts of the body is maintained by multiple homeostatic mechanisms, but because of the sensitivity of the cortical neurons to ionic change, it is not surprising that an additional defense has evolved to protect them. Other suggested functions for the blood–brain barrier are protection of the brain from endogenous and exogenous toxins in the blood and prevention of the escape of neurotransmitters into the general circulation.

3.3 Regulation of cerebral blood flow

Of all the body tissues, the brain is the least tolerant of ischemia. Interruption of cerebral blood flow for as little as 5 seconds results in loss of consciousness, and ischemia lasting just a few minutes results in irreversible tissue damage. Fortunately, regulation of the cerebral circulation is mainly under direction of the brain itself.

3.3.1 Autoregulation

Cerebral blood flow is autoregulated extremely well between the arterial pressure limits of 60 and 140 mmHg. That is, mean arterial pressure can be decreased acutely to as low as 60 mmHg or increased to as high as 140 mmHg without significant change in cerebral blood flow. In people who have hypertension, this autoregulatory range shifts to higher pressure levels, up to maximums of 180 to 200 mmHg. Conversely, if the arterial pressure falls below 60 mmHg, cerebral blood flow then does became severely compromised. Also, if the pressure rises above the upper limit of autoregulation, the blood flow increases rapidly and can cause severe overstretching or rupture of cerebral blood vessels, sometimes resulting in serious brain edema or cerebral hemorrhage.

3.3.2 Effects of PCO_2 and PO_2

The cerebral vessels are very sensitive to carbon dioxide tension. Increases in arterial blood carbon dioxide tension (PCO_2) elicit marked cerebral vasodilation; and decreases in

---

[1] 星形胶质细胞发出的突起，包裹在毛细血管周边。

PCO_2 which can be caused by hyperventilation[1], diminish cerebral blood flow.

Experiments have shown that a decrease in cerebral tissue PO_2 below about 30 mmHg (the normal value is 35 to 40 mmHg) immediately begins to increase cerebral blood flow. This is fortuitous because brain function becomes deranged at lower values of PO_2, especially at PO_2 levels below 20 mmHg. Even coma can result at these low levels. Thus, the oxygen mechanism for local regulation of cerebral blood flow is an important protective response against diminished cerebral neuronal activity and, therefore, against derangement of mental capability.

3.3.3 Neural control

The cerebral vessels are innervated by the cervical sympathetic nerve fibers that accompany the internal carotid and vertebral arteries into the cranial cavity. The sympathetic control of the cerebral vessels appears to be weaker than in other vascular beds. Transection of the sympathetic nerves[2] or mild to moderate stimulation of them usually causes little change in cerebral blood flow because the blood flow autoregulationmechanism can override the nervous effects.

[1] 过度换气。

[2] 切断交感神经：一种研究神经元功能的实验方法。

Chapter 5 RESPIRATION

The goals of respiration are to provide oxygen to the tissues and to remove carbon dioxide. To achieve these goals, respiration can be divided into four major functional events: ① pulmonary ventilation, which means the inflow and outflow of air between the atmosphere and the lung alveoli; ② exchange of O_2 and CO_2 between the alveoli and the blood by diffusion; ③ transport of O_2 and CO_2 in the blood to and from the cells; and ④ exchange of O_2 and CO_2 between blood in tissue capillaries and cells in tissues by diffusion (Figure 5–1).

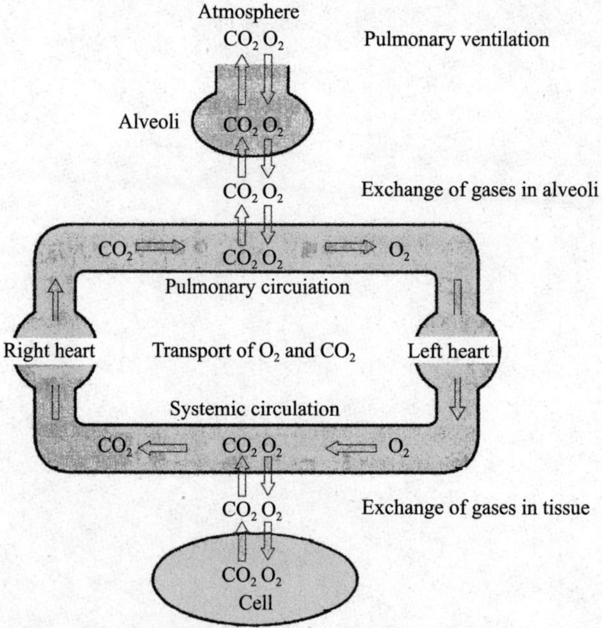

Figure 5–1 The steps of respiration.

Section 1 Pulmonary ventilation

1 The power of pulmonary ventilation

The pressure difference between the pulmonary pressure and the external environment is the direct force of pulmonary ventilation. Respiratory movement is the primary force of pulmonary ventilation. The contraction and relaxation of the respiratory muscles cause enlargement and contraction of the chest and lungs, and change the intrapulmonary pressure.

1.1 Respiratory movement

The lungs can be expanded and contracted in two ways: ① by downward and upward movement of the diaphragm to lengthen or shorten the chest cavity [1] and ② by elevation and depression of the ribs to increase and decrease the anteroposterior [2] diameter of the chest cavity. Figure 5–2 shows these two methods.

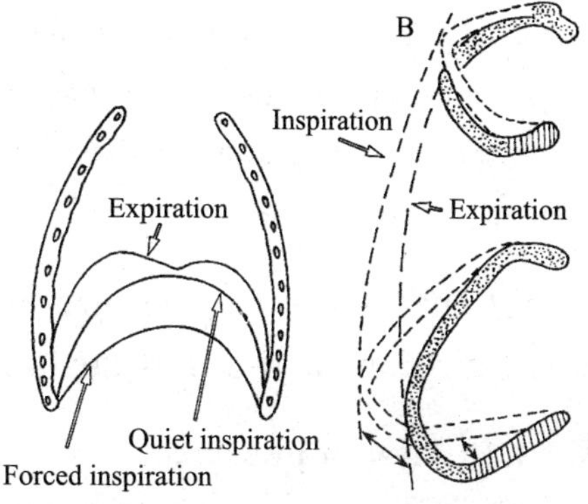

Figure 5–2 Chest volume changes induced by respiratory muscle activity

1.1.1 Muscles that cause lung expansion and contraction

The most important muscles of breathing are the diaphragm and the intercostales externi[3] which responsible of eupnea(quiet breathing)[4]. But for forced breathing(heavy breathing) [5], others muscles are involved which are classified as: ① Accessory inspiratory muscles, such as the sternocleidomastoid [6] muscles, the anterior serrati, and the scaleni[7]. ② Expiratory muscles, such as the abdominal muscles and the intercostales interni. [8]

1.1.2 The process of respiratory movement

In normal quiet breathing, during inspiration, when the diaphragm contract, its dome moves downward into the abdomen, enlarging the chest cage[9]. When the intercostales externi contract, they pull the upper ribs forward in relation to the lower ribs, and this causes leverage on the ribs to raise them upward, making the anteroposterior thickness of the chest about 20 % greater during maximum inspiration than during expiration. Then, during expiration, the inspi-

---

[1] 胸腔。

[2] 前后。

[3] 肋间肌。

[4] 平静呼吸。

[5] 用力呼吸。

[6] 胸锁乳突肌。

[7] 斜角。

[8] 肋间内肌。

[9] 扩大胸廓。

ratory muscles [1] simply relaxes, and the volume of the chest dropped to that of a quiet state.

During forced breathing, however, in addition to the involvement of accessory inspiratory muscles for forced inspiration, the elastic forces are not powerful enough to cause the necessary forced expiration, so that extra force is achieved mainly by contraction of the expiratory muscles [2]. The abdominal muscle pushes the abdominal contents upward against the bottom of the diaphragm and the intercostales interni function exactly oppositely to the intercostales interni, because they angle between the ribs in the opposite direction and cause opposite leverage.

1.2 Difference in pressure between the atmosphere and the alveoli that causes air flow in or out of the lungs.

1.2.1 Alveolar pressure

Alveolar pressure is the pressure of the air inside the lung alveoli. When the glottis is open and no air is flowing into or out of the lungs, the pressures in all parts of the respiratory tree, all the way to the alveoli, are equal to atmospheric pressure, which is considered to be the zero reference pressure in the airways–that is, 0 mmHg. To cause inward flow of air into the alveoli during inspiration, the pressure in the alveoli must fall to a value slightly below atmospheric pressure (below 0). During normal inspiration, alveolar pressure decreases to about –1 centimeter of water. This slight negative pressure is enough to pull 0.5 liter of air into the lungs in the 2 seconds required for normal quiet inspiration.

During expiration, opposite changes occur: The alveolar pressure rises to about +1 mmHg, and this forces the 0.5 liter of inspired air out of the lungs during the 2 to 3 seconds of expiration.

1.2.2 Pleural pressure and its changes during respiration

Pleural pressure [3] is the pressure of the fluid in the narrow space between the lung pleura and the chest wall pleura. This is normally a slight suction , which means a slightly negative pressure.

What has caused the pleural pressure to be subatmospheric [4] ? As the lungs (tending to move inward from their stretched position because of their elastic recoil) and the thoracic wall (tending to move outward from its compressed position because of its elastic recoil [5]) "try" to move ever so slightly away from each other, there occurs an infinitesimal enlargement of the

[1] 吸气肌。

[2] 呼气肌。

[3] 胸腔内压力。

[4] 负压。

[5] 弹性反冲。

fluid–filled pleural space between them. But fluid cannot expand the way air can, and so even this tiny enlargement of the pleural space–so small that the pleural surfaces still remain in contact with each other–drops the pleural pressure below atmospheric pressure.

The normal pleural pressure at the beginning of inspiration is about –5 mmHg, which is the amount of suction that is required to hold the lungs open to their resting level. Then, during normal inspiration, the expansion of the chest cage pulls outward on the lungs with still greater force and creates a still more negative pressure to an average of about –7.5 mmHg. Its changes cause the lungs and thoracic wall to move in and out together during normal breathing.

1.2.3 Transpulmonary pressure

The pressure difference between the alveolar pressure and the pleural pressure is called the transpulmonary pressure. The pressure inside the lungs is the aer pressure inside the alveoli (P_{alv}), and the pressure outside the lungs is from the pressure of the intrapleural [1] fluid surrounding the lungs (P_{ip}).

$$\text{Transpulmonary pressure} = P_{alv} - P_{ip}$$

Between breaths when the respiratory muscles are relaxed and no air is flowing. The P_{alv} is 0 mmHg; that is, it is the same as atmospheric pressure. The P_{ip} is approximately 4 mmHg less than atmospheric pressure—that is, –4mmHg. Therefore, the transpulmonary pressure ($P_{alv} - P_{ip}$) equals [0 mmHg–(– 4 mmHg)]= 4 mmHg. This transpulmonary pressure is a measure of the elastic forces in the lungs that tend to collapse the lungs. Elastic recoil is defined as the tendency of an elastic structure to oppose stretching or distortion. In other words, inherent elastic recoil tending to collapse the lungs is exactly balanced by the transpulmonary pressure tending to expand them, and the volume of the lungs is stable at air is present in the lungs between breaths.

During surgery or trauma, the chest wall is pierced without damaging the lung. Atmospheric air rushes through the wound into the pleural space (a phenomenon called pneumothorax [2]), and the intrapleuralpressure goes from –4 mmHg to 0 mmHg. The transpulmonary pressure acting to hold the lung open is thus eliminated, and the lung collapses.

To summarize, when the respiratory muscles contract or relax, they directly change the dimensions of the chest, which in turn causes the transpulmonary pressure to change. The change in transpulmonary pressure then causes a change in lung size, which causes changes in pressure between the atmosphere and the alveoli. It is this difference in pressure that causes air flow into or out of the lungs.

---

[1] 胸膜腔内的。

[2] 气胸。

2 Resistance of pulmonary ventilation

When breathing, the power produced by respiratory movement must overcome the resistance of pulmonary ventilation to achieve the function of pulmonary ventilation. The resistance to pulmonary ventilation includes both inelastic and elastic resistance. Inelastic resistance includes inertial resistance, viscous drag, and airway resistance. The airway resistance is closely related to the changes in physiological function and the clinic. Elastic resistance includes the elastic resistance of the lungs and the elastic resistance of the thorax. Most of the elastic resistance of the lung comes from the surface tension of alveoli. So here the airway resistance and the surface tension of alveoli are mainly introduced.

2.1 Airway resistance is the most important inelastic resistance for pulmonary ventilation

The volume of air that flows into or out of the alveoli per unit time is directly proportional to the pressure difference between the atmosphere and alveoli and inversely proportional to the resistance to flow offered by the airways. The factors that determine airway resistance are analogous to those determining vascular resistance in the circulatory system: tube length, tube radius, and interactions between moving molecules (gas molecules, in this case). The most important factor by far is the tube radius: Airway resistance is inversely proportional to the fourth power of the airway radii.

Asthma is a disease characterized by intermittent attacks in which airway smooth muscle contracts strongly[1], markedly increasing airway resistance. The basic defect in asthma is chronic inflammation of the airways, the causes of which vary from person to person and include, among others, allergy and virus infections.The important point is that the underlying inflammation causes the airway smooth muscle to be hyperresponsive[2] and to contract strongly.

2.2 Lung compliance reflects the strength of the elastic resistance

The degree of lung expansion at any instant is proportional to the transpulmonary pressure[3]. But just how much any given transpulmonary pressure expands the lungs depends upon the stretchability, or compliance, of the lungs. Lung compliance (C_L) is defined as the magnitude of the change in lung volume (ΔV_L) produced by a given change in the transpulmonary pressure:

[1] 哮喘是一种以间歇性发作为特征的疾病，发病时气管平滑肌强烈收缩。

[2] 气道高反应性。

[3] 在任何时刻，肺扩张程度和跨肺压是成正比的。

$$C_L = \triangle V_L / \triangle (P_{alv} - P_{ip})$$

Thus, the greater the lung compliance, the easier it is to expand the lungs at any given transpulmonary pressure. When lung compliance is abnormally low, pleural pressure must be made more subatmospheric than usual during inspiration to achieve lung expansion. This requires more vigorous contractions of the diaphragm and inspiratory intercostales muscles[1]. Persons with low lung compliance due to disease therefore tend to breathe shallowly and must breathe at a higher frequency to inspire an adequate volume of air.

2.2.1 Surfactant is the most important determinant of lung compliance

There are two major determinants of lung compliance[2]. One is the stretchability of the lung tissues, particularly their elastic connective tissues. The other is the surface tension at the air–water interfaces within the alveoli.

2.2.1.1 Surface tension of the alveolar decreases lung compliance

The surface of the alveolar cells is moist, and so the alveoli can be pictured as air–filled sacs lined with water. At an air–water interface, the attractive forces between the water molecules, known as surface tension, make the water lining like a stretched balloon that constantly tries to shrink and resists further stretching. Thus expansion of the lung requires energy not only to stretch the connective tissue[3] of the lung but also to overcome the surface tension of the water layer lining the alveoli.

2.2.1.2 Surfactants decrease surface tension of the alveolar

Indeed, the surface tension of pure water is so great that were the alveoli lined with pure water, lung expansion would require exhaustion muscular effort and the lungs would tend to collapse. It is extremely important, therefore, that the type Ⅱ alveolar cells secrete a detergent–like substance known as pulmonary surfactant, which markedly reduces the cohesive forces between water molecules on the alveolar surface. Therefore, lung compliance increases and makes it easier to expand the lungs.

Surfactant is a complex of both lipids and proteins[4], but its major component is a phospholipid[5] that forms a monomolecular layer between the air and water at the alveolar surface. The amount of surfactant tends to decrease when breaths are small and constant. A deep breath, which people normally intersperse frequently in their breathing pattern, stretches the type Ⅱ cells , which stimulates the secretion of surfactant. This is why patients who have had thoracic

---

[1] 吸气肋间肌。

[2] 肺顺应性有两个主要影响因素。

[3] 结缔组织。

[4] 表面活性物质是由复杂的脂质和蛋白构成的。

[5] 磷脂。

or abdominal surgery[1] and are breathing shallowly because of the pain must be urged to take occasional deep breaths.

2.2.2 Clinical significance of surfactant

A striking example of what occurs when surfactant is deficient is the disease known as respiratory–distress syndrome of the newborn. This is the second leading cause of death in premature infants, in whom the surfactant–synthesizing cells may be too immature to function adequately. Because of low ling compliance, the infant is able to inspire only by the most strenuous efforts, which may ultimately cause complete exhaustion, inability to breathe, lung collapse, and death. Therapy in such cases is assisted breathing with a mechanical ventilator and the administration of natural or synthetic surfactant via the infant's trachea.

3 Pulmonary volume and capacity[2]

3.1 Pulmonary volume

Four pulmonary lung volumes, when added together, equal the maximum volume to which the lungs can be expanded. The significance of each of these volumes is the following (Figure5–3):

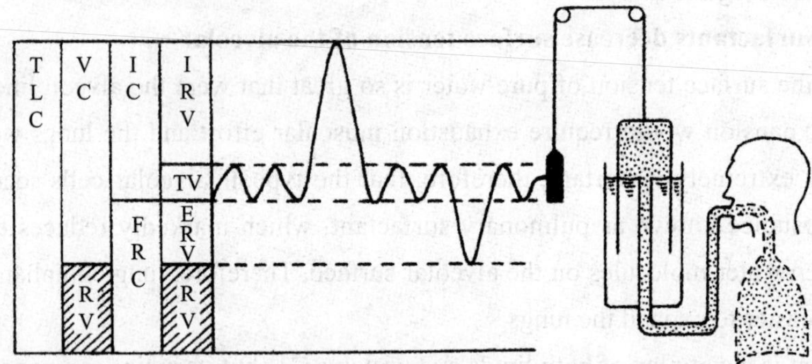

Figure 5–3 Diagram showing respiratory excursions during normal breathing and during maximal inspiration and maximal expiration.

(1) The Tidal Volume (TV) The volume of air inspired or expired with each normal breath[3], it amounts to about 500 ml.

(2) The Inspiratory Reserve Volume (IRV) The maximum extra volume of air that can be

[1] 腹部手术。

[2] 肺容积和肺容量。

[3] 潮气量（TV）是指每一次正常呼吸所吸入或呼出的空气量。

inspired over and above the normal tidal volume[1], it is usually equal to about 3000 ml.

(3) The Expiratory Reserve Volume (ERV) The maximum extra volume of air that can be expired by forceful expiration after the end of a normal tidal expiration[2], this normally amounts to about 1100 ml.

(4) The residual volume (RV) The volume of air remaining in the lungs after the most forceful expiration[3]. This volume averages about 1200 ml.

3.2 Pulmonary capacity

In describing events in the pulmonary cycle, it is sometimes desirable to consider two or more of the volumes together. Such combinations are called pulmonary capacities.

(1) The inspiratory capacity (IC) The amount of air (about 3500 ml) a person can breathe in, beginning at the normal expiratory[4] level and distending the lungs to the maximum amount. IC = TV+IRV

(2) The functional residual capacity (FRC) The amount of air that remains in the lung at the end of normal expiration (about 2300 ml). FRC = ERV + RV

(3) The vital capacity (VC) The maximum amount of air a person can expel from the lungs after first filling the lungs to their maximum extent and then expiring to the maximum extent[5] (about 4600 ml). VC = IRV + TV+ERV = IC + ERV

(4) The total lung capacity (TLC) The maximum volume to which the lungs can be expanded with the greatest possible effort (about 5800 ml). TLC = VC + RV = IC + FRC

(5) Forced vital capacity (FVC) Refers to the maximum amount of air a person can expel from the lungs after first filling the lungs to their maximum extent and then expiring to the maximum extent to the fastest speed in a certain period of time, also called timed vital capacity. It is usually calculated the percentage of (respectively FEV_1%, FEV_2%, FEV_3%) the exhaled gas volume respectively at the 1st s, 2nd s, 3th s end of (respectively showed as FEV_1, FEV_2, FEV_3) expiration in FVC. In normal adults, FEV_1% is about 83%, FEV_2% is about 96%, and FEV_3% is about 99%. The clinical significance of FEV_1 is the greatest, and if less than 65%, it may indicate a certain degree of airway obstruction. The amount of FVC is a dynamic index that reflects not only the maximum ventilation volume but also the change of resistance when breathing. It is a better index to evaluate the pulmonary ventilation function, which is commonly used in clinic.

---

[1] 补吸气量（IRV）：平静吸气末，再尽力吸气所能吸入的气体的量。

[2] 补呼气量（ERV）：平静呼气末，再尽力呼气所能呼出的气体的量。

[3] 余气量（RV）：最大呼气末尚存留于肺内不能呼出的气体量。

[4] 呼气的；吐气的。

[5] 肺活量（VC）：尽力吸气后，从肺内所能呼出的最大气体量。

4 Pulmonary ventilation volume

4.1 Minute ventilation volume

The minute ventilation volume[1] is the total amount of new air moved into the respiratory passages each minute; this is equal to the tidal volume times the respiratory rate. The normal tidal volume[2] is about 500 ml, and the normal respiratory[3] rate is about 12 breaths per minute. Therefore, the minute respiratory volume averages about 6 L/min.

4.2 Dead space and its effect on alveolar ventilation

The space in the respiratory passages where no gas exchange takes place is called the anatomic dead space[4], such as nose, pharynx, and trachea.The normal dead space air in a young adult man is about 150 ml. On occasion, some of the alveoli themselves are nonfunctional or are only partially functional because of absent or poor blood flow through adjacent pulmonary capillaries. Therefore, from a functional point of view, these alveoli must also be considered dead space, the alveolar dead space[5]. The sum of the anatomic and alveolar dead spaces is called physiologic dead space[6]. In a normal person, the alveolar dead space is so small that can be neglected. So the physiologic dead space equals to the anatomic dead space.

4.3 Alveolar ventilation[7]

The ultimate importance of the pulmonary ventilatory system[8] is to continually renew the air in the gas exchange areas of the lungs where the air is in proximity to the pulmonary blood. These areas include the alveoli[9], alveolar sacs[10], alveolar ducts[11], and respiratory bronchioles[12]. However, during normal quiet respiration, the volume of air in the tidal volume

[1] 每分通气量。

[2] 潮气量。

[3] 呼吸的。

[4] 解剖无效腔。

[5] 肺泡无效腔。

[6] 生理无效腔。

[7] 肺泡通气量。

[8] 肺通气系统。

[9] 肺泡。

[10] 肺泡小囊。

[11] 肺泡小管。

[12] 呼吸性细支气管。

is only enough to fill the respiratory passageways down as far as the terminal bronchioles[1], i.e. anatomic dead space , with only a small portion of the inspired air actually flowing all the way into the alveoli.

Alveolar ventilation per minute is the total volume of new air entering the alveoli and adjacent gas exchange areas each minute. It is equal to the respiratory rate times the amount of new air that enters these areas with each breath[2].

$$VA = Freq \times (TV - VD),$$

Where VA is the volume of alveolar ventilation per minute, Freq is the frequency of respiration per minute, TV is the tidal volume, and VD is the dead space volume. Thus, with a normal tidal volume of 500 mL, a normal dead space of 150 ml, and a respiratory rate of 12 breaths per minute, alveolar ventilation[3] equals 12 × (500 – 150), or 4200 mL/min. Increased depth of breathing is far more effective in elevating alveolar ventilation than is an equivalent increase in breathing rate. Conversely, a decrease in depth can lead to a critical reduction in alveolar ventilation(Table 5–1).

Table 5–1 The respective ventilation volume and alveolar ventilation volume corresponding to different the frequency of respiration and tidal volume

Frequency of respiration(times/min)	Tidal volume(mL)	Ventilation volume(mL/min)	Alveolar ventilation volume(mL/min)
16	500	8000	5600
8	1000	8000	6800
32	250	8000	3200

4.4 Rate at which alveolar air is renewed by atmospheric air

The average male functional residual capacity of the lungs[4] is about 2300 ml. Yet only 350 ml of new air is brought into the alveoli with each normal respiration, and this same amount of old alveolar air is expired. Therefore, the volume of alveolar air replaced by new atmospheric air[5] with each breath is only one seventh of the total.

[1] 终末细支气管。

[2] 它等于呼吸率乘以每次呼吸进入这些区域的新空气的数量。

[3] 肺泡通气量。

[4] 男性肺的平均功能剩余容量。

[5] 大气。

Section 2 Exchange of gases

We have now completed our discussion of the lung mechanics that produce alveolar ventilation [1], but this is only the first step in the respiratory process [2]. O_2 must move across the alveolar membranes [3] into the pulmonary capillaries [4], be transported by the blood to the tissues, leave the tissue capillaries and enter the extracellular fluid [5], and finally cross plasma membranes to gain entry into cells. CO_2 must follow a similar path in reverse (Figure 5-4).

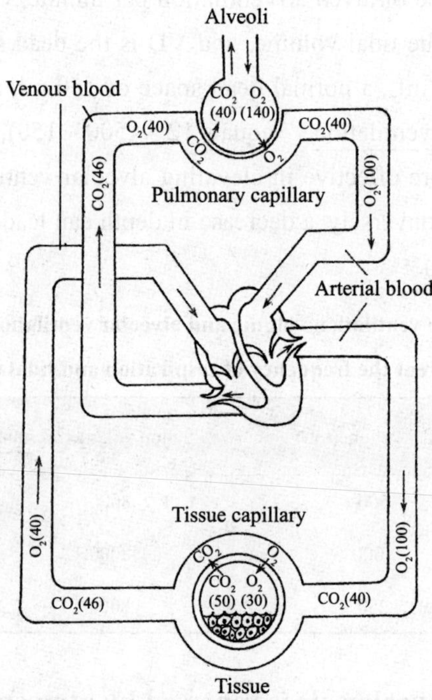

Figure 5-4 Partial pressures of gases in different parts of the body induced by exchange of gases

1 Factors that affect the rate of gas diffusion

All the factors that affect the rate of gas diffusion can be expressed in a single formula, as follows:

---

[1] 肺泡通气量。

[2] 呼吸过程。

[3] 肺泡膜。

[4] 肺毛细血管。

[5] 细胞外液。

$$D \propto \frac{\Delta P \times T \times A \times S}{d \times \sqrt{MW}}$$

D is the diffusion rate.

ΔP is the pressure difference between the two ends of the diffusion pathway. In a mixture of gases, the pressure exerted by each gas is independent of the pressure exerted by the others. The total pressure of the mixture is simply the sum of the individual pressures. These individual pressures istermed partial pressures. The partial pressure of a gas is directly proportional to its concentration[1]. When the pressure of a gas is greater in one area than in another area, there will be net diffusion[2] from the high –pressure area toward the low–pressure area.

T is temperature.

A is the cross–sectional area of the pathway, the greater the cross–sectional area of the pathway, the greater will be the total number of molecules to diffuse.

S is the solubility of the gas in a fluid[3], the greater the solubility of the gas, the greater will be the number of molecules available to diffuse for any given pressure difference.

d is the distance of diffusion, the greater the distance the molecules must diffuse, the longer it will take the molecules to diffuse the entire distance.

MW is the molecular weight of the gas. The greater the velocity of kinetic movement of the molecules, which is inversely proportional to the square root of the molecular weight[4], the greater is the rate of diffusion of the gas.

2 Diffusion of gases through the respiratory membrane

2.1 Respiratory membrane[5]

Gas exchange between the membranes of all the terminal portions of the lungs, not merely in the alveoli themselves. These membranes are collectively known as the respiratory membrane, also called the pulmonary membrane. Respiratory membrane consists of different layers(Figure5–5):

---

[1] 气体的分压正比于它的浓度。

[2] 扩散。

[3] S是气体在液体中的溶解度。

[4] 分子量。

[5] 呼吸膜。

(1) A layer of fluid lining the alveolus and containing surfactant[1] that reduces the surface tension[2] of the alveolar fluid.

(2) The alveolar epithelium[3] composed of thin monolayer epithelial cells.

(3) An epithelial basement membrane.

(4) A thin interstitial space between the alveolar epithelium and the capillary membrane.

(5) A capillary basement membrane that in many places fuses with the alveolar epithelial.

(6) The capillary endothelial membrane[4].

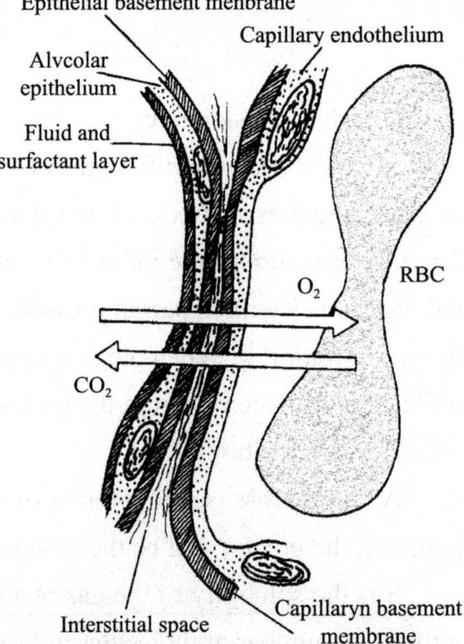

Figure 5–5 Ultrastructure of the alveolar respiratory membrane shown in cross section.

Despite the large number of layers, the overall thickness of the respiratory membrane in some areas is as little as 0.2 mm, and it averages about 0.6 mm.

From histological studies, it has been estimated that the total surface area of the respiratory membrane is about 70 m^2 in the normal adult. The total quantity of blood in the capillaries of the lung at any given instant is 60 to 140 ml. Now imagine this small amount of blood spread over the entire surface of 70m^2, and it is easy to understand the rapidity of respiratory exchange of oxygen and carbon dioxide.

The average diameter[5] of the pulmonary capillaries is only about 5 mm, which means that red blood cells must squeeze through them. Therefore, the red blood cell membrane usually touches the capillary wall so that oxygen and carbon dioxide need not pass through significant amounts of plasma as they diffuse between the alveolus and the red cell. This, too, increases the rapidity of diffusion.

[1] 表面活性剂。

[2] 表面张力。

[3] 上皮细胞。

[4] 内皮细胞。

[5] 直径。

2.2 Factors that affect the rate of gas diffusion through the respiratory membrane

The factors that determine how rapidly a gas will pass through the membrane are ① the pressure difference of the gas between the two sides of the membrane. ② The thickness of the membrane, ③ the surface area of the membrane, ④ the diffusion coefficient of the gas in the substance of the membrane, and ⑤ the ventilation–perfusion [1] ratio.

2.2.1 Pressure difference

The pressure difference across the respiratory membrane is the difference between the partial pressure of the gas in the alveoli and the pressure of the gas in the pulmonary capillary blood. The blood that enters the pulmonary capillaries is systemic venous blood pumped to the lungs via the pulmonary arteries. Having come from the tissues, it has a relatively high PCO_2 (46 mmHg in a normal person at rest) and a relatively low PO_2 (40mmHg). The differences in the partial pressures of oxygen and carbon dioxide on the two sides of the respiratory membrane result in the net diffusion of oxygen from alveoli to blood and of carbon dioxide from blood to alveoli. As this diffusion occurs, the capillary blood PO_2 rises and its PCO_2 falls. The net diffusion of these gases ceases when the capillary partial pressures become equal to those in the alveoli.

2.2.2 The thickness of the respiratory membrane

The thickness of the respiratory membrane occasionally increases–for instance, as a result of edema fluid [2] in the interstitial space of the membrane and in the alveoli —so that the respiratory gases must then diffuse not only through the membrane but also through this fluid. Also, some pulmonary diseases [3] cause fibrosis of the lungs, which can increase the thickness of some portions of the respiratory membrane. Because the rate of diffusion through the membrane is inversely proportional to the thickness of the membrane, any factor that increases the thickness to more than two to three times normal can interfere significantly with normal respiratory exchange of gases.

2.2.3 The surface area of the respiratory membrane

The surface area of the respiratory membrane can be greatly decreased by many conditions. For instance, removal of an entire lung decreases the total surface area to one–half normal. Also, in emphysema [4], many of the alveoli coalesce, with dissolution of many alveolar walls. Therefore, the new chambers are much larger than the original alveoli, but the total sur-

[1] 换气－灌注法。

[2] 水肿液。

[3] 肺病。

[4] 肺气肿。

face area of the respiratory membrane is often decreased as much as fivefold because of loss of the alveolar walls. When the total surface area is decreased to about one–third to one–fourth of normal, exchange of gases through the membrane is impeded to a significant degree, even under resting conditions.

2.2.4 The ventilation–perfusion ratio

The ventilation–perfusion ratio (V_A/Q) is a important concept to help us understand respiratory exchange when there is balance or imbalance between alveolar ventilation and alveolar blood flow. Normally, V_A/Q is 0.84. When V_A is normal for a given alveolus and Q is also normal for the same alveolus, then the V_A/Q is also normal. Whenever V_A/Q is below normal, there is inadequate ventilation to provide the oxygen needed to fully oxygenate the blood flowing through the alveolar capillaries. Therefore, a certain fraction of the venous blood passing through the pulmonary capillaries does not become oxygenated. This fraction is called shunted blood. Whenever V_A/Q is above normal, there may be ventilated alveoli with inadequate or no blood supply, increasing the alveolar dead space.

3 Gas exchange in the tissues

As the systemic arterial blood enters capillaries throughout the body, it is separated from the interstitial fluid[1] by only the thin capillary wall, which is highly permeable to both oxygen and carbon dioxide. The interstitial fluid in turn is separated from intracellular fluid by the plasma[2] membranes of the cells, which are also quite permeable to oxygen and carbon dioxide. Metabolic reactions occurring within cells are constantly consuming oxygen and producing carbon dioxide. Therefore, intracellular PO_2 is lower and PCO_2 higher than that in blood. As a result, there is a net diffusion of oxygen from blood into cells, and a net diffusion of carbon dioxide from cells into blood. In this manner, as blood flows through systemic capillaries[3], its PO_2 decreases and its PCO_2 increases(Figure 5–4).

Section 3 Transport of oxygen and carbon dioxide in the blood

1 The form of breathing gas in the blood

Respiratory gases are transported in the blood in two forms: chemical combination and physical dissolution[4], and most of the gases combine with chemical substances for transport

[1] 组织液。

[2] 血浆。

[3] 全身毛细血管。

[4] 化学结合和物理溶解。

(Table 5–2). Physical dissolution plays an important role in the process of gas exchange. Because gas gets into the blood to be first dissolved in plasma for improving their tension, then chemical combination can occur further when gas exchange. On the contrary, when the gas in the blood is released, physical dissolution is started firstly. The tension of the gas[1] in the plasma is decreased, and then the gas is separated from the combined state to be added in order to continue to release. The conjunctive state of physics and chemistry of the normal gas always keep the dynamic equilibrium[2].

Table 5–2 Content of O_2 and CO_2 in the blood (ml/100ml)

	Arterial blood			Mixed venous blood		
	Physical dissolution	Chemical combination	Total	Physical dissolution	Chemical combination	Total
O_2	0.31	20	20.31	0.11	15.2	15.31
CO_2	2.53	46.4	48.93	2.91	50	52.91

2 Transport of O_2 in the blood

Normally, about 98.5 % of the oxygen transported from the lungs to the tissues is carried in chemical combination with hemoglobin[3]. The remaining 1.5 % is transported in the dissolved state in the water[4] of the plasma and cells. Thus, under normal conditions, oxygen is carried to the tissues almost entirely by hemoglobin.

It should be noted that the oxygen molecule combines just loosely and reversibly with the heme portion of the hemoglobin. Oxygen binds with the hemoglobin when PO_2 is high, as in the pulmonary capillaries, but when PO_2 is low, as in the tissue capillaries, oxygen is released from the hemoglobin. Thus, there are two forms of hemoglobin – deoxyhemoglobin (Hb, tense form)[5] and oxyhemoglobin (HbO_2, relaxed form)[6]. In per 100 ml of blood, the maximal capacity of hemoglobin to bind oxygen is termed oxygen capacity[7], and the actual binding amount of oxygen with hemoglobin is called oxygen content[8]. The oxygen saturation[9]

[1] 气体的张力。

[2] 动态平衡。

[3] 与血红蛋白化学结合。

[4] 水溶解状态。

[5] 血红蛋白。

[6] 氧合血红蛋白。

[7] 血氧容量：每百毫升血液中，血红蛋白的最大氧气结合量。

[8] 血氧含量：每百毫升血液中，血红蛋白的实际氧气结合量。

[9] 血氧饱和度：血氧含量占血氧容量的百分比。

is expressed as the percentage of hemoglobin oxygen content accounting for oxygen capacity in hemoglobin.

2.1 Reversible binding of hemoglobin with O_2

O_2 in the blood exists in the form of oxyhemoglobin (HbO_2). Conjunction and dissociation of O_2 with hemoglobin is a reversible reaction.

$$Hb+O_2 \underset{PO_2\ (low)}{\overset{PO_2\ (high)}{\rightleftharpoons}} HbO_2$$

This reaction is a reversible reaction without enzyme catalysis[1]. When the red cells were treated with high oxygen pressure in lungs, Hb and O_2 rapidly combine as oxyhemoglobin. Oxygenated hemoglobin of tissue cells in the lower partial pressure of oxygen dissociates and releases O_2 to become deoxyhemoglobin. Oxyhemoglobin is bright red and deoxygenated hemoglobin is purple blue.

2.2 Oxygen dissociation curve[2]

In Figure 5-6, the ordinate represents hemoglobin oxygen saturation, and 100% is the mean of highest hemoglobin oxygen saturation. When the percentage is lower, the oxygen saturation is smaller, that is to say the dissociation of oxygen is more. The abscissa represents the oxygen partial pressure. From the oxygen dissociation curve can be seen, the relationship between oxygen partial pressure and hemoglobin oxygen saturation is a "S" curve.The characteristic of the oxygen dissociation curve is extremely important in understanding oxygen exchange.

There is a deep slope when the PO_2 is between 15mmHg and 60mmHg, showing that in the tissue, when the PO_2 slightly drops, oxygen saturation will drop substantially, releasing large amounts of O_2 for tissue utilization. As the tissue activity increases, PO_2 can fall to 15mmHg, then HbO_2 is further dissociated and oxygen saturation drops to around 22%.

Their are a relatively flat portion (or plateau) when the PO_2 is between 60mmHg and 100 mmHg. Thus, the amount of oxygen that combines with hemoglobin increases very rapidly as PO_2 increases from 15 to 60mmHg. At a PO_2 of 60mmHg, 90 % of total hemoglobin is combined with oxygen, indication that, from this point on, a further increase in PO_2 produces only a small increase in oxygen saturation. It shows that people have great tolerance to the decrease

[1] 无酶催化的可逆反应。

[2] 氧解离曲线。

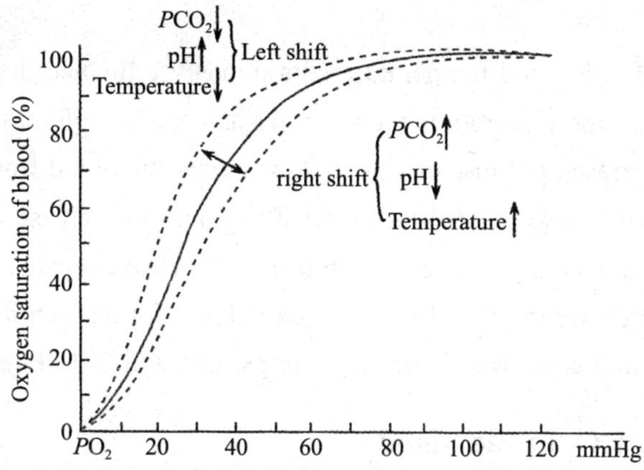

Figure 5-6 The oxygen dissociation curve

of oxygen content in the air or respiratory hypoxia. As in the high altitude plateau, or suffering from certain diseases of the respiratory system, PO_2 of inhaled gas or alveolar will be reduced. But as long as the PO_2 not less than 60mmHg, hemoglobin oxygen saturation will be remained at about 90%, still can guarantee the blood oxygen content in high.

This "S" curve is very beneficial to the use of oxygen in the human body. The reason for the "S" curve is the allosteric effect [1] of hemoglobin. Hb consists of four polypeptide chains (subunits) having a heme at the center of each subunit. The center of each heme contains a Fe^{2+}, each which can combine a O_2, so each Hb molecule can combine up to 4 O_2. As soon as one subunit of hemoglobin combines with O_2, the other three subunits undergo a configuration change that accelerates the binding of O_2. Similarly, as long as there is one subunit dissociated from O_2, the rate of dissociation of the other three subunits and O_2 will also increase.

2.3 Factors that influence the oxygen transport

At any given PO_2, a variety of other factors affect the degree of hemoglobin saturation, including blood PCO_2 [2], H^+ concentration [3], temperature and the concentration of 2,3-diphosphoglycerate (DPG) [4], the product by the erythrocytes in the case of hypoxia. An increase in any of these factors causes the dissociation curve to shift to the right, which means less affinity of hemoglobin for oxygen at any given PO_2. On the contrary, a decrease in any of these factors causes the dissociation curve to shift to the left, which means a greater affinity of hemoglobin for oxygen. The effect of CO_2 on the capacity of hemoglobin transporting O_2 is known as

[1] 变构效应。

[2] 二氧化碳分压。

[3] 氢离子浓度。

[4] 2,3－二磷酸甘油酸（DPG）。

Bohr effect[1].

PCO_2, H^+ concentration and temperature continuously influence the blood in tissue capillaries, because each of these factors is higher in tissue capillary blood than in arterial blood. The blood PCO_2 is increased because carbon dioxide enters the blood from the tissues. The H^+ concentration is elevated because of the elevated PCO_2 and the release of metabolically produced acids such as lactic acid[2]. The temperature is increased because of the heat produced by tissue metabolism. Therefore, the affinity of hemoglobin for oxygen is decreased as it passes through the tissue capillaries, which means more oxygen will be released by hemoglobin.

3 Transport of CO_2 in the blood

CO_2 transport is in the two forms of physical dissolution and chemical combination from tissue to blood. The physical dissolved quantity accounts for 5% of the total, and chemical combination quantity accounts for 95% of the total, mainly in the forms of bicarbonate[3] (88%). and carbamino hemoglobin[4] (7%).

3.1 Bicarbonate

CO_2 produced by tissue metabolism getting into blood combines with H_2O to generate H_2CO_3, which is decomposed into HCO_3^- and H^+. This reaction is carried out mainly in red blood cells. The reaction is as follows:

$$CO_2+H_2O \xrightarrow{\text{carbonic anhydrase}} H_2CO_3 \longrightarrow HCO_3^-+H^+$$

CO_2 enters the erythrocytes from the blood in the tissues and react with water to form bicarbonate. The reversible reaction of CO_2 with H_2O to form H_2CO_3 is rate-limiting, and is very slow unless catalyzed by the carbonic anhydrase (CA)[5].

The most CO_2 that is from tissue into blood finally exists in red blood cells in the form of $KHCO_3$ and exists in the form of $NaHCO_3$ in plasma, namely it is transported from blood to lungs in the form of bicarbonate.

In the lungs, the reaction goes in the opposite direction because PCO_2 in the alveoli is lower than that in the venous blood, and causes release of CO_2 from the blood into the alveoli (Figure 5-7).

---

[1] 波尔效应。

[2] 乳酸。

[3] 碳酸氢盐。

[4] 氨基甲酰血红蛋白。

[5] 碳酸酐酶（CA）催化。

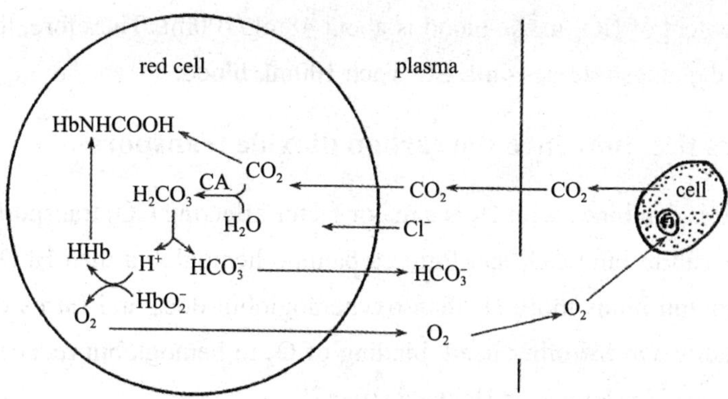

Figure 5–7 Transport pattern of CO_2 in the blood

3.2 Carbamino hemoglobin

The remaining carbon dioxide molecules that enter the blood react reversibly with the amino groups of hemoglobin to form carbamino hemoglobin.

$$HbNH_2 + CO_2 \longrightarrow HbNHCOO^- + H^+$$

This reaction goes rapidly without enzyme assistance. Oxygenation [1] is the main factor to regulate it. This efficiency of transport form for CO_2 is very high. Although CO_2 in the carbaminohemoglobin forms of transportation accounts for only 7%, there are about 17.5% of the total CO_2 released by carbaminohemoglobin in the lungs.The reaction is mainly regulated by the oxygenation effect. Either the oxyhemoglobin or the deoxyhemoglobin can combine with CO_2, but the ability of deoxyhemoglobin combining with CO_2 is stronger.

3.3 Carbon dioxide dissociation curve [2]

The curve reflecting the relationship between PCO_2 and the content of CO_2 in the blood is known as the carbon dioxide dissociation curve which is nearly linear.Figure 5–8 shows that in venous blood, when PO_2 is 40mmHg, and PCO_2 is45mmHg,i.e, point A, the content of CO_2 in the blood is about 52mL/100mL. While in arterial blood, when PO_2 is 100mmHg and PCO_2 is

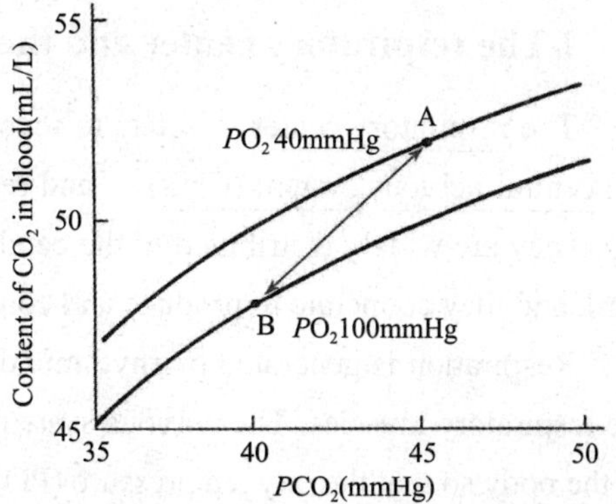

Figure 5–8 Carbon dioxide dissociation curve

[1] 氧合。

[2] 二氧化碳解离曲线。

40mmHg, the content of CO_2 in the blood is about 48mL/100mL.Therefore, the venous blood passing through the lungs releases 4mL CO_2 each 100mL blood.

3.4 Factors that influence the carbon dioxide transport

Whether Hb is combined with O_2 is a major factor affecting CO_2 transport. Deoxygenated Hb is more powerful to bind CO_2 and form carbamino hemoglobin than HbO_2 because deoxygenated hemoglobin binds more H^+ than oxyhemoglobin does and forms carbamino compounds more readily. On the other hand, binding of O_2 to hemoglobin reduces its affinity for CO_2. This phenomenon is known as Haldane effect [1].

Consequently in the tissues, HbO_2 releases O_2 to form Hb, which binds CO_2 to become carbaminohemoglobin. In the lungs, more HbO_2 is produced, causing carbamino hemoglobin to release CO_2 and H^+.

Thus, the transportation of O_2 and CO_2 is not isolated, but interactive. CO_2 affects transport of O_2 through the Bohr effect, whereas O_2 affects transport of CO_2 through Haldane effect.

Section 4 Regulation of respiration

The significance of respiratory movement is to ensure the exchange of gas between the lung and the outside world, thus providing the O_2 needed for metabolism, and discharging the CO_2 produced by metabolism in the body to maintain the relative stability of PO_2, PCO_2 and pH in the environment. Breathing is both a voluntary movement and an automatic rhythmic activity. The depth and frequency of respiration change accordingly with the change of the internal and external environment of the body, so as to meet the needs of the material metabolism of the body.

1 The respiratory center and the formation of respiratory rhythm

The respiratory center [2] refers to several groups of neurons that are located bilaterally in the central nervous system (CNS) [3] and responsible for the generation and control of breathing. They are widely distributed in the cerebral cortex, diencephalon, pons medulla and spinal cord, and they cooperate to produce and control the respiratory rhythm.

Respiration is generated by rhythmic discharge of motor neurons in the brain that control the respiratory muscles. The nervous system controls alveolar ventilation to meet the demands of the body so that the oxygen pressure (PO_2) and carbon dioxide pressure (PCO_2) in the arteri-

---

[1] 何尔登效应。

[2] 呼吸中枢。

[3] 中枢神经系统（CNS）。

al blood remain almost constant even during strenuous exercise.

1.1 Spinal cord

Motor neurons in spinal cord controlling breathing muscle are located in the 3 ~ 5 cervical segment to innervate diaphragmatic muscles and cornuanterius medullae spinalis of thoracic segments to dominate intercostal and abdominal muscles. The spinal cord is just a relay station[1] that receives signals from the brain and then sends impulses to the respiratory muscles. It also functions as the elementary center[2] that is involved in some respiratory reflexes.

1.2 Lower brain stem

The lower brainstem[3] refers to the pons and medulla oblongata[4] which is a involuntary regulatory system[5]. There were respiratory related neurons in the lower brainstem. When inspiratory, the neuron that discharges is called inspiratory neuron[6], the neuron that discharges when expiratory is called expiratory neuron[7]. The respiratory related neurons were mainly distributed in three symmetrical areas: ① Dorsal respiratory group(DRG)[8]. It is located in nuclei tractussolitarii(NST), consisting mainly of inspiratory neurons and their axons cross to the side down to the cervical and thoracic segments of spinal cord to dominate motoneurons of diaphragm and external intercostal muscle. ② Ventral respiratory group(VRG)[9]. They are mainly distributed in the Nucleus posterior, nucleus ambiguous, and nucleus of facial nerve, and their adjacent areas. They contain many types of respiratory neurons. In VRG, there is a region of the so–called 'pre–Botzinger complex(pre–BÖt C)'[10], which may be a critical part of the origin of the mammalian respiratory rhythm. ③ Pontine respiratory group(PRG)[11]. This area is equivalent to the nucleus parabronchial medialis(NPBM)[12] and the adjacent Kolliker–Fuse (KF),

---

[1] 中继站。

[2] 基本中枢。

[3] 低位脑干。

[4] 脑桥和延髓。

[5] 非随意调节系统。

[6] 吸气神经元。

[7] 呼气神经元。

[8] 背侧呼吸组。

[9] 腹侧呼吸组。

[10] 包钦格复合体。

[11] 脑桥呼吸组。

[12] 臂旁内侧核。

two of them are called PBKF, which is the location for the pneumotaxic center (PC) [1], mainly containing expiratory neurons. Its function is to limit the inspiration and to facilitate the conversion of the inspiration to the expiration(Figure 5–9).

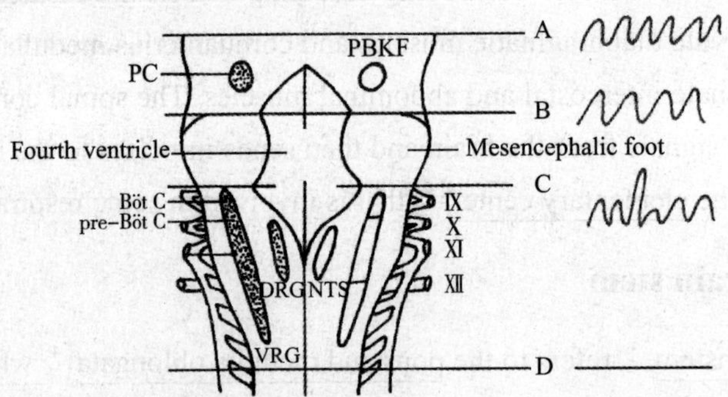

Figure 5–9 Respiratory neurons in the brain stem and changes in respiration after cutting off the brainstem at different planes

Ⅸ, Ⅹ, Ⅺ, Ⅻ represent Ⅸ, Ⅹ, Ⅺ, Ⅻ cranial nerves respectively;

A, B, C and D represent different sections respectively

Control of the respiratory rhythm depends on neurons that are primarily located in the medulla. In several nuclei of the medulla, neurons called medullary inspiratory neurons discharge in synchrony with inspiration and cease discharge during expiration. They provide the rhythmic imput to the motor neurons innervating the inspiratory muscles.

1.3 Cerebral cortex

The cerebral cortex [2] can control breathing to stop breathing or forced respiration within limits. The motor area of cerebral cortex control motor neuron activity of breath through the corticospinal tract andcorticobulbar tract, which is a voluntary regulatory system [3].

2 Respiratory reflex regulation

2.1 Pulmonary stretch reflex

Inspiratory inhibition or excitation caused by expanding or shrinking of lung is called pulmonary stretch reflex [4], which includes pulmonary inflation reflex [5] and pulmonary defla-

[1] 呼吸调整中枢。

[2] 大脑皮层。

[3] 随意调节系统。

[4] 肺牵张反射。

[5] 肺扩张反射。

tion reflex[1].

Pulmonary inflation reflex refers to the process of suppressed inspiration by inflation of the lungs. The pulmonary stretch receptors[2] are located in the airway (from bronchi down to bronchioles) smooth muscle layer, and are activated by lung inflation.

When pneumatic dilation make respiratory tract expand, impulses produced by excitement of stretch receptors pass through crude fiber of vagus nerve[3] to medulla oblongata. The neural connections make inspiratory off switch mechanism exciting, inspiration turn into expiration. The reflection can strengthen the alternation of inspiration and expiration to quicken breathing rate.

In the animal experiment, if the vagi were destructed, prolonged inspiration and deep slow breathing could be observed. In humans, however, this pulmonary stretch–receptor reflex plays a role in setting respiratory rhythm only under conditions of very large tidal volumes, as in rigorous exercise.

Pulmonary deflation is the reflex in which deflation of the lungs enhances inspiration. The associated receptors[4] are also located in the airway smooth muscles. When lung markedly reduce, lung deflation reflex can appear and have little regulation significance in quiet breathing.

It must be noted that the pulmonary stretch reflex does not function during quiet respiration, but occurs only when the lung is markedly dilated or atrophic.

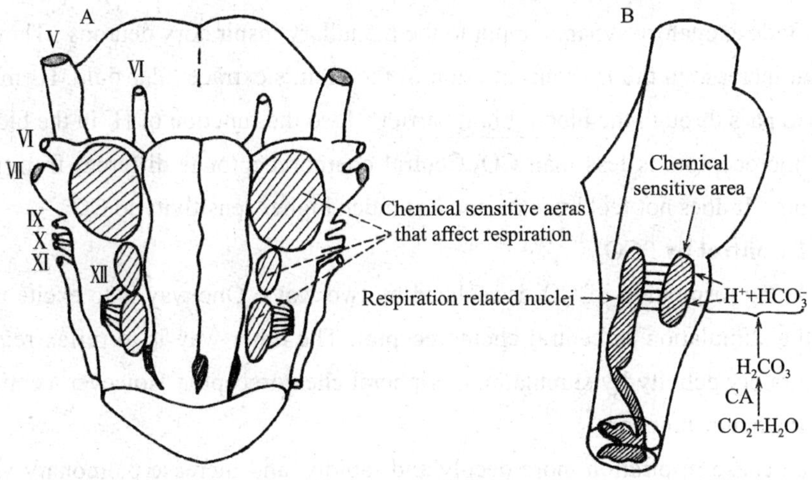

Figure 5–10 Central chemoreceptor

[1] 肺萎缩反射。

[2] 肺牵张感受器。

[3] 粗迷走神经纤维。

[4] 相关受体。

2.2 Respiratory reflex of chemical sensitivity

The ultimate goal of respiration is to maintain proper concentrations of oxygen, carbon dioxide, and hydrogen ions in the body fluid. And respiratory activity is highly responsive to changes in any one of these.The changes of chemical constituents in the blood, especially hypoxemia, carbon dioxide and hydrogen ion concentration increased, can stimulate chemoreceptors to make the respiratory center change so as to adjust the frequency and depth of respiratory movement to ensure the value of PO_2, PCO_2 and pH is relatively constant in the arterial blood(Figure 5–10).

2.2.1 Peripheral chemoreceptors[1] and central chemoreceptors[2]

There are many inputs to the medullary inspiratory neurons, but most important for the automatic control of ventilation are from peripheral chemoreceptors and central chemoreceptors.

The carotid body[3] and aortic body[4] belong to peripheral chemoreceptor, which can feel stimulus for changes of PO_2, PCO_2 and H^+ (pH) in arterial blood and pushes impulses into the medulla by the sinus nerve[5] and vagus nerve, the function of carotid body is far greater than the aortic body. The peripheral chemoreceptor can be affected by stimulation of PO_2 in carotid blood, but not affected by the content of O_2 in arterial blood.

The central chemoreceptors are located in the medulla and, like the peripheral chemoreceptors, provide excitatory synaptic input to the medullary inspiratory neurons . They are stimulated by an increase in the H^+ concentration of the brain's extracellular fluid. H^+ in the blood is not easy to pass through the blood–brain barrier[6], so the function of H^+ in the blood for the central chemoreceptors is less than CO_2.Central chemoreceptor is different from peripheral chemoreceptor. It does not feel hypoxia and has much higher sensitivity to CO_2.

2.2.1.1 Control by PCO_2

Stimulating respiration of CO_2 is realized by two ways. One way is to excite respiratory center by the stimulation of central chemoreceptor. The other way is to reflex regulation of central respiratory activity by stimulating peripheral chemoreceptor. However, central chemoreceptor is the major function.

CO_2 can cause respiration more deeply and rapidly, and increase pulmonary ventilation.

---

[1] 外周化学感受器。

[2] 中枢化学感受器。

[3] 颈动脉。

[4] 主动脉体。

[5] 窦神经。

[6] 血脑屏障。

In the experiment, when the environmental CO_2 concentration increases to 1%, the pulmonary ventilation will be one time than that at rest in order to clear CO_2.CO_2 can rapidly passes through the blood–brain barrier into the cerebrospinal fluid and brain tissue fluid, and under the action of carbonic anhydrase, combines with H_2O to form H_2CO_3, which is dissociated into H^+, which can stimulate the central chemoreceptor. In the presence of a prolonged increase in H^+ generation in the brain extracellular fluid (ECF) as a result of long–standing CO_2 retention, enough HCO_3^- may cross the blood–brain barrier to buffer, or "neutralize," the excess H^+, removing it from solution so that it no longer contributes to free H^+ concentration.CO_2 stimulating chemoreceptor can make the respiratory strengthening through reflex, but direct effect of CO_2 on the respiratory center is inhibition. So a slight increase in PCO_2 can stimulate breathing, but when PCO_2 is severely elevated, breathing is inhibited.This condition is called CO_2 anesthesia. However, when experimental animals inhaled CO_2 whose concentration is 7% or above, headache and dazzle will appear, and even respiration will be inhibited.

2.2.1.2 Control by [H^+]

When the [H^+] in arterial blood increases, the respiration is deeper and rapider[1]. The changes of H^+ (pH changes) regulate respiratory mainly by the peripheral chemoreceptor especially the carotid body. The sensitivity of central chemoreceptor to H^+ is very high and 25 times higher than peripheral chemoreceptor, but H^+ is not easy to pass through the blood–brain barrier, so its role is limited.

2.2.1.3 Control by O_2

When PO_2 decreases, respiration is deeper and rapider. Hypoxia completely relies on the stimulation of peripheral chemoreceptors to strengthen respiration. The lower of PO_2 in arterial blood is, the more the afferent impulses. Like that of CO_2, hypoxia stimulating peripheral chemoreceptor can make the respiratory strengthening through reflex, but direct effect of hypoxia on the respiratory center is inhibition. So a slight hypoxia can stimulate breathing, but a severehypoxia make breathing inhibited. The peripheral chemoreceptors respond to the PO_2 of the blood, not the total O_2 content of the blood. O_2 content in the arterial blood can fall to dangerously low or even fatal levels without the peripheral chemoreceptors ever responding to reflexly stimulate respiration. For example, in patient with CO intoxication, arterial blood O_2 content is down, but PO_2 is normal, so there is no respiratory change.

CO_2 is the strongest breathing stimulus, and normally the body relies mainly on CO_2 stimulation and maintenance of breathing. Inserious emphysema[2], for instance, low PO_2 and retention of CO_2 can be observed because of impaired gas exchange of the lung. Long–term retention of CO_2 would reduce the sensitivity of the central receptors to H^+. in this case, breathing is mainly driven by the effect of low PO_2 via the peripheral receptors. Therefore, if such a

[1] 深快的呼吸。

[2] 严重的肺气肿。

patient were given pure oxygen[1], breathing would cease because of increased PO_2. This must be paid attention to when oxygen treatment is administered clinically[2].

2.2.2 Interaction of PCO_2, H^+ and PO_2 in respiratory regulation

During the three factors of PCO_2, H^+ and PO_2, if only to change one factor and remain other two factors unchanged, PCO_2 and H^+ fluctuating slightly can cause significant changes in pulmonary ventilation, especially the role of PCO_2 is more obvious (Figure5–11).

But under normal physiological conditions, the influence of the three factors on respiration is mutual interference.That is, in these three factors, if one factor is changed, and the other two factors are not limited, the change of ventilation rate is obviously different from the above. The effect of PCO_2 is increased greatly, while the effect of PO_2 is greatly diminished.This is because that the three can be coordinated and strengthened while regulating, and can be also offset by each other.When $PCO_2$was increased, the concentration of H^+ was increased, and the stimulation of both was added, so that the ventilatory volume was increased significantly when compared with PCO_2 alone. When the H^+ stimulation increases the volume of ventilation, the hyperventilation reduces PCO_2 and discharges large amounts of CO_2, which reduces H^+.Thus, the effect of ventilation at this time is less than that of H^+ alone on ventilation.The same is true of the effect of PO_2 levels on ventilation (Figure 5–12) .

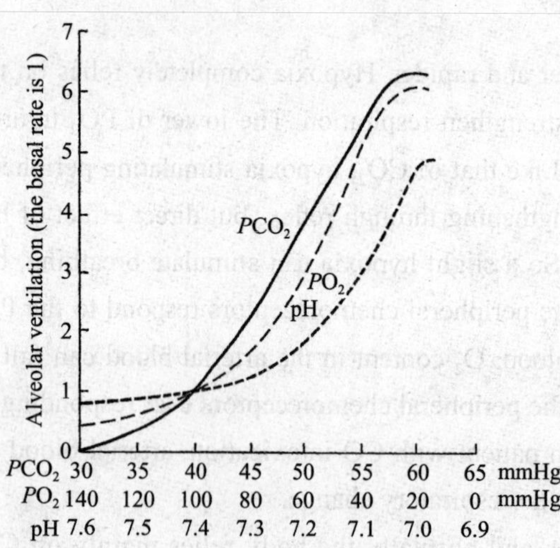

Figure 5–11 The respective effects of O_2, CO_2 and H^+ levels in arterial blood on alveolar ventilation independently

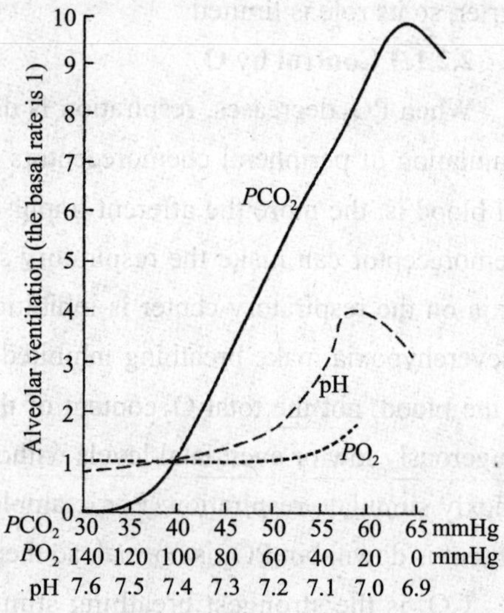

Figure 5–12 Effects of O_2, CO_2 and H^+ levels in arterial blood on alveolar ventilation under normal physiological conditions in vivo

[1] 纯氧。

[2] 临床上。

Chapter 6 DIGESTION AND ABSORPTION

The main physiological function of digestive system is to digest and absorb food to supply matter and energy sources for organism metabolism. Digestion is a process essential for the conversion of food into a form that can be utilized by the body, including mechanical and chemical digestions.

Mechanical digestion[1] is accomplished mainly by the motility of oral cavity, stomach and gut[2] etc. which has three functions: movement of solids and liquids in an oral to anal direction; grinding of food; mixing food with digestive juice. Chemical digestion[3] requires the secretion of special enzymes to catalyze the various complex foodstuff molecules into simple forms. Two ways cooperate with each other to complete digestion of the food.

Absorption[4] is the process of transporting small molecules from the lumen of the gut into blood and lymph[5] stream.

The digestive system consists of digestive tracts and digestive glands[6].

Section 1 General introduction

1 Physiological characteristics of gastrointestinal smooth muscle

1.1 General principles of gastrointestinal smooth muscle

Except for oral cavity, pharynx, proximal esophagus and external anal sphincter, the musculature of alimentary tract is smooth muscle[7]. In addition to the common characteristics of muscle tissue, such as excitability, conductivity, contractility[8] and so on, digestive tract smooth muscle

[1] 机械性消化。

[2] 口腔、胃和肠。

[3] 化学性消化。

[4] 吸收。

[5] 淋巴。

[6] 消化道和消化腺。

[7] 除了口腔、咽、近端食管和肛门外括约肌，消化道肌肉都是平滑肌。

[8] 兴奋性、传导性、收缩性。

also has other characteristics such as tense contraction, slower automatic rhythmicity movement, higher extensibility [1] and sensitivity to chemistry, temperature and mechanical stretch.

1.2 Electrical activity of gastrointestinal smooth muscle

The smooth muscle of gastrointestinal tract [2] undergoes three kinds of bioelectric phenomena: resting potential, basic electrical rhythm and spike potentials [3] (Figure 6–1).

1.2.1 Resting potential

The resting potential of the gastrointestinal smooth muscle is between –50 ~ –65 mV. It is mainly caused by K^+ efflux, while many ions, for instance, Na^+, Cl^-, Ca^{2+}, and the activity of sodium pump are also involved. The resting potential of the gastrointestinal smooth muscle is not stable, and spontaneous depolarization can occur periodically [4].

1.2.2 Basic electrical rhythm

There is spontaneous depolarization periodically in the smooth muscle membrane potential which is called "basic electrical rhythm (BER)" or "slow wave potential" [5]. Their intensity usually varies between 5 and 15 mV, and their frequency ranges in different parts of the human gastrointestinal tract between 3 and 12 per minute. The BER is not action potential, but slow, undulating change in the resting membrane potential, and control the appearance of intermittent spike potential [6], which in turn actually cause the muscle contraction. Most gastrointestinal contractions occur rhythmically, and this rhythm is determined almost entirely by the BER.

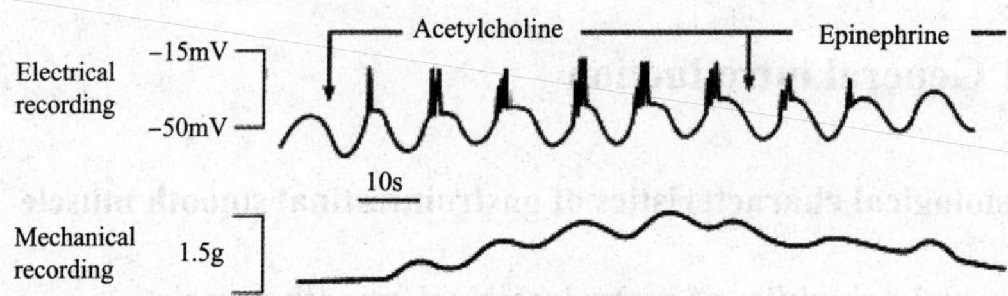

Figure 6–1 Membrane potentials in intestinal smooth muscle.

1.2.3 The spike potentials

The spike potentials [7] are true action potentials that occur automatically when cell mem-

[1] 紧张性收缩，缓慢的节律性运动，很好的伸展性。

[2] 胃肠道。

[3] 静息电位，基本电节律和锋电位。

[4] 周期性地发生自动去极化。

[5] 基本电节律和慢波电位。

[6] 基本电节律是在静息电位的基础上膜电位的起伏变化，它不是动作电位，但是控制着锋电位的间歇性出现。

[7] 锋电位。

brane depolarization reaches the threshold potential [1] (such as –40mV). The higher the slow wave potentials rise above this level, the greater the frequency of the spike potentials, usually ranging between 1 and 10 spikes per second, and the greater the muscle contraction is.

In the gastrointestinal smooth muscle, the entry of large amounts of calcium ions [2] along with smaller amounts of sodium ions [3] is responsible for the action potentials. These channels are much slower to open and also to close than the rapid sodium channels [4].

In conclusion, the contraction of smooth muscle is produced after the spike potential, and spike potentials occurs on the basis of BER. BER is the initial potential of gastrointestinal motility, determines the direction, speed and rhythm of peristalsis from oral to anus direction [5].

2 Innervation of digestive system

The gastrointestinal tract has two nervous systems: one is extrinsic nerve system, also called autonomic nervous system,which includes sympathetic and parasympathetic nerves [6]. The other is intrinsic nervous system of its own, called the enteric nervous system [7] (Figure 6–2).

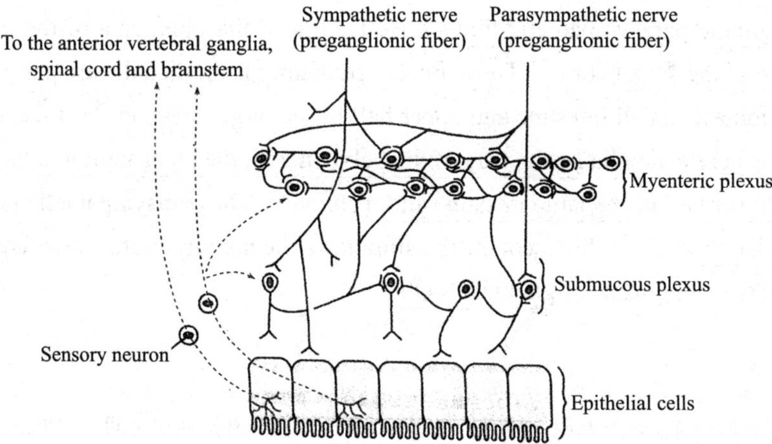

Figure 6–2 The intramural nerve plexus of the gastrointestinal tract and its connection with the external nerve

---

[1] 阈电位。

[2] 大量钙离子的内流。

[3] 钠离子。

[4] 与快钠通道相比，这些通道开放的慢，关闭的也慢。

[5] 蠕动的节律。

[6] 一个是外在神经系统，又叫自主神经系统，包括交感和副交感神经。

[7] 另一个是它本身的内在神经系统，又叫肠神经系统。

2.1 Intrinsic nerves

The intrinsic nerves have Myenteric nerve plexus lying between the longitudinal and circular muscle layers, which has excitatory and inhibitory effects to dominate the cells of smooth muscle, and Meissner's plexus lying between the circular muscle layer and the submucosa, mainly functions to adjust gland cells and epithelial cells[1]. In addition, there are intermediate neurons between the two nerve plexus to interact extensively with each other. The intrinsic neural functions normally are modulated by but independently of extrinsic neural control.

2.2 Extrinsic nerves

The extrinsic nerves include the sympathetic and parasympathetic nerves[2]. The preganglionic fibers of sympathetic nerves to the gastrointestinal tract originate in the spinal cord between the segments T–6 and L–3[3]. The postganglionic fibers[4] spread along with the blood vessels to all parts of the gut, terminating principally on neurons in the enteric nervous system. The sympathetic nerve endings secrete norepinephrine.[5] In general, stimulation of the sympathetic nervous system inhibits activity in the gastrointestinal tract.

Preganglionic parasympathetic fibers arise from medulla oblongata of the brain and the sacral portion of the spinal cord[6]. Those fibers originating from medulla are part of the vagi[7] and supply stomach, small intestine and upper half of the large intestine[8]. Fibers from sacral cord reach the pelvic ganglia by the way of the pelvic nerve, the postganglionic fibers of which innervating lower half of the large intestine and rectum[9]. The parasympathetic nerve endings secrete acetylcholine[10], which, contrarily, stimulates the activity in the gastrointestinal tract, including the smooth muscle or glandular cells[11].

---

[1] 内在神经有肌间神经丛和黏膜下神经丛。前者存在于纵行和环形肌层之间，对平滑肌细胞有兴奋和抑制作用；后者存在于在环形肌和黏膜下层之间，主要功能是调节腺细胞和上皮细胞的作用。

[2] 交感和副交感神经。

[3] 支配胃肠道的交感神经节前纤维起源于脊髓 T6 和 L3 节段之间。

[4] 节后纤维。

[5] 去甲肾上腺素。

[6] 副交感神经节前纤维起源于延髓和骶部脊髓。

[7] 迷走神经。

[8] 大肠。

[9] 从骶髓发出的纤维通过盆神经到达盆腔神经节，其节后纤维支配大肠下半段和直肠。

[10] 乙酰胆碱。

[11] 腺细胞。

3 Digestive gland secretion

There are several types of exocrine glands, such as salivary gland, liver, pancreas, etc. or exocrine cells, which are dispersed in the wall of digestive tract, such as intestinal gland cells, gastric gland cells, in the digestive system[1]. They provide different types of secretion into the gut to assist food digest. The constitutions of secretion include water, electrolytes and organic substances such as enzymes, mucus, etc. Most digestive secretions are formed only in response to the presence of food in the alimentary tract. The types of enzymes and other constituents of the secretion vary in accordance with the types of food present. Table 6–1 shows the quantity of secretion by different digestive glands in a day.

Table 6–1 Daily secretion quantities of digestive glands

	Daily volume (ml)	pH
Saliva	1,000	6.0 ~ 7.0
Gastric secretion	1,500	1.0 ~ 3.5
Pancreatic secretion	1,000	8.0 ~ 8.3
Bile	1,000	7.8
Small intestinal secretion	1,800	7.5 ~ 8.0
Large intestinal secretion	200	7.5 ~ 8.0

4 Gastrointestinal hormones

Gastrointestinal tract produces many hormones. When food is ingested, these hormones are released. Each hormone is found in a ultrastructurally distinctive type of cell[2]. These cells are scattered among the non-endocrine epithelial cells[3] in the mucosa of the stomach and intestine. Their release activates or inhibits secretory and motor activity of various digestive organs[4]. All known gastrointestinal hormones are peptides with molecular weights in most cases ranging between 2,000 and 5,000. The main function of gastrointestinal hormones is shown in Table 6–2.

[1] 在消化系统，有不同种类的外分泌腺体，如唾液腺、肝脏、胰腺等，或外分泌腺细胞，这些细胞分散存在消化道管壁，如小肠腺细胞、胃腺细胞。

[2] 每一种激素都是由超微结构不同的特定的内分泌细胞所分泌。

[3] 没有内分泌功能的上皮细胞。

[4] 它们的释放要么刺激、要么抑制消化器官的分泌和运动。

Table 6–2 The main function of gastrointestinal hormones

	Gastrin	Secretin	Cholecystokinin(CCK)
Gastric acid	++	–	+
Pancreatic HCO_3^-	+	++	+
Pancreatin	++	+	++
Hepatic bile	+	+	+
Small intestine fluid	+	+	+
Esophago–Gastric sphincter	+	–	–
Stomach smooth muscle	+	–	+–
Small intestinal smooth muscle	+	–	+
Gallbladder smooth muscle	+	+	++

"+" represents "activate", "–" represents "inhibit"

Section 2 Oral cavity digestion

The process of digestion begins in the mouth. The food stays in oral cavity for a short time by chewing to be crushed and mixing with saliva, forming the alimentary bolus to be swallowed[1]. Saliva has a weak chemical digestion of food.

1 The secretion of saliva

Saliva is secreted primarily by three pairs of large glands: submandibular glands, sublingual glands and parotid glands, and the abundant small buccal glands also contribute to the total volume of this fluid by their mucous secretion[2]. In saliva, water accounts for 99%. Organic compounds include mucin, salivary amylase, lysozyme and immunoglobulin[3] and so on. Inorganic compounds are mainly K^+, HCO_3^-, Na^+, Cl^- and so on.

Saliva has a number of functions as follows: ① moistens the cavity and thus facilitates swallowing, ② assists in keeping the mouth and teeth clean, ③ may have antibacterial effects, ④ salivary amylase plays a minor part in digestion of starch[4].

[1] 食物在口腔内停留很短的时间，在口腔通过咀嚼被碾碎，与唾液混合，形成可被吞咽的食团。

[2] 唾液是三对大唾液腺颌下腺、舌下腺和腮腺分泌的，另外丰富的小颊腺也分泌黏液成为唾液的一部分。

[3] 黏蛋白、唾液淀粉酶、溶菌酶和免疫球蛋白。

[4] 淀粉。

2 Chewing and swallowing

2.1 Chewing

Chewing is a mechanical process of digestion in the oral cavity. Moreover, it can chop the food and mix it with saliva, thus make full contact of food with saliva amylase to cause chemical digestion. Much of the chewing process is caused by the chewing reflex, and can also reflectively cause the digestive activity of stomach, pancreas, liver and gallbladder and the insulin secretion [1], which can provide preparation conditions for subsequent digestion.

2.2 Swallowing

Swallowing is a reflection process of moving food from mouth into stomach, which can be divided into three stages: ① Oral stage, the bolus is squeezed into the pharynx. ② Pharyngeal stage, which refers to the process of bolus from pharynx into the upper end of the esophagus. It is a rapid series of reflex action caused by bolus stimulating soft palate. ③ Esophageal stage, in which the bolus is propelled down through esophagus into the stomach by esophageal peristalsis [2] (Figure 6–3).

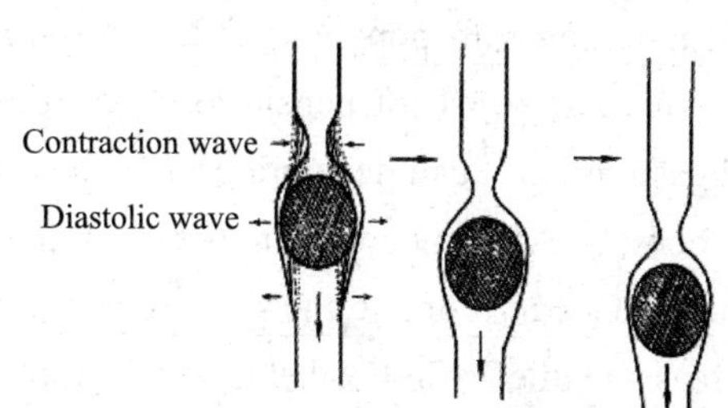

Figure 6–3 Esophageal peristalsis

Esophageal peristalsis is the sequential relaxation and contraction of esophageal muscle which opens a passage ahead of the bolus through muscle relaxation and closes the esophagus behind the bolus through muscle contraction, thus creating a pressure gradient and moves the content downward [3]. The most distal 2 ~ 4 cm of the esophagus forms a zone of high pressure which serves as a barrier preventing reflux of acidic gastric content into the esophagus [4]. The esophageal muscle at distal segment with a high pressure is called the lower esophageal sphincter.

---

[1] 胃、胰、肝、胆的消化活动及胰岛素的分泌。

[2] ①口腔期：将食团挤入咽内。②咽期：指食团从咽到食管上端的过程。这是由于食团刺激软腭引起的一系列快速反射过程。③食管期：通过食管蠕动将食团经食道推进入胃内。

[3] 食管蠕动是食管肌肉的顺序放松和收缩，通过肌肉放松打开食团前面的通道，同时通过肌肉收缩关闭食团后面的食道，从而产生压力梯度使食团向下移动。

[4] 食管最远端的 2 ~ 4cm 形成高压，可以防止酸性胃内容物反流到食管。

Section 3 Stomach digestion

1 The secretion of gastric juice

The cells of the gastric glands secrete about 2,000ml of gastric juice daily. Gastric juice is transparent aqueous solution, with its pH being 0.9 ~ 1.5. The juice contains a variety of substances, mainly including hydrochloric acid, pepsinogen, mucus, and intrinsic factor.

1.1 Hydrochloric acid (HCl)

The parietal cell of oxyntic gland [1] is responsible for the secretion of HCl which has several functions : ① It can activate pepsinogen into pepsin [2] ; ② It provides the necessary pH for pepsin to start protein digestion; ③ It can denature protein and microbes; ④ After it enters into the small intestine, HCl can promote the secretion of pancreas and bile [3]; ⑤ It is helpful in promoting the absorption of calcium and ferrum(Fe).

The HCl secretion process is shown in Figure 6–4. The parietal cells are polarized, with an apical membrane facing the lumen of the gastric glands and a basolateral membrane in contact with the interstitial fluid [4].

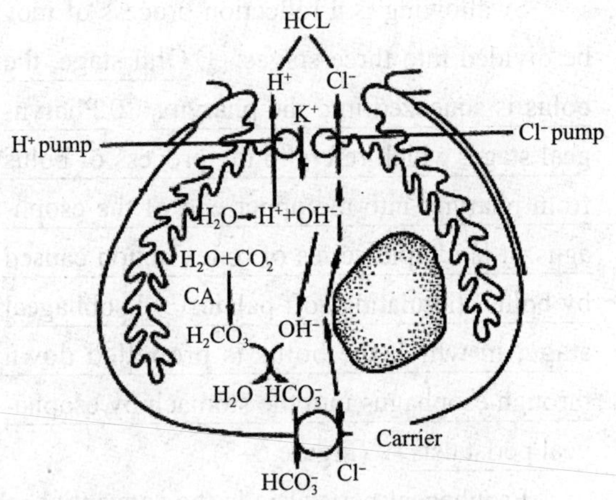

Figure 6–4 HCl secretion by parietal cells

Hydrochloric acid secretion is an active process of energy dissipation. The active secretion of H^+ is related to the function of proton pump on apical membrane of the cell. Proton pump is a transporter embedded in the membrane with the function of transporting H^+ and K^+ and hydrolyzing ATP. In the cytoplasm H_2O is resolved into H^+ and OH^- . Under the action of the proton pump, H^+ is actively transported to the small lumen, and $OH^-$is combined with CO_2 to generate HCO_3^- by carbonic anhydrase catalyzing. In the basal side of the cell, HCO_3^- and Cl^- exchange, HCO_3^- get out, and Cl^- get into the cell. In the cells, Cl^- get into the lumen through the specific channel of the apical membrane. In the lumen Cl^- combines with H^+ to

[1] 泌酸腺。

[2] 盐酸可以激活胃蛋白酶原成胃蛋白酶。

[3] 胰液和胆汁。

[4] 壁细胞是极性细胞，顶膜面面向细胞的小管腔，基底膜与细胞间液接触。

form HCl. When needed, HCl is secreted into the gastral cavity by parietal cells.

1.2 Pepsinogen

The chief cells[1] secrete pepsinogen. Pepsinogen can be activated into pepsin by contacting HCl or previously formed pepsin. Pepsin is a proteolytic enzyme, which is active in a highly acid medium (optimal pH 2.0). Pepsins hydrolyze the protein in the food into polypeptides of very diverse sizes. Because pepsins have a pH optimum of 1.6 ~ 3.2, their action is terminated when the gastric contents are mixed with alkaline pancreatic juice in the duodenum and jejunum[2].

1.3 Mucus and gastric barrier

Mucus is secreted by the epithelial cells, mucus neck cells, cardiac gland and pyloric gland[3] which are all on the gastric mucosa. Its main ingredient is glycoprotein. The viscous mucus is easy to form gel on the gastric mucosal surface, thus can protect the mucosa from mechanical damage from food. In the slime layer, the HCO_3^- can neutralize H^+ of the surface of gastric mucosa. When the gastric H^+ in the gastral cavity diffuses to epithelial cells of gastric mucosa through the mucus layer, its diffusion velocity slows down significantly. At the same time, H^+ is neutralized by HCO_3^- in layer of mucus, which not only avoid the direct erosion of H^+ to the gastric mucosa, also make pepsinogen not be activated in the side of epithelial cells to effectively prevent the digestion of gastric mucosa from pepsin.

This anti damage barrier composed of mucous barrier and HCO_3^- is known as mucus–bicarbonate barrier[4] (Figure 6–5).

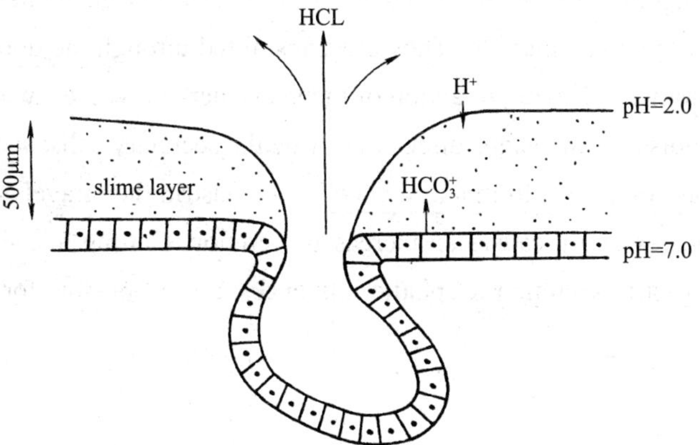

Figure 6–5 mucus bicarbonate barrier

[1] 主细胞。

[2] 十二指肠和空肠里的碱性胰液。

[3] 上皮细胞、颈黏液细胞、贲门腺和幽门腺。

[4] 由黏液和碳酸氢盐构成的抗损伤屏障成为黏液—碳酸氢盐屏障。

1.4 Intrinsic factor

Intrinsic factor is a glycoprotein secreted by the parietal cell. It is essential to the absorption of vitamin B_{12}. Intrinsic factor owns two active sites[1], one binding to vitamin B_{12} to protect them not to be destroyed, and the other binding to epithelial cells of the ileum[2] to promote vitamin B_{12} absorption. Lacking of intrinsic factors will lead to megaloblastic anemia[3].

2 Regulation of gastric secretion

Gastric secretion is regulated by both nervous and hormonal mechanisms. The nervous regulation is effected through the parasympathetic fibers of the vagus nerves as well as through local enteric nervous system reflexes[4]. Hormone regulation is mainly through the hormone gastrin. For convenience, the physiological stimulation of gastric secretion is usually discussed in terms of cephalic, gastric, and intestinal influences (or phases)[5] (Figure 6–7), although these overlapping. The cephalic influences are vagus mediated response induced by activity in the central nervous system. The gastric influences are primarily local reflex responses and responses to gastrin. The intestinal influences are the reflex and hormonal feedback effects on gastric secretion initiated from the mucosa of the small intestine.

2.1 Cephalic phases

The gastric secretion occurs even before food enters the stomach, which can be verified by a sham feeding test as shown in the Figure 6–6. It results from the sight, smell, thought, or taste of food. Neurogenic signals causing gastric secretion may originate in the appetite centers of the amygdala or hypothalamus[6]. They are transmitted through the dorsal motor nuclei of the vagi[7] to the stomach. The motor action of the vagus nerve involves two mechanisms: first, postganglionic impulses of the vagus directly activate the secretary cells; secondly, vagal activity causes the release of gastrin from antral G cells[8]. Gastrin then travels in the blood stream to the gastric glands, where it causes an increased secretion. Cutting of the vagi abolishes the cephalic phase of gastric secretion. Cephalic influences are responsible for one–third to one–

[1] 活性位点。

[2] 回肠。

[3] 巨幼红细胞性贫血。

[4] 神经调节是通过迷走神经的副交感神经纤维及局部肠神经系统反射来实现的。

[5] 头、胃和肠的影响（期）。

[6] 杏仁体和下丘脑。

[7] 迷走神经背核。

[8] 迷走神经的活动可以引起胃窦部 G 细胞分泌胃泌素。

half of the acid secreted in response to normal meal(Figure 6–7).

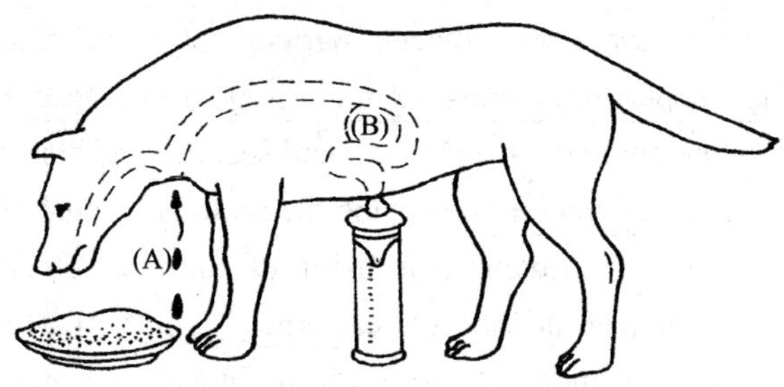

A: Esophageal fistula; B: Gastric fistula

Figure 6–6 Sham feeding experiment

2.2 Gastric phases

When foods get into the stomach, theycontinuetocausethegastric secretionthroughme-chanical(by distension) and chemical stimuli. At least three different mechanisms are involved: distension initiating a vago–vagal reflex; distension initiating a local reflex; chemical stimulation of gastrin release [1]. Many substances especially the digestive products of protein can cause gastrin release.

2.3 Intestinal phases

When the food come into duodenum [2], gastric secretion can also be initiated. It was postulated that the food causes the intestine to release one or more hormones which stimulate the gastric secretion. Gastrin is thought to be the most important hormone of all.

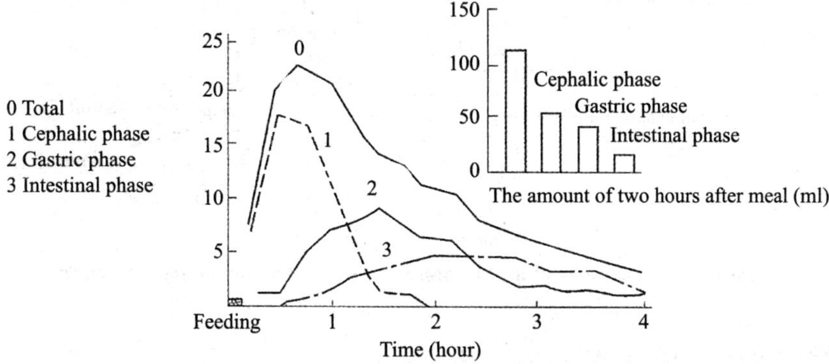

Figure 6–7 The relative relation between three phases of gastric juice secretion

[1] 胃扩张引起迷走－迷走神经反射，胃扩张引起肠神经系统反射，化学刺激引起胃泌素的释放。

[2] 十二指肠。

There are still many other influences of gastric secretion. For example, The gastric mucosa secretes a chemical substance called histamine through the way of paracrine[1], which can bind to the H_2 histamine receptor on the adjacent parietal cell membrane, causing gastric acid secretion. Clinically, H_2 receptor antagonists (cimetidine) can be used as a kind of treatment drug of peptic ulcer[2],by antagonize the effect of acid secretion of histamine, reducing gastric acid secretion. In addition, hypoglycemia[3] acts via the brain and vagal efferent nerves to stimulate acid and pepsin secretion. Intravenous infusion of amino acids can also stimulate acid secretion. Other stimulants include alcohol and caffeine[4], both of which act directly on the mucosa. The beneficial effects of moderate amounts of alcohol on appetite and digestion, as a result of this stimulatory effect on gastric secretion, have been known since ancient times.

Conversely, some factors can inhibit the secretion of gastric acid, such as hydrochloric acid in the stomach and somatostatin secreted by D cells in the antrum, stomach floor, and small intestine mucosa[5]. They can directly inhibit the secretion of gastric acid by parietal cells, and can also reduce the secretion of gastric acid by inhibiting the secretion of gastrin and other indirect pathways. In addition, the release of prostaglandins[6] in the gastric mucosa, the hydrochloric acid, fat digestion products and hypertonic solution of the duodenum and the upper jejunum also inhibit the secretion of gastric juice.The neurological and humoral factors affecting gastric secretion are shown in Figure 6–8.

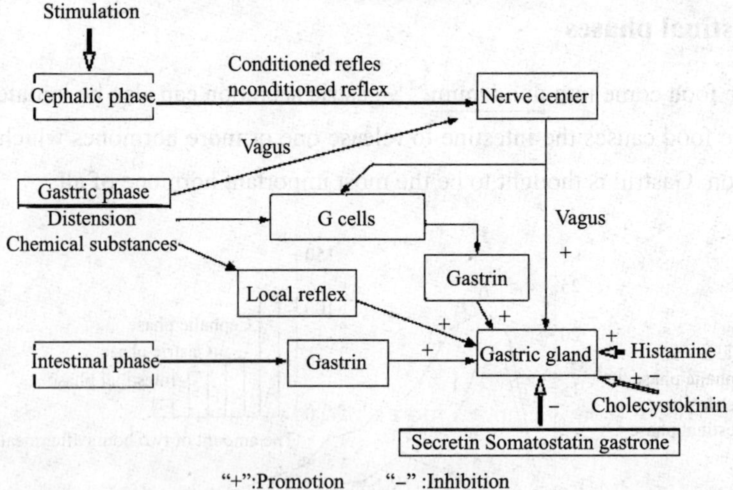

Figure 6–8 Neurological and humoral factors affecting gastric secretion

[1] 胃黏膜通过旁分泌释放一种称作组织胺的化学物质。

[2] 临床上，H_2 受体阻断剂（甲氰咪胍）被用作消化性溃疡的治疗药物。

[3] 低血糖。

[4] 咖啡因。

[5] 由胃窦、胃底及小肠黏膜内的 D 细胞分泌的生长抑素。

[6] 前列腺素。

3 Gastric movement and regulation

It is generally accepted that there are three types of gastric motility:receptive relaxation, tense contraction and gastric peristalsis.

3.1 The main forms of gastric motility

3.1.1 Receptive relaxation

With each swallow of food, there is a slight receptive relaxation of the body of the stomach. The stomach thus accommodates itself to the meal with little rise of pressure in intragastric pressure. Receptive relaxation is a reflex mediated by the vagus nerves. Afferent vagal impulses arise from the stretch receptors in the pharynx and esophagus[1]. The vagal efferent nerres involved in this reflex are neither adrenergic nor cholinergic[2]. It may act through the release of some peptides.

3.1.2 Tense contraction

Tense contraction refers to the constant contraction of the gastric smooth muscle. It can maintain the shape and position of the stomach, and make the stomach have a certain pressure, so as to helping digestion in the stomach. If the stomach tensity is too low, it can cause gastric ptosis and gastric dilatation[3], leading to digestive dysfunction.

3.1.3 Gastric peristalsis

When the stomach is full, peristaltic waves begin at the middle part of the stomach and spread down the antrum[4] at a rate of three times per minute. The gastric peristalsis helps to grind the food and mix the stomach contents. It also propell the food through the pyloric sphincter[5] to empty the stomach of its contents.

3.2 Gastric emptying

The process of gastric chyme entering the duodenum is called gastric emptying[6].The rate at which gastric contents pass into the duodenum depends on their chemical and physical characteristics. Coarse food is emptied more slowly than finely ground or mashed food. Solid food remains in stomach longer than liquids. Chemical compositions of the solid food affect its emptying rate, with sugar faster than protein, and protein faster than fat

---

[1] 咽和食管的牵张感受器。

[2] 参与该反射的迷走神经传出纤维既非肾上腺素能和胆碱能的。

[3] 胃下垂和胃扩张。

[4] 胃窦部。

[5] 胃幽门括约肌。

[6] 胃食糜进入十二指肠的过程称为胃排空。

3.3 Regulation of gastric motility

The movement of the stomach is also regulated by nerves and hormones. Stimulation of the vagus nerve promotes movement of the stomach, and hormones such as gastrin and motilin [1] also strengthen the movement of the stomach. On the contrary, the excitement of sympathetic movement [2], secretin and gastric inhibitory peptide decrease the stomach movement.

3.4 Vomiting

Vomiting[3] refers to the strong reflection process of contents in the stomach and intestines being ejected from the oral. Vomiting is a protective defense reflex that can release harmful substances from the stomach. The vomiting center is closely related to the respiratory center and cardiovascular center, so vomiting often leads to respiratory and cardiovascular reactions.

Section 4 Small intestine digestion

Digestion in small intestine is the most important stage in the process of digestion. Chyme in the intestine remains about 3 to 8 hours. After the chemical digestion of pancreatic juice, bile and intestinal fluid and the mechanical digestion of intestinal movement, chyme turns into small molecules to be absorbed by the small intestine, the undigested food get into the large intestine.

1 The secretion of pancreatic juice

1.1 The nature, composition and function of pancreatic juice

Pancreatic juice is mainly secreted by pancreatic acinar cells and ductal cells [4]. It is colorless and transparent and a kind of alkaline liquid (pH 7.8 ~ 8.4). Daily secretion of normal adults is 1 ~ 2 L. In pancreatic juice, the main inorganic substances are water, bicarbonate ions [5], Na^+, K^+, Cl^- and so on, which are mainly secreted by ductal cells. The main organic matters are a variety of digestive enzymes (pancreatic amylase, lipase, proteolytic enzymes [6], etc.) secreted by acinar cells. Pancreatic juice can neutralize gastric acid in the duodenum to

[1] 胃动素。

[2] 交感神经活动。

[3] 呕吐。

[4] 胰液主要由胰腺腺泡细胞和导管细胞分泌。

[5] 碳酸氢根离子。

[6] 胰淀粉酶、脂肪酶、蛋白酶。

provide the weak alkaline environment for activities of various enzymes in the small intestine. All kinds of enzymes in pancreatic juice decompose various substances in food.

(1) Carbohydrate digestive enzyme

The pancreatic enzyme for digesting carbohydrates is amylase which hydrolyzes starches, glycogen, and most other carbohydrates except cellulose into disaccharides and trisaccharides.[1]

(2) Fat digestive enzymes

The main enzymes for fat digestion are pancreatic lipase capable of hydrolyzing neutral fat into fatty acids and monoglycerides, cholesterol esterase capable of hydrolyzing cholesterol esters, and phospholipase which splits fatty acids from phospholipids.[2]

(3) Proteolytic enzymes

When synthesized in the pancreatic cells, the proteolytic enzymes are in the forms of trypsinogen, chymotrypsinogen, and procarboxypeptidase[3], which are all enzymatically inactive. They become activated only after being secreted into the intestinal tract.Trypsinogen is activated by an enzyme called enterokinase[4], which is secreted by the intestinal mucosa. Trypsinogen can also be autocatalytically activated by trypsin that has already been formed. Chymotrypsinogen is activated by trypsin to form chymotrypsin, and procarboxypolypeptidase is activated in a similar manner.

By far the most abundant of these is trypsin. The trypsin and chymotrypsin split whole and partially digested proteins into peptides of various sizes. Carboxypolypeptidase splits individual amino acids from the carboxyl ends of the peptides, thus completing the digestion of much of the proteins all the way to the amino acid state. In addition, the nuclease split the two types of nucleic acids: ribonucleic and deoxyribonucleic acids[5].

1.2 Control of pancreatic secretion

As with gastric acid secretion, there are cephalic, gastric and intestinal phase of pancreatic secretion. The cephalic phase involves the activation of the vagi by conditioned reflex and unconditioned reflex[6]. The gastric and intestinal phase both involve food in the gut. Food entering the stomach causes an increased pancreatic secretion (gastric phase). Two mechanisms are involved:

---

[1] 水解淀粉、糖原和除了纤维素以外的大多数其他碳水化合物成为双糖和三糖。

[2] 胰脂肪酶能够水解中性脂肪转化为脂肪酸和单甘酯，胆固醇酯酶能水解胆固醇酯，磷脂将脂肪酸从磷脂上水解下来。

[3] 胰蛋白酶原、糜蛋白酶原、羧基肽酶原。

[4] 肠致活酶。

[5] 核酸酶分裂了两种类型的核酸：核糖核酸和脱氧核糖核酸。

[6] 条件反射和非条件反射。

One is the reflex response to distension involving both vagal afferent and efferent nevves[1]; The other is the release of gastrin from the antral mucosa in response to protein digestion products. Gastrin evokes a pronounced increase in pancreatic enzyme output. The main stimulant for pancreatic secretion is the presence of food and acid in the small intestine (intestinal phase.) The strongest stimulants of secretion are fatty acids, monoglyceride, protein digestion products and acid. The response is mediated by the release of secretin and cholecystokinin[2] (Figure 6-9).

There are many hormones can inhibit the secretion of pancreatic juice. For example, the pancreatic polypeptide[3] inhibits the basal secretion of the pancreas and the pancreatic secretion caused by vagal nerve stimulation. Somatostatin is the strongest known hormone suppressing the secretion of the pancreas, through inhibiting secretin and cholecystokinin stimulation of pancreatic secretion.

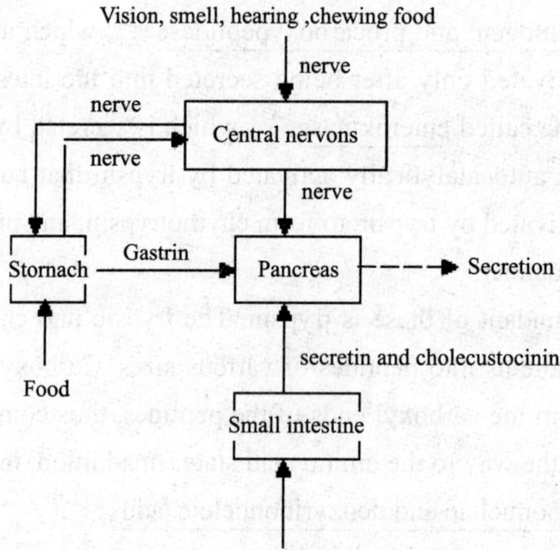

Figure 6–9 Control of pancreatic secretion

2 Bile secretion and discharge

2.1 The nature, composition and function of bile

Bile is secreted continuously by the liver cells but is normally stored in the gallbladder until needed in the duodenum. Bile is bitter and colored. The inorganic substances in bile are Na^+, K^+, Cl^-, HCO_3^- and so on. The main organic matters are bile salts, bile pigment, choles-

[1] 迷走的传入和传出神经。

[2] 促胰液素和缩胆囊素。

[3] 胰多肽。

terol and lecithin [1], but without digestive enzymes. The bile salt may be related to absorption and digestion of fat (Table 6–3). Bile pigment is a decomposition product of hemoglobin. Its type and concentration determine the color of bile. Bile salt, lecithin and cholesterol in the bile maintain appropriate proportion to keep the cholesterol being in dissolved state, otherwise cholesterol may be deposited to form stones.

Table 6–3 Composition of bile

	Liver bile	Gallbladder bile
Water	97.5g/dl	92g/dl
Bile salts	1.1 g/dl	6g/dl
Bilirubin	0.04 g/dl	0.3 g/dl
Cholesterol	0.1 g/dl	0.3 to 0.9 g/dl
Fatty acids	0.12 g/dl	0.3 to 1.2 g/dl
Lecithin	0.04 g/dl	0.3 g/dl
Na^+	145mEq/L	130mEq/L
K^+	5 mEq/L	12 mEq/L
Ca^{2+}	5 mEq/L	23 mEq/L
Cl^-	100 mEq/L	25 mEq/L
HCO_3^-	28 mEq/L	10 mEq/L

Bile salts play an important role in the digestion and absorption of fat. It can reduce the surface tension of the fat and turn the fat into droplets dispersing in the aqueous solution to increase the functionary area of pancreatic lipase and fat. When the concentration of bile salt reaches a certain degree, it can conglomerate micelles [2]. Fatty acid and monoglyceride can seep into the micelles to form the water soluble complex, which can promote the absorption of cholesterol, fatty acid and fat soluble vitamin A, D, E, K. Bile salt deficiency may affect the digestion and absorption of fat, even cause the fatty diarrhea [3].

2.2 The regulation of bile secretion and discharge

The maximum volume of the gallbladder is 50 ~ 70 ml. In the bile, water, sodium, chloride, and most other small electrolytes are continuously absorbed by the gallbladder mucosa, which caused the other bile constituents, including the bile salts, cholesterol, and bilirubin [4], are concentrated. Bile is stored in the gallbladder. When the presence of food in the duodenum,

[1] 胆盐、胆色素、胆固醇和卵磷脂。

[2] 微胶粒。

[3] 脂肪性腹泻。

[4] 胆红素。

the bile can be emptied.

Two basic conditions are necessary for the gallbladder to empty: the sphincter of Oddi [1] must relax to allow bile to flow from the common bile duct into the duodenum, and the gallbladder itself must contract to provide the force required to move the bile along the common duct.

The emptying of the gallbladder is controlled by two factors: Fat and protein in the food entering the small intestine elicit the release of CCK which is absorbed into the blood and transported to the gallbladder, causing its contraction; Vagal stimulation causes contraction of the gallbladder muscle and inhibition of the sphincter of Oddi. .

Approximately 94% of the bile salts are reabsorbed by the intestinal mucosa in the distal ileum[2]. They enter the portal blood and return to the liver. On reaching the liver, the bile salts are absorbed from the venous sinusoids[3] into the hepatic cells[4] and then re-secreted into the bile. This process is called enterohepatic circulation of bile salts [5].The quantity of bile secreted by the liver each day is highly dependent on the enterohepatic circulation of bile salts.

3 Small intestinal secretion

Small intestinal fluid is a weak alkaline liquid (pH 7.6) secreted by the duodenum, intestinal gland. It contains enterokinase and a variety of digestive enzymes (sucrase, maltase, isomaltase and lactase [6]). Daily secretion is about 1 ~ 3L for adults. Small intestine fluid can protect duodenal mucosa from acid erosion and provide suitable pH environment for a variety of digestive enzymes. A large number of small intestinal fluid can dilute the digestion products of intestines to reduce the osmotic pressure [7] and be conducive to digestion and absorption of digestion products.

The secretion of small intestine is regulated by the local mechanical and chemical stimuli through local intrinsic plexus [8] reflexes and by hormones such as gastrin, secretin and others. The principal components and functions of various digestive juices are shown in Table 6-4.

[1] 奥迪括约肌。

[2] 回肠末端。

[3] 静脉窦。

[4] 肝细胞。

[5] 这个过程称作胆盐的肠肝循环。

[6] 蔗糖酶、麦芽糖酶、异麦芽糖酶、乳糖酶。

[7] 渗透压。

[8] 内在神经丛。

Table 6–4 The principal components and functions of various digestive juices

Digestive juice	Secretory volume (L)	pH	Main components	Enzyme substrates	Hydrolysis products of enzymes
Saliva	1.0 ~ 1.5	6.0 ~ 7.1	Mucus		
			Salivary amylase	Amylum	Barley sugar
Gastric juice	1.5 ~ 2.5	0.9 ~ 1.5	Mucus		
			HCl		
			Pepsin (Pepsinogen)	Protein	Proteose, Peptone, Polypeptide
			Intrinsic factor		
Pancreatic juic	1.0 ~ 2.0	7.8 ~ 8.4	HCO_3^-		
			Amylopsin	Amylum	Barley sugar
			Trypsinogen (Trypsin)	Protein	Amino acid, Oligopeptide
			Chymotrypsin (proto)	Protein	Amino acid, Oligopeptide
			Pancreatic lipase	Triacylglycerol	Fatty acid, Glycerin, Monoglyceride
Bile	0.8 ~ 1.0	6.8 ~ 7.4	Bile salt, Cholesterol, Bile pigment		
Intestinal fluid	1.0 ~ 3.0	7.5 ~ 8.0	Mucus		
			Enterokinase	Trypsinogen	Trypsin
Colorectal fluid	0.5	8.3 ~ 8.4	Mucus, HCO_3^-		

4 The movement of small intestine

4.1 The movement type

4.1.1 Tonic contractions

The tonic contraction[1] of the smooth muscle is the basis for the small intestine to maintain its basic shape and perform other forms of motion. When the tonic contraction of the small intestinal smooth muscle increases, it is beneficial to the mixing and delivery of small intestinal contents

4.1.2 Segmental motility[2] (Mixing contractions)

When a portion of the small intestine becomes distended with chyme, circular smooth

[1] 紧张性收缩。

[2] 分节运动。

muscle[1] of the small intestine begin to rhythmically contract and relax.These rhythmic contractions occur at rate of 11 to 12 per minute.These contractions cause "segmentation" of the small intestine, dividing the intestines into regularly spaced segments looking like a chain of sausages.Each section alternates between contraction and relaxation.Therefore, the segmental contractions "chop" the chyme many times a minute, in this way promoting the progressive mixing of the solid food particles with the secretions of the small intestine. Segmental motility can also promote the reflux of blood and lymph, as well as being conducive to absorption(-Figure 6–10).

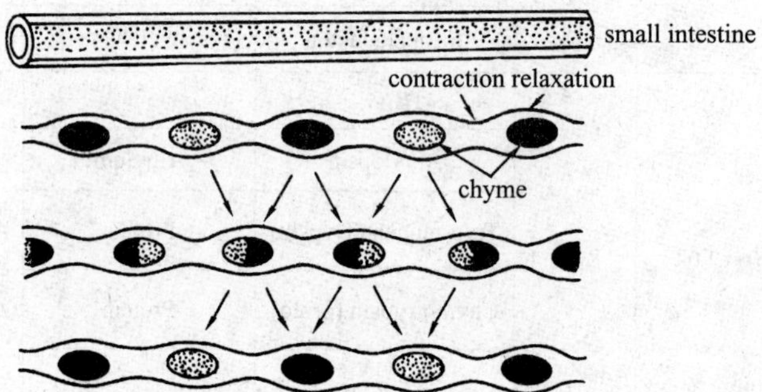

Figure 6–10 A pattern of segmental movements in the small intestine

4.1.3 Peristalsis (propulsive movements)

The bowel contents are pushed slowly through peristalsis. The usual cause of peristalsis in the small intestine is distention. They can move at velocity of 0.5 ~ 2 cm per second. Peristalsis activity of the small intestine is greatly increased after a meal. Peristalsis in the small intestine is normally very weak, intense irritation of the intestinal mucosa, as occurs in some sever cases of infections diarrhea, can cause both very powerful and rapid peristalsis called the peristaltic rush[2].

The intestinal peristalsis can promote intestinal gas movement, and make a sound, which is called 'bowel sound'[3]. Bowelsound can be used to evaluate the intestinal motor function.

4.2 The movement regulation

Parasympathetic nervous stimulation strengthens the small intestine movement, sympathetic nerve excitation produces the inhibitory effect. The myenteric plexus also plays an important regulatory role in the movement of small intestine. Gastrin, motilin, CCK and 5–HT can strengthen the intestinal movement; however, secretin, glucagon, vasoactive intestinal pep-

[1] 环形平滑肌。

[2] 蠕动冲。

[3] 肠鸣音。

tide, epinephrine and gastric inhibitory peptide inhibit the movement of small intestine

4.3 The function of the ileocecal sphincter

At the junction of the terminal ileum and cecum, the annular muscle is markedly thickened and has sphincter function called the ileocecal sphincter. Normally, ileocecal sphincter maintains mild contraction, can prevent the content from the ileum too quickly into the large intestine, thereby prolonging the residence time of chyme in the small intestine, which is conducive to the full digestion and absorption of the contents in the small intestine. When the peristaltic waves reach the terminal ileum , ileocecal sphincter relaxes, and about 4ml chyme is emptied from the ileum into the colon. In addition, ileocecal sphincter also has a kind of valve function, which can prevent colon contents flowing backwards into the ileum, protecting intestinal from germs.

Section 5 Colon digestion

1 The secretion of large intestine and the role of bacteria in the large intestine

A small amount of alkaline viscous liquid (pH 8.3 ~ 8.4) is secreted by large intestine mucosa. Its main ingredients are mucus and bicarbonate and its main function is to protect the intestinal mucosa and lubricate feces[1].

There are many kinds of bacteria in the large intestine, such as Escherichia coli, Staphylococcus[2], etc. Bacteria produce enzymes that can break down food residues. Generally,the decomposition on sugar and fat by bacteria is called fermentation[3], the decomposition on the protein by bacteria is known as corruption[4]. Bacteria can also use food residues to synthesize vitamin B complex and vitamin K, which are used by the human body after absorption through the intestinal wall.

[1] 润滑粪便。

[2] 大肠杆菌、葡萄球菌。

[3] 发酵。

[4] 腐败。

2 Large intestine movement and defecation reflex[1]

2.1 Mixing movements[2]

In the same manner that segmentation movements occur in the small intestine, large circular constrictions occur in the large intestine.At the same time, the longitudinal muscle[3] of the colon contracts.They also at times move slowly toward the anus[4] during contraction, especially in the cecum and ascending colon[5], and thereby provide a minor amount of forward propulsion of the colonic contents. In this way, all the fecal material is gradually exposed to the mucosal surface of the large intestine, and fluid and dissolved substances are progressively absorbed until only 80 to 200 milliliters of feces are expelled each day.

2.2 Propulsive movements–'mass movements[6]'

A mass movement is a modified type of peristalsis.It is a simultaneous contraction of the smooth muscle over large confluent areas. These contractions occur in the descending colon and sigmoid[7] and serve to empty the colon rapidly. They are the predominant propulsive force during defecation. Now the movement forms of main digestive organs and their physiological significance are shown in Table 6–5.

Table 6–5 Movement forms of main digestive organs and their physiological significance

Digestive organs	Movement forms	Physiological significance
Oral cavity	Mastication	Chops the food and mixes it with saliva
	Swallowing	Bolus is propelled down through esophagus into the stomach
Stomach	Receptive relaxation	Accommodates itself to the meal
	Tonic contraction	Maintain the shape and position of the stomach, and make the stomach have a certain pressure
	Peristalsis	Helps to grind the food and mix the stomach contents.
		It also propels the food through the pyloric sphincter to empty the stomach

[1] 排便反射。

[2] 复合运动。

[3] 纵行肌。

[4] 肛门。

[5] 盲肠和升结肠。

[6] 集团运动。

[7] 降结肠和乙状结肠。

续表

Digestive organs	Movement forms	Physiological significance
Small intestine	Tonic contraction	Being the basis for the small intestine to maintain its basic shape and perform other forms of motion
	Peristalsis	Pushing the bowel contents slowly
	Segmental motility	Promoting the progressive mixing of the solid food particles with the secretions of the small intestine.
		Promoting the reflux of blood and lymph.
		Being conducive to absorption.
Large intestine	Mixing movements	Providing a minor amount of forward propulsion of the colonic contents.
		All the fecal material is gradually exposed to the mucosal surface of the large intestine, and fluid and dissolved substances are progressively absorbed.
	Mass Movements	Ampty the colon rapidly
	Peristalsis	Pushing the bowel contents slowly

2.3 Defecation reflex

Ordinarily, defecation is initiated by defecation reflexes. One of these reflexes is an intrinsic reflex mediated by the local enteric nervous system in the rectal wall[1].To be effective in causing defecation, it usually must be fortified by another type of defecation reflex, a parasympathetic defecation reflex that involves the sacral segments of the spinal cord[2].

When it becomes convenient for the person to defecate, the defecation reflexes can purposely be activated by taking a deep breath to move the diaphragm downward and then contracting the abdominal muscles to increase the pressure in the abdomen, thus forcing fecal contents into the rectum[3] to cause new reflexes. Reflexes initiated in this way are almost never as effective as those that arise naturally, for which reason people who too often inhibit their natural reflexes are likely to become severely constipated[4].

[1] 一种反射是直肠壁上由内在神经系统介导的局部反射。

[2] 一种由骶髓发出的副交感神经介导的排便反射。

[3] 直肠。

[4] 便秘的。

Section 6 Absorption

1 Sites and ways of absorption

1.1 Sites and ways of absorption

In different parts of the digestive tract, the absorption of the material and the ability is not the same(Figure 6–11). In mouth and esophagus, food nearly can not be absorbed. The absorption ability of the stomach is very weak, only can absorb a small amount of water, alcohol and some drugs (such as aspirin). Large intestine mainly absorbs water and inorganic salt, can also absorb some drugs slowly.

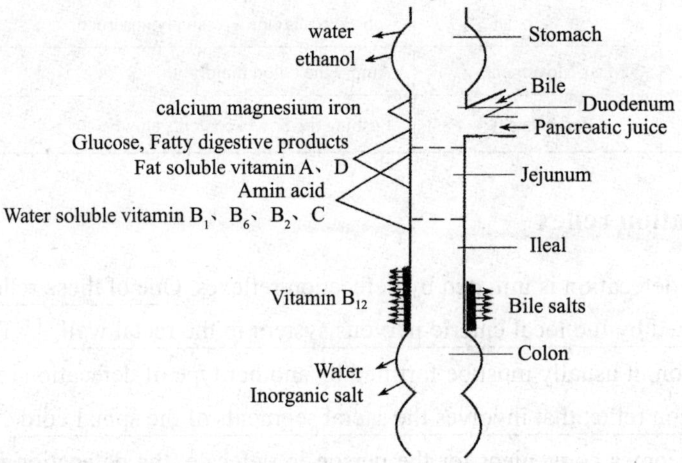

Figure 6–11 The absorption sites of various nutrients in the digestive tract

The small intestine is the main site of absorption. The digested products of carbohydrate, protein and fat are mostly absorbed in the duodenum and jejunum. Small intestine is very long and has large plicae circulares, villus and microvilli in mucosa on the free surface of each villus epithelial cells[1], thus having a huge area to be conducive to the absorption of small intestine(Figure 6–12). Food retention time is about 3 ~ 8 hours, which is sufficient for absorption. When food reaches the ileum, the absorption is usually over. The ileum can only absorb bile salts and vitamin B_{12}.

[1] 小肠很长，而且有大的环状皱襞，在每个绒毛上皮细胞游离面有黏膜绒毛和微绒毛。

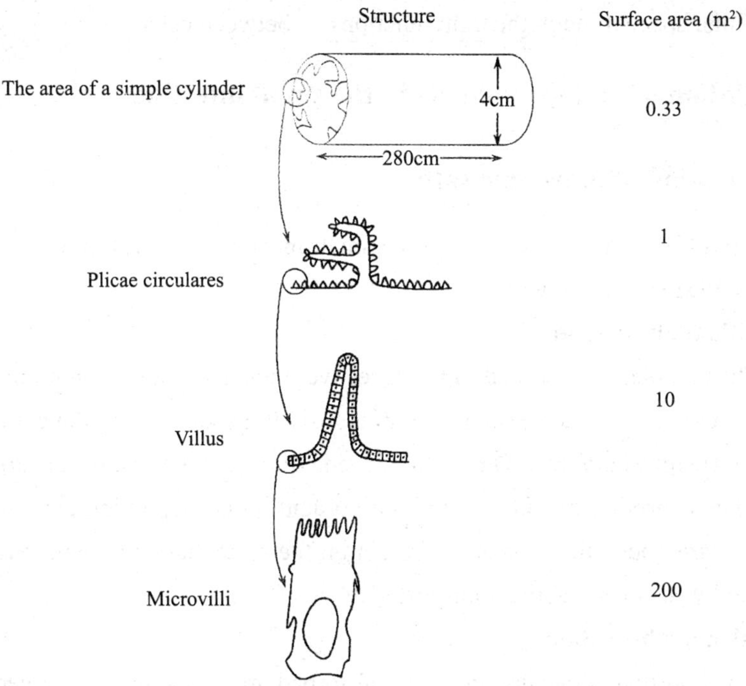

Figure 6–12 The relationship between the structure of the small intestine and the increase of the surface area of the small intestine

1.2 Ways of absorption

Absorption through the gastrointestinal mucosa occurs by active transport, simple diffusion, and facilitating diffusion [1]. The physical principles of these processes were explained in chapter two. Briefly, active transport imparts energy to the substance as it is being transported against a concentration gradient, or moving it against an electrical potential. On the other hand, the term diffusion means simply transport of substances through the membrane as a result of molecular movement along an electrochemical gradient [2].

There are two main approaches for small molecules to be absorbed into the blood or lymph : ① Transcellular pathway [3]: small molecules get into the cell through the cavosurface membrane of villous columnar epithelial cells [4], and then get into the blood or lymph through bottom side of the cell. ② Paracellular pathway [5]: small molecules get into the blood or lymph

[1] 主动转运、单纯扩散和协助扩散。

[2] 电化学梯度。

[3] 跨细胞途径。

[4] 绒毛柱状上皮细胞的管腔面膜。

[5] 细胞旁途径。

in the intercellular space through the tight junctions [1] between cells.

2 Absorption of major nutrients in the small intestine

2.1 Absorption of inorganic salts

Salts have different absorption rate in the small intestine. Absorption of NaCl is the fastest, absorption of $MgSO_4$ is slowest.

2.1.1 Sodium absorption

Na^+ can be completely absorbed in the digestive tract. The sodium pump in the epithelial cells on the bottom side of the membrane continuously transports Na^+ to the extracellular fluid against electro–chemical gradient. On the lumen side of digestive tract, the absorption of Na^+ is related with the absorption of glucose and amino acid. Glucose, amino acid and Na^+ in the intestinal cavity are bound to transporter protein on the epithelial cell membrane, and are absorbed together by secondary active transport way.

2.1.2 Calcium absorption

Only a small portion of calcium in food is absorbed, most calcium is excreted in the feces. Calcium salt in the acid solution is soluble and only the aqueous solution of calcium salts can be absorbed. Calcium can be absorbed against electro–chemical gradient in the small intestine and colon. On the cell surface of intestinal mucosa, there is a kind of calcium binding protein which has high affinity with calcium, participating in the active transport of calcium and promoting calcium absorption. Vitamin D and fat can promote calcium absorption in the small intestine.

2.1.3 The absorption of iron

The amount of iron absorbed normally is 1 mg in the adult every day. Iron is more readily absorbed in the ferrous state (Fe^{2+}), but most of the dietary iron is in the ferric form (Fe^{3+}). Vitamin C and acidic environment can turn ferric iron into ferrous iron, and promoting the absorption of iron.Iron is absorbed in the upper part of small intestine. Iron absorption is increased when body iron stores are depleted or when erythropoiesis [2] is increased, and decreased under the reverse conditions.

2.1.4 The absorption of negative ion

The negative ions for absorption in the small intestine are mainly Cl^- and HCO_3^-. The electric potential changes caused by intraluminal [3] Na^+ absorption can promote negative ions migrating into the cell.

---

[1] 紧密连接。

[2] 红细胞生成。

[3] 管腔内的。

2.2 Absorption of sugar

Sugar that is only decomposed into monosaccharide can be absorbed. The main parts of absorption are the duodenum and jejunum. Glucose accounts for about 80% in the monosaccharide of absorption.

Monosaccharide absorption can be carried out with inverse concentration difference, so it is an active transport process of consuming energy which comes from the sodium pump and belongs to a secondary active transportion the same direction with Na^+. The carrier protein combined with Na^+ can increase the affinity to glucose, so glucose binding to the carrier protein is transported into the cell. Two Na^+ and one monosaccharide can be transported into the cell by the transporter every time. The absorbteb Na^+ is transported into the lateral intercellular spaces, and the glucose is transported by glucose transporter into the interstitium and thence to the capillaries [1] (Figure 6–12).

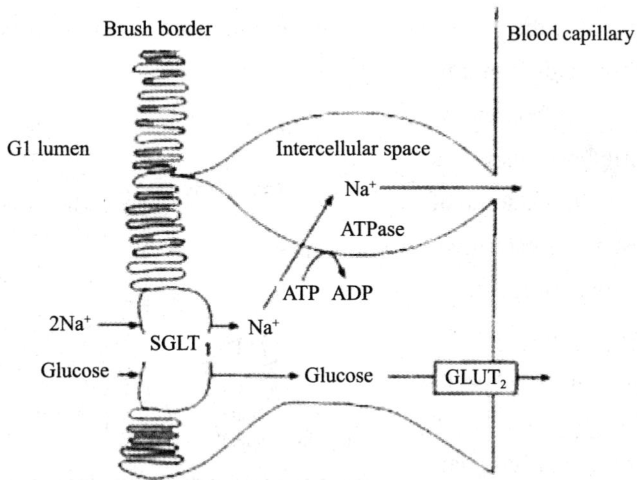

Figure 6–12 The mechanism of glucose absorption of intestinal epithelial cells
GI: gastrointestinal; SGLT: sodium–glucose–linked;
transporter; $GLUT_2$: glucose transporter 2

2.3 Protein absorption

Proteins need to be decomposed into amino acids to be absorbed.Absorption of amino acids is rapid in the duodenum and jejunum but slow in the ileum.Amino acid absorption is an active transport process, similar to glucose, coupling with $Na^+$and carrying out coordinated

[1] 被吸收的钠离子被转运到细胞外侧间隙，葡萄糖被葡萄糖转运蛋白转运到细胞间质，然后转运至毛细血管。

transport. There are three different kinds of special carrier systems of amino acids in the small intestine wall to respectively transport neutral amino acids、alkaline amino acids and acidic amino acids[1].

2.4 Fat absorption

More than 95% of the fat in food is triglycerides, in addition to cholesterol esters and phospholipids. The digestive products of triglycerides are fatty acid, monoglyceride and glycerol[2].

Hydrolysis[3] products of the fat have different ways of absorption. Glycerol dissolving in water is absorbed along with monosaccharide. Short and medium chain fatty acids can be directly diffused into the epithelial cells of small intestine from the intestinal lumen, thus into the blood. Only long chain fatty acids, monoglyceride and cholesterol can be absorbed by binding to bile salt together to form mixed micelle[4]. The fate of the fatty acids in enterocytes[5] depends on their size. Fatty acids containing less than 10 ~ 12 carbon atoms pass from the mucosal cells directly into the portal blood[6], where they are transported as free (unesterified) fatty acids. The fatty acids containing more than 10 ~ 12 carbon atoms are reesterified to triglycerides in the mucosal cells[7]. In addition, some of the absorbed cholesterol is esterified. The triglycerides and cholesteryl esters are then coated with a layer of protein, cholesterol, and phospholipids to form chylomicrons[8]. These leave the cell and enter the lymphatics (Figure 6–13).

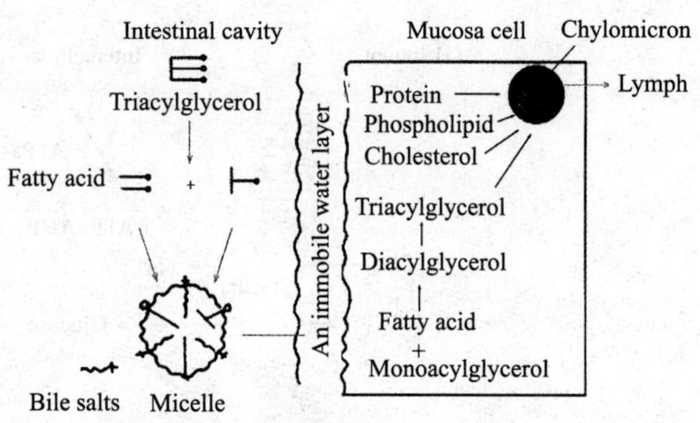

Figure 6–13 Digestion and absorption of fat in the small intestine

---

[1] 中性氨基酸、碱性氨基酸和酸性氨基酸。

[2] 食物中除了胆固醇酯和磷脂，95% 以上的脂肪是甘油三酯。甘油三酯的消化产物是脂肪酸、单甘酯和甘油。

[3] 水解。

[4] 只有长链脂肪酸、单甘油酯和胆固醇可以和胆盐结合在一起形成混合胶束而被吸收。

[5] 肠上皮细胞。

[6] 门静脉血。

[7] 超过 10 ~ 12 碳原子的脂肪酸在肠黏膜细胞再酯化为甘油三酯。

[8] 甘油三酯和胆固醇酯外被一层蛋白、胆固醇和磷脂形成乳糜微粒。

2.5 Vitamin absorption

Vitamins are divided into two types:water soluble vitamins and fat soluble vitamins. Water soluble vitamins are absorbed by diffusion, but vitamin B_{12} can only be absorbed by being combined with internal factor into compound in the terminal ileum. Due to soluble in fat, the mechanism of fat soluble vitaminabsorptionmay be similar to that of lipids, most absorbed into the blood through the lymph.

2.6 Water absorption

Most of the water in the digestive tract is absorbed in the small intestine. Only small amounts of water move across the gastric mucosa and large intestine. Water moves in both directions across the mucosa of the small and large intestines in response to osmotic gradients[1]. Osmotic pressure caused by various solutes, especially NaCl, is the mainly driving force to promote water absorption.

[1] 由于渗透梯度的作用，水在小肠和大肠黏膜两侧可以向两个方向上运动。

Chapter 7 ENERGY METABOLISM AND BODY TEMPERATURE

Section 1 Energy metabolism

In the metabolism process, the living organism takes in materials for energy, growth, and repair. Therefore, different chemical compounds are synthesized and destroyed, cellular structures are continuously formed, renewed and destroyed. When the chemical compounds are split, their potential energy is released and converted into the kinetic energy, mainly thermal and mechanical, partly–electrical. Usually, the metabolism process of the energy storage, release, transfer and utilization is known as the energy metabolism[1]. This section mainly discusses the source and utilization of human energy, the determination of energy metabolism, the main factors affecting the energy metabolism and the basic metabolism.

1 The source and use of body's energy

1.1 Energy sources

Energy is required in the life processes of each individual human being. Since the human body cannot produce its own energy, therefore, it must continuously take in foods to supply that energy to carry on the life processes to withstand environmental adversity and better survival. This food also provides materials for growth and repair of the cells and tissues.

1.2 Transformation and utilization of body's energy

The energy for all physiological activities comes from the conversion of higher–energy adenosine triphosphate (ATP)[2] to lower–energy phosphates ADP. When ATP releases its energy, a high–energy bond is split away, which contains about 33.47KJ of energy, and ade-

[1] 生物体内物质代谢过程中能量代谢伴随发生的能量的释放、转移、贮存和利用称为能量代谢。
[2] 腺苷三磷酸。

nosine diphosphate (ADP) [1] is formed. This released energy is used to energize virtually all of the cells' other functions and perform various physiological activities, such as synthesis of substances and muscular contraction. Therefore, ATP is not only an important energy storage material, but also a direct energy supply material.

In addition to ATP, there is a kind of energy storage material containing high energy phosphate bond is creatine phosphate(CP) [2], it mainly exists in the muscle and brain tissues, When the material oxidation energy released too much, ATP transfers high energy phosphate bonds to creatine to generate CP and store energy. When the ATP is consumed and reduced, the CP can transfer the stored energy to ADP and generate ATP to supplement the consumption of ATP. This supplement is faster than the direct release of energy from food oxidation, just a fraction of a second, which can meet the energy needs of the body in the event of emergency physiological activities. Therefore, CP can be regarded as the repository of ATP, but it can not directly provide the energy needed for cell life activities. From the whole process of energy metabolism, the synthesis and decomposition of ATP is the key link of energy conversion and utilization.

The ultimate way for the released energy of material decomposition: ① Turn into heat energy; ② Stored in the high–energy phosphate bonds of energetic compounds(ATP, ADP, CP, et al), to be used for the body to complete the various physiological activities, such as muscle contraction and relaxation, transmembrane active transport and glandular secretion.

1.3 Energy metabolism measurement

1.3.1 Some concepts in energy metabolism measurement

(1)Thermal equivalent of food [3] The caloric value of food is the energy released by 1g of a kind of food which is oxidized. Thermal equivalent of food is usually measured in units of joules (J). Thermal equivalent of food is divided into bio thermal and physical thermal equivalent. The former refers to the energy produced by the oxidation of food in the body; The latter refers to the energy released when the food is burned in vitro. Sugar and fat in the body can be completely oxidized into CO_2 and H_2O, so their physical thermal equivalent [4] and biological thermal equivalent [5] are equal. The protein in the body cannot be completely oxidized, because some of ehe energy in urea, uric acid, creatinine and other molecules is discharged from urine. Therefore, the biological thermal equivalent is less than physical thermal equivalent for

[1] 腺苷二磷酸。

[2] 磷酸肌酸。

[3] 食物的热价：1 克某种食物氧化时所释放的能量。

[4] 物理热价。

[5] 生物热价。

protein (table 7–1).

Table 7–1 Data on the oxidation of three nutrients

Nutrients	Heat production(kJ/g)			Oxygen consumption	Carbon dioxide production (L/g)	Thermal equivalent of oxygen (kJ/L)	Respiratory quotient (RQ)
	Physical thermal equivalent	Biological thermal equivalent	Nutritional thermal equivalent *				
Sugar	17.15	17.15	16.7	0.83	0.83	21.00	1.00
Fat	39.75	39.75	37.7	2.03	1.43	19.70	0.71
Protein	23.43	17.99	16.7	0.95	0.76	18.80	0.80

*This data is used to calculate the thermal equivalent of food in nutrition[1]

(2)Thermal equivalent of oxygen [1] Means that the quantity of energy liberated per liter of oxygen used in the body.Thermal equivalent of oxygen reflects the relationship between the amount of O_2 consumed and the heat output of a kind of food. Because of the different proportion of carbon, hydrogen and oxygen in the molecular structure of the different nutrients, their Thermal equivalent of oxygen is also different(Table 7–1).

(3)Respiratory quotient, RQ [2] The respiratory quotient (RQ) is the ratio in the steady state of the volume of CO_2 produced to the volume of O_2 consumed in a certain period of time .In RQ, CO_2 and $O_2$are expressed in terms of the molar number (mol), However, in the same temperature and pressure conditions, Any of various gases of equal number, whose volume is equal, the volume number (ml or L) of CO_2 and O_2 can be used to compute RQ.

The amount of CO_2 produced by glucose oxidation is equal to the amount of O_2 consumed, so the RQ is 1 for carbohydrates. The RQ of fat and protein are respectively 0.71 and 0.80(Table 7–2). In daily life, the food is mixed with sugar, fat and protein which are in the decomposition in the body at the same time.Therefore, the overall RQ changes between 0.71 ~ 1. Normal people with mixed food RQ is generally about 0.85.

It is generally believed that RQ can reflect the proportion of oxidative decomposition of the three kinds of nutrients in the whole body, but the actual situation is not completely consistent. This is because that the body's tissues and cells not only can simultaneously oxidize and break down all kinds of nutrients, but also can change one nutrient into another.

(4)Non–protein respiratory quotient(NPRQ) [3] Under normal circumstances, the body's energy comes mainly from the oxidation of sugar and fat, the protein factor can be ignored. The ratio of the amount of CO_2 produced by the oxidation of sugar and fat to the amount of O_2

[1] 氧热价：某种食物氧化时消耗 1 升氧气所产生的热量。

[2] 呼吸商。

[3] 非蛋白呼吸商：由糖和脂肪氧化时产生的 CO_2 量和消耗的 O_2 量的比值。

consumed is called non–protein respiratory quotient. There is a certain proportion between the non–protein respiratory quotient and the thermal equivalent of oxygen (Table 7–2).

Table 7–2 Non–protein respiratory quotient and thermal equivalent of oxygen

Non–protein respiratory quotient	Oxidation percentage(%)		Thermal equivalent of oxygen(kJ/L)
	Sugar	Fat	
0.70	0.00	100.0	19.61
0.71	1.10	98.9	19.62
0.73	8.40	91.6	19.72
0.75	15.6	84.4	19.83
0.77	22.8	77.2	19.93
0.79	29.9	70.1	20.03
0.80	33.4	66.6	20.09
0.82	40.3	59.7	20.19
0.84	47.2	52.8	20.29
0.86	54.1	45.9	20.40
0.88	60.8	39.2	20.50
0.90	67.5	32.5	20.60
0.92	74.1	25.9	20.70
0.94	80.7	19.3	20.82
0.96	87.2	12.8	20.91
0.98	93.6	6.37	21.01
1.00	100.0	0.0	21.12

1.3.2 Principle and method of measuring the energy metabolism

The energy metabolism of the body follows the law of conservation of energy, that is, in the process of energy conversion from one form to another, the energy does not increase or decrease. Therefore, in the process of energy metabolism, The body's consumption of energy which is contained in energy substances should be equal to the heat and external work, such as skeletal muscle contraction. Therefore, if no external work, measuring the amount of heat emitted by the body within a certain period of time can reflect the energy consumed by the body at the same time.

Energy metabolism rate[1]: Energy metabolism rate is the amount of energy metabolism in unit time, and it is a common index to evaluate the level of energy metabolism. There are three methods to measure the energy generated in per unit time, they are direct calorimetry, indirect calorimetry and simplified determination.

[1] 能量代谢率：是指机体在单位时间内的能量代谢量，是评价机体能量代谢水平的常用指标。

(1) Direct calorimetry[1] Direct calorimetry is a method of directly measuring the heat dissipation of the subjects in a quiet state for a certain period of time. The equipment and its operation are too complicated, so this method is rarely used.

(2)Indirect calorimetry[2] The indirect calorimetry is based on the calculation of heat production in the organism, taking into consideration the volume of the consumed oxygen and the volume of carbon dioxide which is given off. The oxygen, consumed by the organism, is used for oxidation of proteins, fats and carbohydrates. Different amounts of oxygen are required to oxidize 1g of different of substances and is different amounts of the heat are produced. The chemical reaction for glucose is as follows:

$$C_6H_{12}O_6+6O_2=6CO_2+6H_2O+\Delta H$$

The steps of indirect calorimetry: ① Measure the body O_2 amount consumed and CO_2 producted in a certain period of time. ② Measure urinary nitrogen discharged in a certain period of time. According to the urine nitrogen(1g urinary nitrogen is equivalent to the oxidative decomposition of 6.25g protein), the protein oxidation amount can be calculated. According to the thermal equivalent of protein,the heat produced by protein is calculated. ③ Based on the amount of oxygen consumed and carbon dioxide produced during the oxidation of 1g proteins, the amount of oxygen consumed and carbon dioxide produced when the protein is oxidized is calculated.Then the remaining O_2 consumption amount and the amount of CO_2 produced and NPRQ can be calculated. According to Table 7–2, thermal equivalent of oxygen corresponding to the NPRQ is found out, then the heat production for non–protein food is calculated. ④ The total heat production can be calculated, namely the sum of heat production of protein food and non–protein food.

(3)Simplified determination[3] In clinical practice, the heat output of proteins can be neglected.Soa convenient method is used. O_2 consumption and CO_2 production by subjects are measured in a certain period of time, and the respiratory quotient will be calculated. Consulting non protein respiratory quotient (Table 7–2) , the corresponding thermal equivalent of oxygen can be found. The thermal equivalent of oxygen is multiplied by oxygen consumption is the produced heat amount at this period of time.

(4) More simplified determination Usually, O_2 consumption of subjects is determined within a certain period of time (usually 6 minutes). Respiratory quotient of mixed diet is 0.82, thermal equivalent of oxygen at this time is 20.20kJ, and the heat production is equal to the O_2 consumption multiplied by thermal equivalent of oxygen

[1] 直接测热法。

[2] 间接测热法。

[3] 简化测定法。

Heat production (kJ) =20.20 (kJ/L) ×VO_2 (L)

2 The main factors affecting energy metabolism

2.1 Muscle activity

The most significant effect on energy metabolism is muscle activity. Any minor activity can improve the metabolism rate. Oxygen consumption increases significantly when people are in exercise and labor. This is because the muscles need to be supplied energy. This will inevitably lead to the increase of the body's oxygen consumption. The strength of muscle activity is also called labor intensity, is usually expressed in terms of the heat output per unit of time. Table 7–3 shows the changes of energy metabolism rate in different intensity of labor or exercise.

Table 7–3 Energy metabolism during rest, labor and exercise

Muscle activity form	Average heat production[kJ/(m^2·min)]
Rest	2.73
Attend meeting	3.40
Clean the window	8.30
Wash clothes	9.89
Sweep the floor	11.36
Play volleyball	17.04
Play football	24.96

2.2 Spiritual activities

The metabolic level of brain tissue is very high. In general spiritual activities, even central nervous system increased metabolic rate itself, the degree is negligible. But when the mind is in a state of tension, such as worry, fear, because of muscular tension, increased hormone which stimulating the metabolism and other factors, the heat production can significantly increase.

2.3 Specific dynamic action of food [1]

After eating food(from 1 hours after eating, until 7 ~ 8 hours), a person will generate heat somewhat more than before eating, though he is in quiet. This shows that the additional energy consumption is caused by eating. This action that food stimulates the body to produce the extra calories is called the specific dynamic action of food.

The specific dynamic action of protein is the most significant, which could reach 30%; sugar and fat about 4% ~ 6%; and mixed food about 10%. Therefore, in order to to keep revenue and expenditure balance, this part of consumption must be taken into account.

[1] 食物的特殊动力效应。

2.4 Environmental temperature

When people are in the quiet state and with a environment temperature of 20 ~ 30℃ , the energy metabolism is the stablest. When the environment temperature is below 20℃ , metabolic rate will increase, mainly due to reflexed shivering and muscle tension caused by the cold stimulation. When the environment temperature is higher than 30℃ , metabolic rate will also increase. It is because that the speed of the chemical reactions in the body is enhanced, which is due to the accelerated rate of chemical reaction in vivo.

3 Basal metabolism

3.1 Concept of basal metabolism

Basal metabolism [1] refers to energy metabolism under basal conditions. The so-called basic state, is a state in which meeting the following conditions: early in the morning, waking, not muscle activity; good Eve sleep, no stress; at least fasting for 12 hours; room temperature being at 20 ~ 25℃ . In this state, energy consumption is only used to maintain basic life activities and energy metabolism is relatively stable. So the energy metabolism per unit time in this state is called basal metabolism rate (BMR) [2] . It should be pointed out that BMR should be lower than that in the quiet, but not the lowest, because the sleeping metabolism rate is lower (8% ~ 10% lower than that in the quiet, but when dreaming that can increases).

Energy metabolism rate means the generated heat in per unit time(1 hour) and body surface area in per square metre. Energy metabolism rate and body weight are disproportionate, but being proportional to the surface area. No matter big or small, the heat production per square meter of body surface area is basically the same. So, the unit of energy metabolism rate is kJ ($m^2 \cdot h$).The body surface area can be got by the following formula:

Surface area (m^2) =0.0061×height (cm) +0.0128×weight (kg)–0.1529

The body surface area can also be got by Figure 7–1.

In addition to body surface area, BMR is also different from the subjects by gender and age (Table 7–4). When other conditions are the same, the average BMR of males is higher than that of the females in the same age group.The average BMR value of children is higher than that of adults.The older

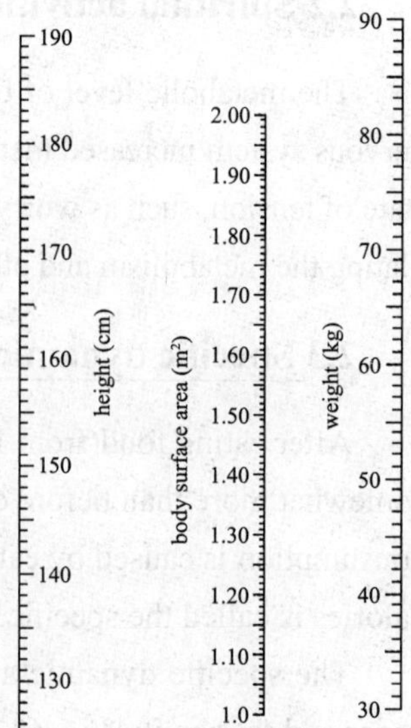

Figure 7–1 Body surface area calculation chart

[1] 基础代谢：是指基础状态下的能量代谢。

[2] 基础代谢率：是指在基础状态下单位时间内的能量代谢，是评价机体能量代谢水平的常用指标。

the age is, the lower the metabolism rate is.

Table 7–4 Average basal metabolism rate in China [kJ/ (m^2·h)]

Age	11 ~ 15	16 ~ 17	18 ~ 19	20 ~ 30	31 ~ 40	41 ~ 50	More than 51
Male	195.5	193.4	166.2	157.8	158.6	154.0	149.0
Female	172.5	181.7	154.0	146.5	146.9	142.4	138.6

3.2 Measurement and change of basal metabolism rate

Computational method of basal metabolic rate[1]: Indirect calorimetry is usually used for the determination of BMR. The NPRQ is considered 0.82, and the corresponding thermal equivalent of oxygen is 20.20 KJ/L. Therefore, only by measuring the oxygen consumption and body surface area in a certain period of time under the basic condition, the BMR can be calculated.

In order to exclude the effects of age and gender, Clinically, the basal metabolic rate is expressed as a percentage of the difference between the measured value and the average value:

BMR(relative value)=(measured value – the average value)/ average value×100%

In general, it is normal that the relative value is about ±10% ~ ±15%. When the relative value is more than 20%, it is thought that there are pathological changes.

Changes in thyroid function produce a noticeable effect. With hyperthyroidism, BMR can be higher than the normal value of 25% ~ 80%; and with hypothyroidism, BMR can be lower than the normal value of 20% ~ 40%. BMR will also change with the changes of adrenal cortex, hypophysis cerebri, and so on.

Section 2 Body temperature

1 The normal body temperature and physiological changes

1.1 Concept of body temperature and its normal value

The human body can be divided into two levels of shell temperature[2] and core temperature.[3] Shell temperature is the temperature of the body surface and the structure under the body surface, such as the skin and subcutis. The shell temperature is not stable, which can be changed by environment temperature or heat loss, and has big differences among various parts.

[1] 基础代谢率计算方法。

[2] 体表温度：是指体表及体表下结构（如皮肤、皮下组织等）的温度。

[3] 体核温度：是指人体深部（如内脏）的温度，比体表温度高且相对稳定。

Core temperature is the temperature of the human deep body temperature(such as the viscus). Core temperature is relatively stable and higher than shell temperature, which has the small differences among various parts. Although the core temperature is relatively stable, the temperature is little difference among internal organs, due to different metabolic levels. Liver temperature is about 38℃ , the highest in the body; brain heat production is up to38℃ ; kidney, and duodenum temperature is slightly lower; rectal temperature is lower. Blood circulation is an important way to transfer heat in the body. Due to the continuous blood circulation, each organ deep temperature often tends to be the same. The relative proportion of the core temperature range and the shell temperature range can change with the change of the environment temperature. In cold environment, the core temperature range is reduced; in the hot environment, the core temperature can be extended to the limbs (Figure 7–2).

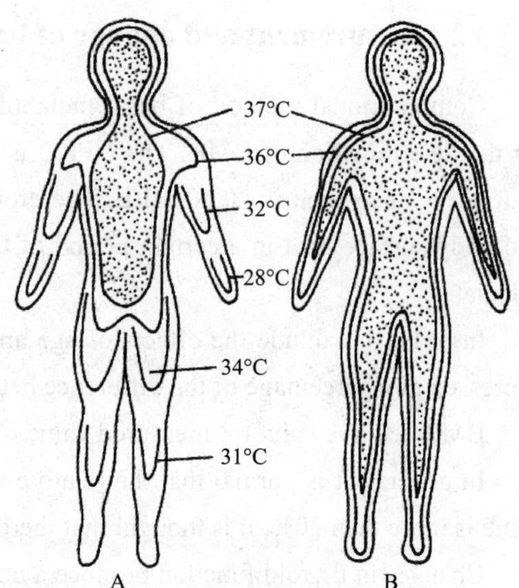

A: environmental temperature 20℃ ; B: environmental temperature 35℃

Figure 7–2 Human body temperature distribution under different environmental temperature

Physiology temperature (body temperature[1])refers to the average temperature of the deep body, namely the core temperature. Because the core temperature is not easy to test, so in clinic, the temperature in recta, oral cavity and axillar[2] etc. is commonly used to represent the body temperature. To measure the rectal temperature:the themometer is inserted into the rectum more than 6cm,the measured temperature value is close to the core temperature, whose normal value is 36.9 ~ 37.9℃ . Oral cavity(the underside of the tongue)is widely used for temperature measurement site.Its advantage is that the measured temperature values are accurate,and the measurement is more convenient.Normal oral temperature is 36.7 ~ 37.7 ℃ . Under axillar, the skin surface temperature is low, so it can not correctly reflect the temperature.Only under the condition that the upper arm clings to the chest , the internal heat can be gradually conducted to the armpit, the temperature gradually increases to being close to the core temperature. Therefore, when the axillary temperature is measured, the required time is at least 10 minutes, and the armpit should be kept dry. Its normal value is 36.0 ~ 37.4℃ .

[1] 体温：是指机体深部的平均温度，即体核温度。

[2] 直肠、口腔和腋窝。

1.2 Normal body temperature variation

The temperature is relatively stable. But in physiological conditions, temperature will change with day and night, age, gender and other factors. The maximum range of body temperature change should not exceed 1℃.

1.2.1 Circadian rhythm of body temperature

The temperature often fluctuates periodically in a day and night: at 2 ~ 6 in the morning, the temperature is the lowest, and at 1 ~ 6 in the afternoon, the temperature is the highest. This circadian fluctuation is called circadian rhythm [1]. A lot of research results show that muscle activity and oxygen consumption are not involved in circadian rhythm of body temperature.It is an internal biological rhythm. Animal experiments indicated that biological rhythm phenomenon is controlled by hypothalamic biological clock.

1.2.2 The influence of gender

Women's average temperature is 0.3℃, higher than that of men. This may be because of more subcutaneous fat in women, so less heat released. Women's basal body temperature varies with the menstrual cycle [2](Figure 7–3). In the menstrual cycle, the body temperature in the follicular phase [3] is low, and is the lowest at ovulation day [4]. After ovulation, it is increased 0.3 ~ 0.6 ℃. Therefore, at women's childbearing age by measuring the basic body temperature every day, it help to understand whether ovulation and the ovulation date. At present, it is thought that the rise in body temperature after ovulation is due to the progesterone [5]'s action to hypothalamus secreted by metoarion.

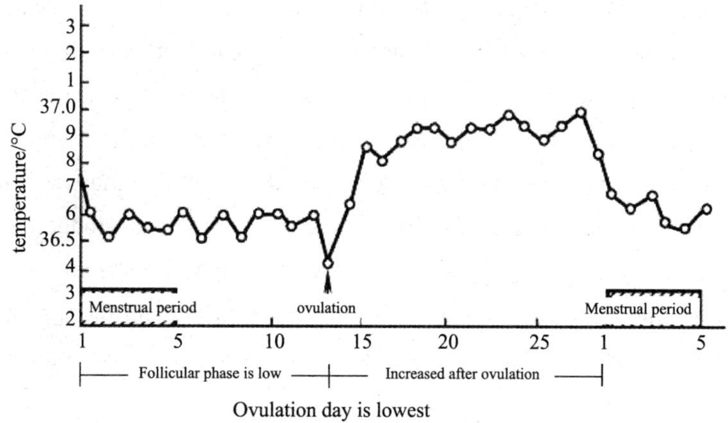

Figure 7–3 Basal body temperature curve during the menstrual cycle

[1] 昼夜节律：在一昼夜中，人体体温呈周期性波动。清晨2 ~ 6时体温最低，午后1 ~ 6时最高，体温的这种昼夜周期性波动称为昼夜节律。

[2] 月经周期。

[3] 卵泡期。

[4] 排卵期。

[5] 孕激素。

1.2.3 The influence of age

The children's body temperature is considerably higher than adults' and it is lower in elderly age. The body temper ature of the newborn, especially premature infant, because of his or her imperfect body temperature regulation, is easily affected by environmental factors. Therefore the infant should keep warm.The elderly has lower basal metabolism rate, so his or her temperature is low, and should also keep warm.

1.2.4 Physical activity and other factors

Physical labor,will raise the body temperature by 1 ~ 2℃ . Other factors, including emotional, mental stress, eating and environmental temperature can affect the body temperature. Sleep temperature is slightly lower. During the sleep the body temperature is decreased by 10%. And anesthetics usually can lower the body temperature.

2 Heat production and heat loss

By the temperature regulating system, the body maintains the dynamic balance of heat production[1] and heat dissipation[2], to keep the stability of core temperature.

2.1 Heat production

2.1.1 The main heat producing organs

The body heat comes from the catabolism of three major nutrient substances in human organs and tissues, especially in the liver, brain, heart, and skeletal muscles during exercise. Due to the different metabolic levels, the heat production in different tissues and organs is not the same. In quiet, skeletal muscle heat production is not great. But, because the total weight of skeletal muscle accounts for about 40% of body weight, it has great potential for heat production. Skeletal muscle tension slightly increases, heat production can be changed obviously. In the strenuous exercise, heat production can be increased 40 times as much as that in the quiet state. Its heat production can account for 90% of the total body heat production when strenuous exercise occurs. In the quiet state, the main heat producing organs are viscera and brain. Among the viscera, the liver is the most exuberant organ, producing the maximum heat. The temperature of the liver is higher than that of the aorta. Liver blood temperature is 0.4 ~ 0.8℃ higher than that of aorta(Table7–5).

---

[1] 产热：体内的热量是由三大营养物质在各组织器官中进行分解代谢及机体利用 ATP 时产生的。机体产热的形式包括基础代谢产热、骨骼肌运动产热、食物特殊动力作用产热及战栗和非战栗产热等。

[2] 散热：人体的主要散热部位是皮肤，体内大部分热量可通过皮肤的辐射、传导和对流等方式向外界发散。

Table 7–5 Percentage of heat production in several tissues and organs

Tissue organ	Percentage of body weight	Heat production(%)	
		Quiet state	Labor or exercise
Brain	2.5	16	1
Viscera	34.0	56	8
Skeletal muscle	56.0	18	90
Others	7.5	10	1

2.1.2 Heat production way

When the body is in a cold environment, heat loss significantly increased. Through shivering thermogenesis [1] and non–shivering thermogenesis [2], the body increases the heat production to maintain its body temperature.

2.1.2.1 Shivering thermogenesis

Shivering is that skeletal muscle, either flexor or extensor, undergoes involuntary rhythmic contraction. When shivering, metabolic rate can be increased by 4 ~ 5 times. In a cold environment, people usually undergoes muscle tension before shiver occurred. Metabolism rate increases at this time.

2.1.2.2 Non–shivering thermogenesis

Non–shivering thermogenesis is also called metabolic heat production. At this moment, the body will generate large heat by the metabolism. Although all organs have metabolic heat production function, but brown fat tissue has the largest heat production function, accounting for about 70% of the total non–shivering thermogenesis. Non–shivering thermogenesis is of considerable importance to newborn children who have brown fat storage, producing heat without shivering.

2.1.3 Regulation of heat production

Regulation of heat production in the body includes humoral regulation and nervous regulation.

2.1.3.1 Humoral regulation:

Participation of thyroid gland in temperature control is the most important humoral factors by the fact that the level of thyroid hormones will rise, and increase the metabolic rate by 20% to 30%when the body has been in the cold for a long time. Adrenalin, noradrenaline and growth hormone can also cause rise of body temperature.

2.1.3.2 Nerve regulation

Sympathetic nervous system can be excited by cold stress, then can increase activity of adrenal medulla, and ultimately lead the release of norepinephrine and epinephrine, which in

[1] 战栗：是指骨骼肌发生不随意的节律性收缩，其节律为 9 ~ 11 次 / 分。

[2] 非战栗产热又称代谢产热，是一种通过提高组织代谢率来增加产热的形式。

turn increase metabolic activity and heat generation.

2.2 Heat loss

2.2.1 The part of losing heat

The main part of losing heat is the skin. As long as skin temperature is greater than that of the surroundings, heat can be lost by radiation, conduction and convection. But when the temperature of the surroundings is greater than that of the skin, the only means by which the body can rid itself of heat is evaporation. In addition, some of the heat can also be with the breath, urine excretion in vitro.

2.2.2 Heat loss way

2.2.2.1 Hermal radiation[1]

It means the human body transfers heat to the outside world in the form of heat ray. When people are in bare case, stand at temperature 21℃ , about 60% of the heat is lost in this way. The amount of radiation depends mainly on the temperature difference between skin and the surrounding environment; secondly depends on the effective radiating area.

2.2.2.2 Thermal conduction[2]

Heat conduction refers to that the body's heat is directly transferred to the cold body contacting with it. How much heat can be transferred is related to the area of the object, the temperature and the thermal conductivity. If the adjacent object is cold, then the heat conduction is large; otherwise, the heat transfer is little. Due to the poor thermal conductivity of fat, clothes, quilts or other, heat loss is little. Because of the better thermal conductivity of the water, in clinical practice, ice bag and ice cap are good thermal conduction way for patients with high fever to reduce temperature.

2.2.2.3 Thermal convection[3]

Heat convection is a way to exchange heat with gas or fluid. The human body surrounded with a thin layer of air, so the body heat is transfered to this layer of air. Due to continuous flow of air, the layer of air will diffuse heat into space. Convection is a special form of conducting heat. Thermal convection is affected by the air convective velocity and temperature.

2.2.2.4 Evaporation[4]

It means that the body surface evaporates water to dissipate body heat. When the temperature of the surroundings becomes greater than that of the skin, instead of losing heat, the body gains heat by both radiation and conduction. Under these conditions, the only mean by which

[1] 辐射散热：是指机体通过热射线的形式将体热传给外界较冷物质的一种散热方式。

[2] 传导散热：是指机体的热量直接传给相接触的较冷物体的一种散热方式。

[3] 对流散热：是指通过气体的流动来交换热量的一种散热方式。对流散热是传导散热的一种特殊形式。

[4] 蒸发散热：是指水分子从体表汽化时吸收热量而发散体热的一种方式。

the body can rid itself of heat is by evaporation. According to the determination, in the normal body temperature, evaporation of 1g water can make the body to loss heat 2.43kJ. Evaporation can be divided into insensible evaporation [1] and sweating [2] .

Even people are in the low temperature environment, water can ooze from skin and respiratory tract and be evaporated, and this water evaporation is insensible evaporation. When a person is not sweating, water still evaporates insensibly from the skin and lungs at a rate of about 1000 mL daily. The insensible evaporation is insensible for us, which has nothing to do with the sweat gland activity. Insensible evaporative is nearly independent of thermoregulatory control when ambient temperature is below 30℃ .

Sweating is that sweat glands secrete sweat which can be felt, so it is called sensible evaporation. When the environmental temperature reaches 30℃ in a quiet state, or when a person is moving, the person begins to sweat. Evaporation of sweat can effectively removes heat. As the ambient temperature increases, the body depends more and more on the evaporation of sweat to achieve heat balance.

2.2.3 Regulation of heat loss

2.2.3.1 Sweating

Sweating refers to the process of secretion of sweat gland through nervous reflex. Sweat glands are divided into apocrine glands and eccrine glands[3]. Apocrine glands are concentrated at the armpits and genital area [4] . Eccrine glands are in systemic skin, which are more important in human thermoregulation. When the surrounding temperature rises or persons are during severe exercise, the heat stimulates eccrine sweat glands, through sympathetic nervous system, to secrete water to the skin surface, where it cools the body by evaporation. This is called thermal sweating. They are controlled through post ganglionic sympathetic nerves that release acetylcholine (ACh). It is well known that the preoptic–anterior hypothalamus area (PO/AH) [5] is the heat regulating center of homeotherm.

2.2.3.2 Changes of skin blood flow

The relationship between skin temperature and heat dissipation is very close. The body can control the caliber of skin blood vessels through the sympathetic nerve, regulating the blood flow of the skin, and changing the temperature of the skin to control the heat dissipation. In the hot environment, sympathetic nervous tension is reduced. Skin arteries and arterio–ve-

---

[1] 不感蒸发：是指机体中水分直接渗透到皮肤和黏膜（主要是呼吸道黏膜）表面不断被汽化蒸发的过程。由于这种蒸发不被人们所觉察，与汗腺活动无关，故得此名。

[2] 发汗：是指汗腺主动分泌汗液的活动，通过汗液蒸发可有效地带走体热。由于发汗可被感觉到，故又称可感蒸发。

[3] 大汗腺和小汗腺。

[4] 腋窝和生殖器区域。

[5] 视前区下丘脑前部。

nous anastomoses are open to the flow of blood to the skin, so more heat is brought to the body surface from the deep body, thus skin temperature is increased, the cooling effect is enhanced. At the same time, the increased skin blood flow strengthens the sweat gland activity. On the contrary, in cold environment, sympathetic nervous tension and skin arteriole contraction are enhanced. Thus, arterio-venous anastomosises close, leading to skin blood flow and skin temperature decrease. This weakened heat dissipation can preserve body temperature.

3 Regulation of body temperature

There are two ways to regulate temperature: autonomic thermoregulation and behavioral thermoregulation. Autonomic thermoregulation refers to a series of regulation activities under the central control, such as adjusting blood flow in skin, sweating, trembling and changing the physiological metabolism, to maintain the dynamic balance of heat production and heat dissipation, so that the temperature is maintained at a relatively stable level. Behavioral thermoregulation refers to a series of conscious regulation activities, such as changing postures, increasing clothing, and improving climatic conditions artificially. Based on the autonomic thermoregulation, the human body can adapt itself to the change of the natural environment through the coordination of the two regulating mechanisms.

3.1 Autonomic thermoregulation

The autonomic thermoregulation is accomplished by temperature receptors, temperature regulating center and effectors.

3.1.1 Thermal receptor

Temperature receptors can be divided into peripheral thermo receptors and central temperature receptors, the former are free nerve endings, and the latter are the neurons.

3.1.1.1 Peripheral thermal receptor [1]

This receptors exist in the skin, mucous membrane and viscera, divided into thermosensitive receptors and cold sensitive receptors. When the local temperature rises, thermosensitive receptors are excited, conversely, cold sensitive receptors are excited. The two types of receptors are sensitive to changing in a certain range of temperature. Peripheral temperature receptors are more sensitive to cold stimulation, to prevent the temperature decreasing.

3.1.1.2 Central thermal receptor

The central thermal receptor refer to those neurons which exist in the central nervous system and are sensitive to temperature changing, including warm-sensitive neurons and cold-sensitive neurons. Spinal cord, reticular formation of brain stem and hypothalamus all contain such temperature sensitive neurons. When the temperature in the local tissue ris-

[1] 外周温度感受器：广泛分布于皮肤、黏膜和内脏中的对温度变化敏感的游离神经末梢，包括热感受器和冷感受器。

es, warm–sensitive neurons are excited; when the temperature in the local tissue decreases, cold–sensitive neurons are excited.

3.1.2 Body temperature regulation center

There are central structures to regulate the body's temperature throughout the central nervous system, from the spinal cord to the brain cortex. The main centers of thermoregulation are situated in PO/AH. This is proved by the fact that destruction of hypothalamus causes loss of ability to control the body temperature, and the animal becomes poikilothermal. Whereas the removal of cerebral cortex, striate body and optic thalamus is not reflected noticeably in the processes of heat production and heat loss. PO/AH can either feel the local brain temperature, or response to temperature informations which occur in areas other than the hypothalamus. After the integration these messages, the body correspondingly responses toward the temperature changes. In addition, these neurons also receive stimulation of heat producing substances, 5–, serotonin, norepinephrine and various peptides directly, and cause corresponding thermoregulation responses.

3.1.3 Temperature set point [1] theory

Temperature set point theory thinks that the regulation of body temperature is similar to a thermostat. A set poin is set in the PO/AH, namely the specified temperature value, such as 37℃. PO/AH regulates body temperature following this temperature. When a person is infected by bacteria, the pyrogen will increase the threshold of thermo sensitive neurons in PO/AH, while the threshold of cold sensitive neuron will be decreased, namely the set point rises. He or she will increase heat production activities and reduce heat dissipation and get fever. As long as the thermal factors are not eliminated, heat and cooling process will continue to maintain a balance in the new temperature level. That is to say, there is no obstacle to temperature regulating function, but only because the set point is upward, so body temperature is elevated to the level of fever. While, elevated body temperature by heatstroke is due to thermoregulatory dysfunction.

3.2 Behavioral thermoregulation [2]

The body changes its posture and behavior in different environments, in particular, it adopts artificial heat preservation and cooling measures to keep body temperature relatively stable, which is called behavioral thermoregulation. Behavioral thermoregulation is the process by which a person's body temperature does not rise too high or too low by means of his or her behavior. For example, people in the cold by, running to keep warm. According to the different environmental temperature, humans can change clothing. But creating artificial climate environment in the cold can be regarded as the more complex behavior adjustment.

---

[1] 体温调定点。

[2] 行为性体温调节。

Chapter 8 FORMATION AND DISCHARGE OF URINE

Section 1 Functional anatomy and blood circulation of the kidney

1 Function structure of the kidney

1.1 Nephron

The nephron is the functional unit of kidney. Each kidney in the human contains about one million nephrons, each capable of forming urine. The nephron consists of a renal corpuscle and a renal tubule[1]. The renal corpuscle consists of a tuft of capillaries, the glomerulus[2], surrounded by Bowman's capsule[3]. The renal tubule is divided into several segments. The part of the tubule nearest the glomerulus is the proximal tubule. This is subdivided into a proximal convoluted tubule and proximal straight tubule. The straight portion heads toward the medulla, away from the surface of the kidney. The loop of Henle includes the proximal straight tubule, thin limb, and thick ascending limb[4]. The next segment, the short distal convoluted tubule, is connected to the collecting duct system by connecting tubules. Several nephrons drain into a cortical collecting duct, which passes into an outer medullary collecting duct. In the inner medulla, inner medullary collecting ducts unite to form large papillary ducts. The collecting ducts perform the same types of functions as the renal tubules, so they are often considered to be part of the nephron[5] (Figure 8-1).

[1] 肾单位由肾小体和肾小管构成。

[2] 肾小球：由肾动脉分支形成的毛细血管网。

[3] 肾小囊：其脏层紧贴毛细血管壁包裹肾小球，壁层与肾小管相连，囊腔与肾小管连通。

[4] 髓袢包括近端小管直段、髓袢细段、髓袢升支粗段。

[5] 集合管发挥着与肾小管同样的作用，因而通常将其认为是肾单位的一部分。

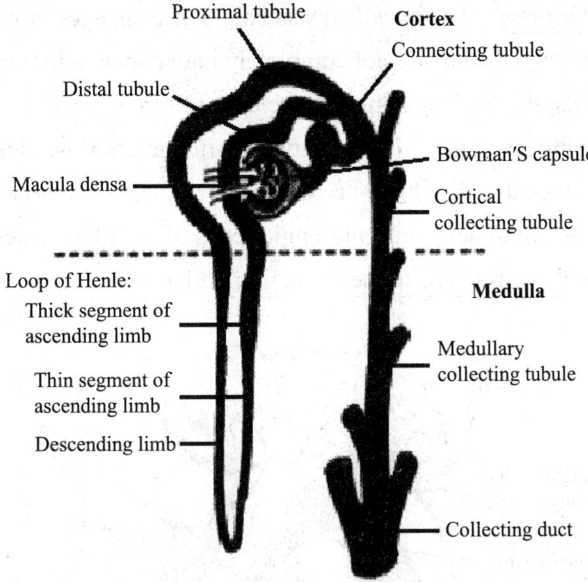

Figure 8–1 Basic tubular segments of the nephron

Characteristics of nephrons are somewhat different depending on how deep they lie within the kidney mass. Those nephrons of which the glomeruli lie close to the surface of the kidney are called cortical nephrons [1]. Their loops of Henle penetrate only a very short distance into the outer portion of medulla. About 20 to 30% of the nephrons have glomeruli that lie deep in the renal cortex near the medulla and are called juxtamedullary nephrons [2]. Their loops of Henle penetrate deeply into the inner zone of the medulla. The juxtamedullary nephrons differ from ordinary ones also by the equal diameter of afferent and efferent arterioles. Then, efferent arterioles of juxtamedullary nephrons do not form a capillary network around tubules, but flows into venous system.

1.2 Juxtaglomerular apparatus [3]

The juxtaglomerular apparatus consists of macula densa cells, extraglomerular mesangial cells and juxtaglomerular cells [4] (Figure 8–2). The macula densa is a specialized group of epithelial cells [5] in the initial portion of the distal tubule that comes in close contact with the af-

[1] 皮质肾单位。

[2] 髓肾单位。

[3] 肾小球旁器。

[4] 球旁器由致密斑细胞、球外系膜细胞、球旁细胞等三部分组成。

[5] 上皮细胞。

ferent and efferent arterioles[1]. The macula densa cells sense changes in volume delivery to the distal tubule by way of signals that are not completely understood, and transfer the information to juxtaglomerular cells, thereby regulating the release of renin[2]. The Juxtaglomerular cells are specialized myoepithelial cells[3] in the media of afferent arteriole close to the glomerulus. The cells contain granules that appear to be composed of the enzyme renin. The extraglomerular mesangial cells are continuous with mesangial cells of the glomerulus; they may transmit information from macula densa cells to the Juxtaglomerular cells[4].

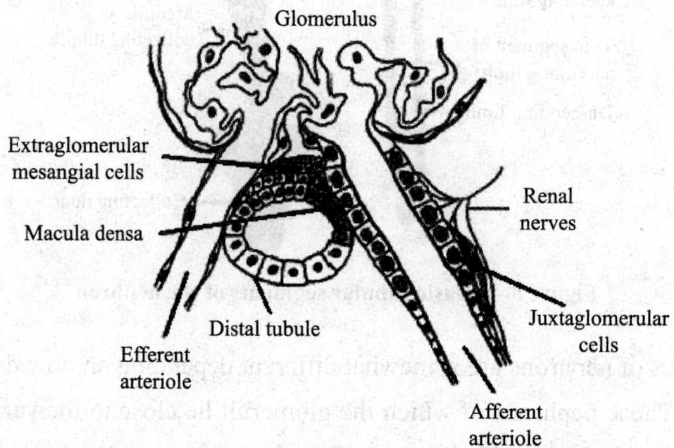

Figure 8–2 Structure of the juxtaglomerular apparatus

2 The renal blood flow

2.1 Characteristics of renal blood flow

(1)Larger renal blood flow Blood flow to the two kidneys is normally about 22 percent of the cardiac output, or 1100 ml/min. The renal artery enters the kidney through the hilum and then branches progressively to form the interlobar arteries, arcuate arteries, interlobular arteries(also called radial arteries) and afferent arterioles[5], which lead to the glomerular capillaries, where large amounts of fluid and solutes(except the plasma proteins) are filtered to begin urine formation. The distal ends of the capillaries of each glomerulus coalesce to form the efferent

[1] 入球动脉和出球动脉。

[2] 肾素：球旁细胞合成、释放的一种酸性蛋白酶，能作用于血浆中的血管紧张素原。

[3] 内皮细胞：一种特殊分化的平滑肌细胞，内含分泌颗粒。

[4] 它们可将致密斑信息传递给球旁细胞。

[5] 肾动脉经肾门进入肾脏，逐渐分支形成叶间动脉、弓状动脉、小叶间动脉（也叫径向动脉）和入球动脉。

arteriole, which leads to a second capillary network, the peritubular capillaries[1], that surrounds the renal tubules. Venous vessels, in general, lie parallel to the arterial vessels (Figure 8–3).

(2)Two capillary beds The renal circulation is unique in having two capillary beds, the glomerular and peritubular capillaries[2]. The blood supply to the medulla is derived from the efferent arterioles of juxtamedullary glomeruli. These vessels give rise to two patterns of capillaries: peritubular capillaries, which are similar to those in the cortex[3], and vasa recta, which are straight, long capillaries. Some vasa recta reach deep into the inner medulla. In the outer medulla, descending and ascending vasa recta are grouped in vascular bundles and are in close contact with each other. This arrangement greatly facilitates the exchange of substances between bloods flowing in and out of the medulla[4].

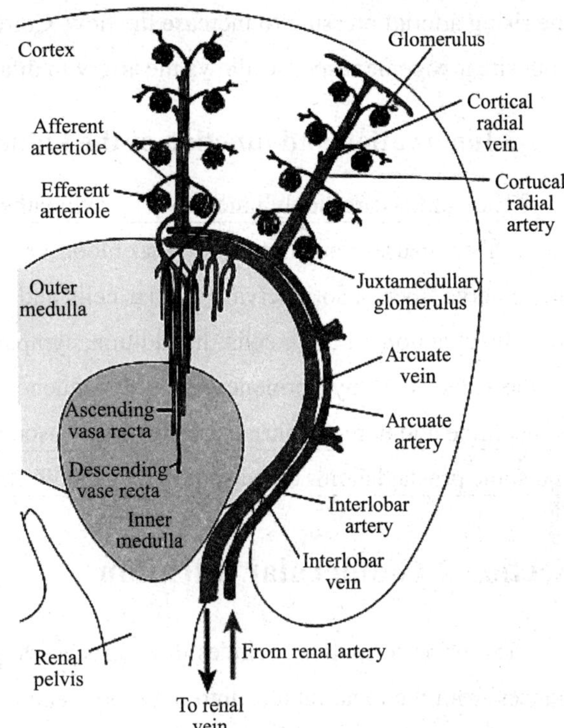

Figure 8–3 The blood supply in the kidney

2.2 Regulation of renal blood flow

The renal blood flow can remain near the normal level despite considerable change in the arterial pressure may occur, which is called autoregulation of renal blood flow[5]. For instance, the renal blood flow of both kidneys remains very near the normal level of 1,200 ml per minute even when the arterial pressure falls as low as 80 mmHg or rises to as high as 160 mmHg. There is a myogenic mechanism[6] to explain this phenomenon. When the arterial pressure rises, it stretches the wall of the arteriole, and this in turn causes a secondary contraction of the arteriole. This decreases the renal blood flow back toward normal, thus opposing the effect of

[1] 肾小管周围毛细血管网。

[2] 肾脏的血液循环的持点是有两套毛细血管网，即肾小球毛细血管网和肾小管周围毛细血管网。

[3] 肾皮质。

[4] 这种排列结构有利于直小管内血流在流入和流出髓质时的物质交换。

[5] 肾脏血流量的自身调节。

[6] 肌源性机制。

the rising arterial pressure to increase the flow. Conversely, when the pressure falls too low, an opposite myogenic response allows the artery to dilate and therefore increases the flow.

3 Innervation and function of the kidney

The kidneys are richly innervated by sympathetic nerve fibers [1]. Stimulation of sympathetic fibers causes constriction of renal blood vessels and a fall in renal blood flow. Sympathetic nerve fibers also innervate tubular cells and may cause an increase in Na^+ reabsorption by a direct action on these cells. In addition, sympathetic nerves increases the release of renin by the kidneys. Many hormones can also influence renal blood flow. Such as Angiotensin II, epinephrine and norepinephrine are powerful vasoconstrictor agents, while the bradykinin, NO and some prostaglandins are vasodilator agents for the renal blood vessels [2].

Section 2 Glomerular filtration

The urine formation includes three processes: glomerular filtration, reabsorption of substances from the renal tubules into the blood, and excretion of substances from the blood into the renal tubules.

The initial step in the formation of urine is production of a plasma filtrate within the glomerulus. Urine formation begins when a large amount of fluid that is virtually free of protein is filtered from the glomerular capillaries into Bowman's capsule. Most substances in the plasma, except for proteins, are freely filtered, so their concentration in the glomerular filtrate in Bowman's capsule is almost the same as in the plasma, and the fluid that filters into Bowman's capsule is called ultrafiltrate or initial urine and the process of the fluid filtering into Bowman's capsule is called glomerular filtration [3].

1 The glomerular filtration rate and the filtration fraction

Glomerular filtration involves the ultrafiltration [4] of plasma in the glomerulus. The quantity of glomerular filtrate formed each minute in all nephrons of both kidneys is called the glo-

[1] 肾脏由肾交感神经支配。

[2] 如血管紧张素 II、肾上腺素和去甲肾上腺素等均有很强的血管收缩作用，使肾血流减少，而缓激肽、NO 和某些前列腺素等则具有血管扩张作用，使肾血流增加。

[3] 从肾小球毛细血管滤过进入肾小囊的液体称为超滤液或原尿，液体由肾小球毛细血管滤过进入肾小囊的过程称为肾小球滤过。

[4] 超滤：除蛋白质外，血浆中所有成分均能滤过进入肾小囊的过程。

merular filtration rate (GFR)[1]. In the normal person this averages approximately 125 ml/min. To express this, the total quantity of glomerular filtrate formed each day averages about 180 L, or more than two times the total weight of the body. Over 99 % of the filtrate is normally reabsorbed in the tubules, with the remainder passing into the urine.

The plasma clearance is a measure of the effectiveness of the kidney to remove substances from the extracellular fluid. Plasma clearance[2] for any substance can be calculated by the formula below:

$$\text{Plasma clearance}=\frac{\text{Quantity of urine}\times\text{Concentration in urine}}{\text{Concentration in plasma}}$$

Inulin is a polysaccharide that has the specific attributes of not being reabsorbed or secreted by the renal tubules and it passes through the glomerular membrane as freely as the crystalloids and water of the plasma[3]. Consequently, glomerular filtrate contains the same concentration of inulin as does plasma, and as the filtrate flows down the tubules all the filtered inulin continues on into the urine. Thus, all the glomerular filtrate formed is cleared of inulin. Therefore, the plasma clearance per minute of inulin is equal to the GFR. For example, let us assume that the inulin concentration in the plasma is 0.1 mmol/L, 12.5 mmoL/L in the urine, and urine volume is 0.001 L/min, so glomerular filtrate (X)=0.001 L/min×12.5 mmoL/L)/0.1 mmoL=125 mL/min.

The filtration fraction (FF)[4] is the fraction of the renal plasma flow that becomes glomerular filtrate. The filtration fraction is calculated as follows:

$$\text{fractionFiltration}=\frac{\text{GFR}}{\text{flowplasmaRenal}}$$

Since the normal plasma flow through both kidneys is 650mL/min and the normal glomerular filtration rate in both kidneys is 125mL, the average FF is approximately 1/5 or 19 %.

2 The filtration membrane

Glomerular filtration involves the ultrafiltration of plasma. The filtration membrane is similar to that of other capillaries, except that it has three major layers: the endothelium of the capillary, a basement membrane, and a layer of epithelial cells (podocytes) surrounding the outer surface of the capillary basement membrane (Figure 8–4). Together, these layers make

---

[1] 肾小球滤过率。

[2] 血浆清除率。

[3] 菊糖是具有特定属性的多糖，它不被肾小管重吸收和分泌，却能与血浆中晶体和水一样自由通过滤过膜。

[4] 滤过分数。

up the filtration barrier [1], which filters several hundred times as the usual capillary membrane. Even with this high rate of filtration, the glomerular capillary membrane normally prevents filtration of plasma proteins.

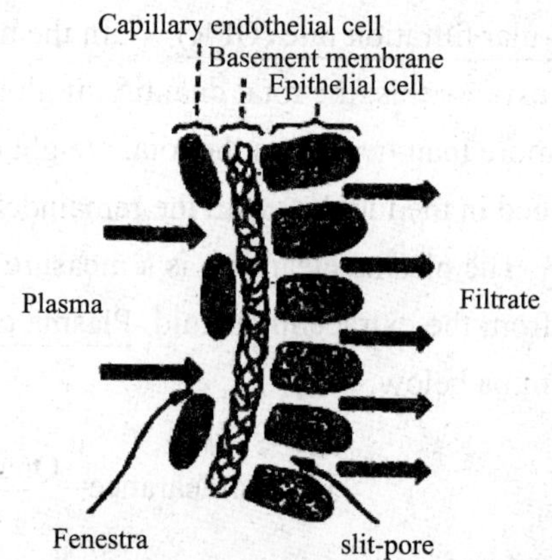

Figure 8–4 Basic structure of the glomerular filtration barrier

The capillary endothelium is perforated by thousands of small holes called fenestrae. The high filtration rate across the glomerular capillary membrane is due partly to these fenestrations [2]. Although the fenestrations are relatively large, endothelial cells are richly endowed with fixed negative charges that hinder the passage of plasma proteins. The basement membrane consists of a meshwork of collagen and proteoglycan fibrillate that have large spaces through which large amounts of water and small solutes can filter. The basement membrane effectively prevents filtration of plasma proteins, in part because of strong negative electrical charges associated with the proteoglycans. The final part is a layer of epithelial cells that line the outer surface of the glomerulus. These cells are not continuous but have foot like processes (podocytes) [3] that encircle the outer surface of the capillaries. The foot processes are separated by gaps called slit pores [4] through which the glomerular filtrate moves. The podocytes, which also have negative charges, provide additional restriction to filtration of negative charged essential for blood e. g. plasma proteins. Thus, all layers of the glomerular capillary wall provide a barrier to filtration of plasma proteins [5].

So, there are two barriers for filtration. First is the mechanical barrier from the pores of the membrane are large enough to allow molecules with diameters up to about 8 nm to pass through;The second is the electrical barrier from electrostatic repulsion of the protein molecules by the proteoglycans keeping these proteins from passing through.

3 Dynamics of glomerular filtration

Glomerular filtration is determined by the sum of the hydrostatic and colloid osmotic forces across the glomerular membrane, which gives the effective filtration pressure (Figure

[1] 滤过屏障：滤过膜三层结构构成的屏障作用。

[2] 窗孔：滤过膜内层的毛细血管内皮细胞上 70 ~ 90 nm 的小孔。

[3] 足突（足细胞）：滤过膜外层的肾小囊上皮细胞上相互交错对插排列的突起。

[4] 裂孔：足突间形成滤过裂隙，裂隙表面覆盖的薄膜上直径 4 ~ 11 nm 的小孔。

[5] 肾小球毛细血管的滤过膜结构对血浆蛋白的滤过具有屏障作用。

8–5). The effective filtration pressure (P_{UF})[1] represents the sum of the hydrostatic and colloid osmotic forces that either favor or oppose filtration across the glomerular capillaries. These forces include ① hydrostatic pressure inside the glomerular capillaries (glomerular hydrostatic pressure, P_{GC})[2], which promotes filtration; ② the hydrostatic pressure in Bowman's capsule (P_B)[3] outside the capillaries, which opposes filtration; ③ the colloid osmotic pressure of the glomerular capillary plasma proteins (π_{GC})[4], which opposes filtration; and ④ the colloid osmotic pressure of the proteins in Bowman's capsule (π_B)[5], which promotes filtration. Under normal conditions, the concentration of protein in the glomerular filtrate is so low that the colloid osmotic pressure of the Bowman's capsule fluid is considered to be zero (π_B=0).

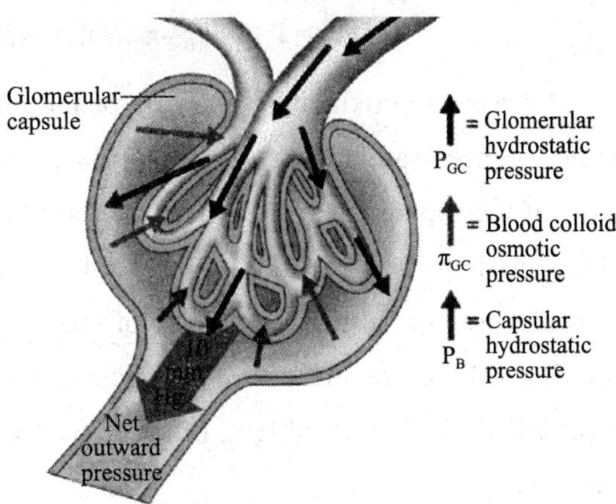

Figure 8–5 Summary of forces causing glomerular filtration

The effective filtration pressure can therefore be expressed as

$$P_{UF} = P_{GC} - P_B - \pi_{GC} + \pi_B \qquad (\pi_B=0)$$

Although the normal values for the determinants of glomerular filtration have not been measured directly in humans, they have been estimated in animals such as dogs and rats. At the arteriolar side of the capillary[6], the normal forces favoring and opposing glomerular filtration in rats are as follows:

Forces favoring filtration (mmHg)	
Glomerular hydrostatic pressure (P_{GC})	45
Bowman's capsule colloid osmotic pressure (π_B)	0
Forces opposing filtration (mmHg)	
Bowman's capsule hydrostatic pressure in (P_B)	10
Glomerular capillary colloid osmotic pressure (π_{GC})	25

[1] 有效滤过压。

[2] 肾小球毛细血管静水压（P_{GC}）。

[3] 肾小囊内的静水压（P_B）。

[4] 肾小球毛细血管内血浆的胶体渗透压（π_{GC}）。

[5] 肾小囊内超滤液的胶体渗透压（π_B）。

[6] 肾小球毛细血管的动脉端。

$$P_{UF} = P_{GC} - P_B - \pi_{GC} + \pi_B = 45 - 10 - 25 + 0 = 10(\text{ mmHg})$$

Because approximately one fifth of the plasma in the capillaries filter into capsule, the protein concentration increase about 20% as the blood passes from the arterial to the venous ends of the glomerular capillaries. The colloid osmotic pressure of the blood plasma rises along the length of the glomerular capillary from 25 mmHg to 35 mmHg. The effective filtration pressure at the venule side of the capillary[1] is equal to $P_{UF} = 45 - 10 - 35 + 0 = 0$ (mmHg). Therefore, most filtration occurs in the first half along the length of the glomerular capillary. In the kidney of rate, filtration has ceased by or perhaps even before the end of the capillary.

4 Factors influencing the glomerular filtration

There are three factors that can affect glomerular filtration: glomerular permeability, effective filtration pressure and renal plasma flow.

(1)Glomerular permeability Normally the permeability of the filtration membrane is stable, and changes very little. But when in nephritis[2], the negative charges in the glomerular wall are dissipated, the permeability will increase, and the albumin can go through the filtration membrane. As a result, albuminuria can occur.

(2)Area of filter membrane Under normal physiological conditions, bilateral glomeruli are sufficient for the kidneys to maintain constant and steady filtration. When acute glomerulonephritis, due to glomerular capillary lumens stenosis or completely blocked, so that the effective filtration area decreased, thus resulting in reduced glomerular filtration rate, showing oliguria or even anuria.

(3)Effective filtration pressure It is determined by P_{GC}, P_B and π_{GC}. If any of them changed, the effective filtration pressure would change, resulting in glomerular filtration change. For example, long-term malnutrition[3] can cause decrease in π_{GC}, leading to increase in effective filtration pressure.

(4)Renal blood flow An increase in the rate of blood flow through the nephrons greatly increases the glomerular filtration[4]. This is that the increasing flow increases the glomerular pressure, which obviously enhances filtration. During sympathetic stimulation of the kidneys, the afferent arterioles are constricted preferentially, thereby decreasing the glomerular

[1] 肾小球毛细血管的静脉端。

[2] 肾炎：肾脏炎性改变可导致滤过膜电学屏障减弱，出现蛋白尿。

[3] 长期营养不良。

[4] 流经肾单位血浆流量增多，肾小球滤过增加。

filtration rate. With very strong sympathetic stimulation, glomerular filtration can decrease to only a few per cent of normal, and urinary output actually can fall to zero for as long as 5 to 10 minutes.

Section 3 Renal tubule and collecting tube reabsorption and secretion

As glomerular filtrated fluid leaves Bowman's capsule and pass through the tubules, it flows sequentially through the successive parts of the tubules–the proximal tubule, the loop of Henle, the distal tubule, the collecting tubule, and, finally, the collecting duct–before it is excreted as urine. Along this course, some substances are selectively reabsorbed[1] from the tubules back into the blood, whereas others are secreted from the blood into the tubular lumen. For many substances, tubular reabsorption[2] plays a much more important role than secretion in determining the final urinary excretion rate. Tubular secretion[3] accounts for significant amounts of potassium ions, hydrogen ions, and a few other substances that appear in the urine.

1 Characteristics of the renal tubule and collecting duct reabsorption

1.1 Tubular reabsorption is quantitatively large

The total length of tubules is 70 ~ 100 km. On the tubular border of the epithelial cell is an extensive brush border[4] that multiplies the surface of area of luminal exposure about 20–fold. So, the total surface tubules is 40 ~ 50 sqm. Daily 150 ~ 180 litres of glomerular filtrate, that is, primary urine is formed and only 1 ~ 1.5 litres of definitive urine is removed from the organism. The rest of the glomerular filtrate is reabsorbed in tubules. Table 8–1 shows the renal handing of several substances that are all freely filtered in the kidneys and reabsorbed at variable rates. From Table 8–1, two things are immediately apparent. First, the processes of glomerular filtration and tubular reabsorption are quantitatively large relative to urinary excretion[5] for many substances. This means that a small change in glomerular filtration or tubular reabsorption can potentially cause a relatively large change in urinary excretion.

---

[1] 选择性重吸收。

[2] 肾小管和集合管的重吸收。

[3] 肾小管和集合管的分泌。

[4] 刷状缘：肾小管上皮细胞顶端膜的微绒毛结构，可增大膜的表面积。

[5] 尿液排泄。

Table 8–1 Filtration, reabsorption, and excretion rates of different substances by the kidneys

	Amount of filtered	Amount of reabsorbed	Amount of excreted	Reabsorption rate (%)
Glucose(g/day)	180	180	0	100
Bicarbonate(mEq/day)	4320	4318	2	> 99.9
Sodium(mEq/day)	25560	25410	150	99.4
Chloride(mEq/day)	19440	19260	180	99.1
Potassium(mEq/day)	756	664	92	87.8
Urea(g/day)	46.8	23.4	23.4	50
Creatinine(g/day)	1.8	0	1.8	0

1.2 Tubular reabsorption is highly selective

Unlike glomerular filtration, tubular reabsorption is highly selective. Some substances, such as glucose and amino acids[1], are almost completely reabsorbed from the tubules, so the urinary excretion rate is essentially zero. Many of the ions in the plasma, such as sodium, chloride, and bicarbonate, are also highly reabsorbed, but their rates of reabsorption and urinary excretion are variable, depending on the needs of the body. Waste products, such as urea and creatinine[2], conversely, are poorly reabsorbed from the tubules and excreted in relatively large amounts. Therefore, by controlling the rate at which they reabsorb different substances, the kidneys regulate the excretion of solutes independently of one another, a capability that is essential for precise control of the body fluid composition[3].

2 Ways and means of the renal tubule and collecting duct reabsorption

2.1 Ways of the renal tubule and collecting duct reabsorption

Water and solutes can be transported through the cell membranes themselves (transcellular path[4]) or through the spaces between the cell junctions (paracellular pathway[5]). Then, after absorption across the tubular epithelial cells into the interstitial fluid, water and solutes are transported through the peritubular capillary walls into the blood by ultrafiltration (bulk flow) that is mediated by hydrostatic and colloid osmotic forces.

---

[1] 葡萄糖和氨基酸。

[2] 尿素和肌酐。

[3] 体液成分。

[4] 跨细胞途径。

[5] 细胞旁途径。

2.2 Means of the renal tubule and collecting duct reabsorption

The basic mechanisms for transport through the tubular membrane are essentially the same as those for transport through other membranes of the body. These are divided into active and passive transport [1] which have been discussed in chapter 2. (Figure 8–6).

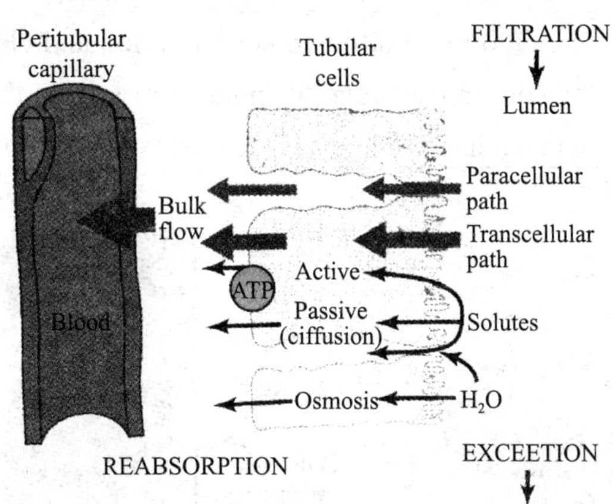

Figure 8–6 Tubular reabsorption mechanisms

The movement of sodium, bicarbonate, chloride, glucose and amino acid from the cells into the interstitial space, particularly the lateral spaces, reduces the osmolality of the tubular fluid and increases the osmolality in the lateral spaces. This causes net osmotic flow of water from the lumen into the lateral space by transcellular and paracellular routes.

3 Reabsorption of several major substances

Tubular transport is selective, different substances are transported by different mechanisms. The amount excreted in the urine depends in large measure on the magnitude of tubular transport. Transport of various solutes and water differs in the various renal tubular segments [2].

3.1 Tubular transport in the proximal tubule

In the proximal tubule, about 60% ~ 70% of the filtered load of water and solutes is reabsorbed. Studies on isolated tubules in vitro indicate [3] that the proximal tubule is responsible for re–absorbing all of the filtered glucose and amino acids, most of the filtered Na^+, K^+, Ca^{2+}, Cl–, HCO_3^- , and about 70% of the filtered water and secreting various organic anions and organic cations (Figure 8–7).

3.1.1 Sodium reabsorption

In the anterior segment of the proximal tubule, reabsorption of sodium ions is via transcellular path and is accompanied by the secretion of hydrogen ions and reabsorption of glucose and amino acids The proximal tubular cells have a Na^+–K^+ pump on the basolateral mem-

[1] 重吸收的机制分为主动转运和被动转运。

[2] 在不同肾小管各段，各种溶质和水的转运机制不同。

[3] 离体肾小管体外研究表明。

brane[1] which pumps sodium out of the cell into the interstitial fluid. This keeps the intracellular concentration of sodium low relative to the lumen. The cell interior also has a membrane potential of −70 mV relative to the lumen[2]. Thus, sodium ions move passively from the lumen into the cell, down concentration and electrical gradients and are actively pumped out of the cell, in exchange for potassium ions at the basolateral membrane. Much of the sodium is pumped into the lateral spaces between the epithelial cells[3].

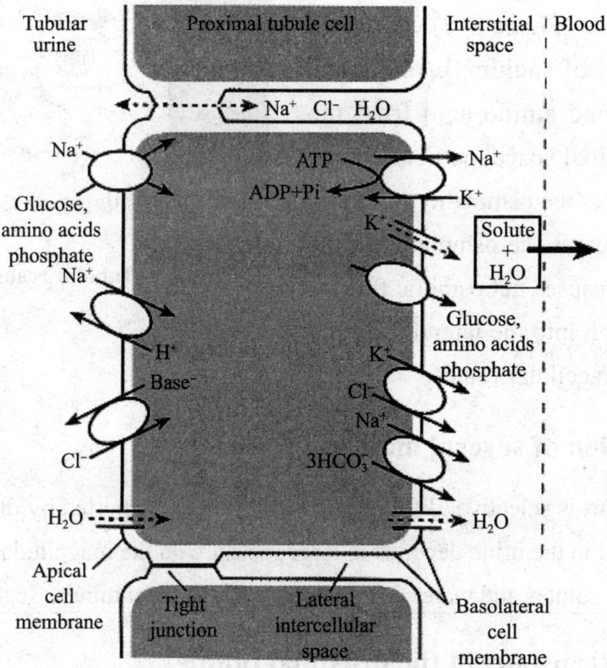

Figure 8–7 Transport in the proximal tubule

In the latter half of the proximal tubule, because of the reabsorption of chloride ions, the potential difference between the inside and outside of the tube causes the sodium ion to undergo passive reabsorption along the potential gradient via the paracellular pathway.

3.1.2 Chloride reabsorption

In the early part of the proximal tubule, sodium reabsorption is, most importantly, accompanied by water. This results in chloride concentration in the tubular lumen increasing along the length of the proximal tubule[4]. In the final two–thirds of the proximal tubule the chloride gradient generated is so large that chloride moves passively into the cell via paracellular path-

[1] 基底侧膜：小管上皮细胞周壁和底部的细胞膜。

[2] 细胞内较小管腔也存在着 −70mV 的膜电位梯度。

[3] 泵入上皮细胞之间的侧面细胞间隙。

[4] 结果导致 Cl^- 在近端小管后段管腔内的浓度不断升高。

way and thence into the interstitial fluid.

3.1.3 Glucose and amino acidreabsorption

Glucose and amino acid are normally entirely re–absorbed[1] from the tubular fluid so that none appears in the urine. It is cotransported with sodium at the luminal membrane, when sodium moves down its electrochemical gradient using the sodium gradient as a source of energy. Glucose and amino acid then are transported from the cell into the interstitial fluid by secondary active transportand thence to the peritubular capillaries.

The ability of renal tubules to reabsorb glucose is limited, and the maximum translocation capacity of each renal unit is different. When the concentration of glucose in plasma is increased, glucose is presented to the tubule at increasing rates. Glucose is absent from urine until the transport process is saturated, i. e. the transport maximum(*Tmax*) for glucose reabsorption[2] is reached. From then on glucose appears in urine at a rate which increases linearly with the filtered load.

The renal threshold for glucose[3] is the plasma glucose concentration at which glucose first appears in urine which is about 0.2 mg/ml (11 mmol/L). Glucose appears in the urine (glycosuria) for diabetic[4] when plasma glucose concentration is over the renal threshold.

3.1.4 Bicarbonate reabsorption

In the proximal tubule, hydrogen ions that enter the lumen in exchange for sodium or are secreted by H^+ ATPase, combine with the bicarbonate ions[5] that were filtered at the glomerulus and form H_2CO_3. This leads to the formation of H_2O and CO_2. This reaction is catalysed by carbonic anhydrase[6] present in the luminal brush border. The CO_2 diffuses into the cell and, by the reverse reaction, forms H^+ and HCO_3^-. These hydrogen ions replace those that entered the lumen. HCO_3^- then diffuses across the basolateral cell membrane, in association with Na^+, into the interstitial space, to be reabsorbed into the peritubular capillaries.

3.1.5 Potassium reabsorption

The proximal tubule reabsorbs about 80% of filtered potassium, but the mechanisms responsible are not fully understood. Potassium is freely filtered at the glomerulus and so is present in the filtrate at a concentration equal to that in plasma. It appears to be reabsorbed passively into the cells of the proximal tubule. The reabsorption of sodium and water into the lateral spaces also tends to cause an increase in potassium concentration in the lumen so that some

---

[1] 完全重吸收。

[2] 葡萄糖重吸收最大转运率。

[3] 肾糖阈。

[4] 糖尿病患者。

[5] 与 HCO_3^-结合。

[6] 碳酸酐酶：存在于小管上皮细胞顶端膜表面，催化 H^+ 和 HCO_3^-生成 CO_2 和 H_2O。

potassium probably diffuses passively through paracellular pathways. In addition, it seems that there is an active transport mechanism for potassium at the luminal border[1].

3.1.6 Other substances reabsorption

The products of protein metabolism include phosphate, sulphate and urea. Phosphate is freely filtered at the glomerulus and is cotransported with sodium at the luminal border of the proximal tubules. The rate of phosphate reabsorption is regulated hormonally[2]; it is decreased by parathyroid hormone and increased by calcitriol, the active form of vitamin D. Like sulphate is reabsorbed by cotransport with sodium.

In plasma 40% ~ 50% of calcium is bound to protein[3] and cannot be filtered by the glomerulus. The remainder is ionized Ca^{2+}, and is freely filtered by the glomerulus. Ca^{2+} is reabsorbed from the proximal tubule in parallel with sodium and water so that its concentration in the tubule remain relatively constant. Ca^{2+} enters tubule cells passively, down concentration and electrical gradients, but probably leaves the cell by a Ca^{2+}–Na^+ countertransport mechanism or via a Ca^{2+} ATPase mechanism[4].

3.2 Tubular transport in the loop of Henle

The descending limb of the loop of Henle has high water permeability and low solute permeability, and the thin and thick ascending limbs have a low permeability to water and the thick ascending limb actively reabsorbs sodium from the tubular fluid.

The active reabsorption of Na^+ that occurs in the thick ascending limb is dependent on the Na^+–K^+ pump in the basolateral membrane, just as it is in the proximal tubule. It mainly occurs via a Na^+–Cl^-–K^+ symporter[5], which couples the movement of these three ions in the ratios 1: 2: 1. In addition, some Na^+ also moves in via a Na^+–H^+ antiporter, thereby leading to H^+ secretion and HCO_3^- reabsorption. The Cl^-, HCO_3^- and some of the K^+ leave the cell via the basolateral membrane, but much of the K^+ that enters the cell leaves again via a K^+ channel in the luminal membrane. This K^+ is probably responsible for generating a positive charge[6] in the lumen of the thick ascending limb, which drives the movement of Na^+, K^+, Ca^{2+} and Mg^{2+} out of the tubule via the paracellular route.

In the thick part of the ascending limb of the loop of Henle, there is reabsorption of Ca^{2+}. Entry of Ca^{2+} into the cells is passive, as in the proximal tubule. Exit from the cells at the baso-

---

[1] 管腔膜上存在有 K^+ 的主动重吸收机制。

[2] 磷酸盐的重吸收率受激素调节。

[3] 血浆中 40% ~ 50% 钙与血浆蛋白结合。

[4] Ca^{2+}–Na^+ 交换或 Ca^{2+} 泵转运机制。

[5] Na^+–Cl^-–K^+ 同向转运体。

[6] K^+ 可能产生正电位作用。

lateral membrane is by a Na^+–Ca^{2+} countertransport mechanism and, more importantly, by an active Ca^{2+} pump.

3.3 Tubular transport in the distal tubule and collecting duct

3.3.1 Transport in the early distal tubule

In the early distal tubule, Na^+ also moves into the cell via a Na^+–Cl^- symporter, then Na^+ is pumped out of the cell into interstitial fluid by Na^+–K^+ pump and the Cl^- leaves the cell again via the basolateral membrane. There is also reabsorption of Ca^{2+} in the distal tubule as the same way of that in the thick part of the ascending limb of the loop of Henle.

3.3.2 Transport in the posterior distal tubule and collecting duct

In the posterior segment of the distal tubule and collecting duct there are two types of cells: the principal cells[1], which can actively reabsorb Na^+ and secrete K^+ and, in the presence of ADH, also absorb water; the intercalated cells[2], which can secrete H^+ and reabsorb HCO_3^-.

(1)The principal cells: In the principal cells, the Na^+–K^+ pump on the basolateral membrane is responsible for the reabsorption of Na^+ and for producing a high concentration of K^+ in the cell, which then causes K^+ to diffuse out of the cell, through K^+ channels, into the luminal fluid where the K^+ concentration is low. The fact that the permeability of the luminal membrane to K^+ is higher than that of the basolateral membrane favors the movement of K^+ into the lumen. Both the reabsorption of Na^+ and the secretion of K^+ in this segment of the tubule are affected by ALD (aldosterone)[3]. In the presence of ADH, water channels are incorporated into the luminal membrane of the principal cells. The basolateral membrane is freely permeable to water. Therefore in the presence of ADH, water passes through the cell, from the lumen to the interstitial fluid down the osmotic gradient caused by the high osmotic concentration of the interstitial fluid.

(2)The intercalated cells: In the intercalated cells, H^+ is generated from the dissociation of H_2CO_3[4] and, as in the proximal tubule, the formation of H_2CO_3 is facilitated by carbonic anhydrase. However, in contrast to the proximal tubule, it is thought that all of the H^+ leaves the intercalated cells via an H^+ pump[5] in the luminal membrane, rather than via countertransport with Na^+. The HCO_3^- that is formed from the dissociation of H_2CO_3 diffuses out of the intercalated cells across the basolateral membrane. These cells also reabsorb K^+ from the tubule, but the mechanism is not known.

---

[1] 主细胞。

[2] 闰细胞。

[3] 醛固酮：调节远曲小管和集合管对 Na+ 的重吸收和 K+ 的分泌。

[4] H_2CO_3 的解离。

[5] H^+ 泵：管腔膜分泌 H^+ 的一种机制。

4 Secretion function of renal tubule and collecting duct

In the renal tubules and collecting ducts, hydrogen ions, ammonia and potassium are secreted helpful for maintaining the acid–base balance.

4.1 Hydrogen ions

The epithelial cells of the proximal tubules, thick segment of the ascending limb of the loop of Henle, distal tubules, collecting tubules, and collecting ducts all secrete hydrogen ions into the tubular fluid [1]. The mechanism by which this occurs is illustrated in Figure 8–8.

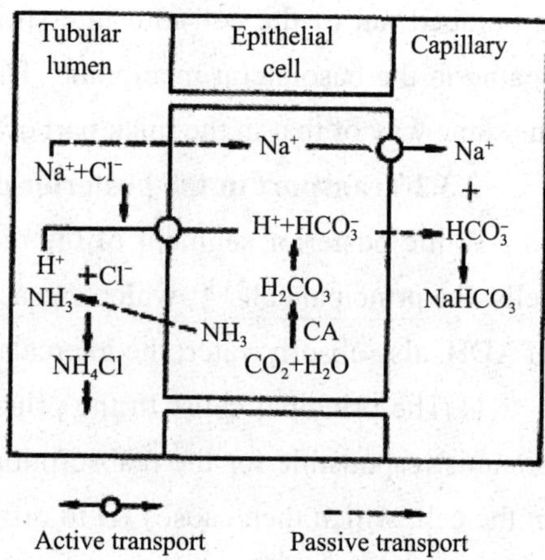

Figure 8–8 H^+, NH_3 secretions and H^+–Na^+ exchange

The secretory process begins with carbon dioxide that either diffuses into or is formed by metabolism in the tubular epithelial cells. The carbon dioxide, under the influence of the enzyme carbonic anhydrase combines with water to form carbonic acid. This then dissociates into bicarbonate ion and hydrogen ion. Finally, the hydrogen ions are secreted by a mechanism of Na^+–H^+ countertransport [2]. That is, when sodium moves from the lumen of the tubule to the interior of the cell, it first combines with a carrier protein in the luminal border of the cell membrane, and at the same time a hydrogen inside the cell combines with the opposite side of the same carrier protein. Then, because the concentration of sodium is much lower inside the cell than in the tubular lumen, this causes movement of the sodium down the concentration gradient to the interior, providing at the same time that energy for moving the hydrogen ion in the opposite direction into the tubular lumen. This process can even transport the hydrogen ion against their concentration gradient [3].

4.2 Ammonia

The epithelial cells of all the tubules continually synthesize ammonia, and ammonia diffuses into the tubules. The ammonia then reacts with hydrogen ion [4], as illustrated in Fig-

---

[1] H^+ 分泌进入小管液。

[2] 通过 Na^+ – H^+ 交换机制。

[3] 逆着 H^+ 浓度梯度。

[4] NH_3 与 H^+ 发生反应。

ure 8–9, to form ammonium ion [1]. This is then excreted into the urine in combination with chloride ion and other tubular anion. Note in the figure that the net effect of these reactions is, again to increase the bicarbonate concentration in the intracellular fluid.

This ammonium ion mechanism for transport of excess hydrogen ions in the tubules is especially important for two reasons: ① Each time an ammonia molecule combines with a hydrogen ion to form an ammonium ion, the concentration of ammonia in the tubular fluid becomes decreased, which caused still more ammonia to diffuse [2] from the epithelial cells into the tubular fluid. Thus, the rate of ammonia secretion into the tubular fluid is actually controlled by the amount of excess hydrogen ions to be transported. ② Most of the negative ions of the tubular fluid are chloride ions[3]. Only a few hydrogen ions could be transported into the urine in direct combination with chloride. Because hydrochloric acid is a very strong acid, the tubular pH [4] would fall rapidly. However, when hydrogen ions combine with ammonia and the resulting ammonium ions then combine with chloride, the pH does not fall significantly because ammonium chloride is only very weakly acidic [5].

4.3 Potassium

Normally, considerable amounts of potassium are secreted into the distal tubules, and some also into the collecting tubules and ducts. Figure 8–9 illustrates this secretion process. It shows that as sodium is transported from the cytoplasm of epithelial cell into the peritubular fluid, potassium is simultaneously transported in the opposite direction to the interior of the cell [6]. It is believed that this inward transport of potassium is not rigidly coupled with the outward transport of sodium. Instead, either all or most of the potassium movement

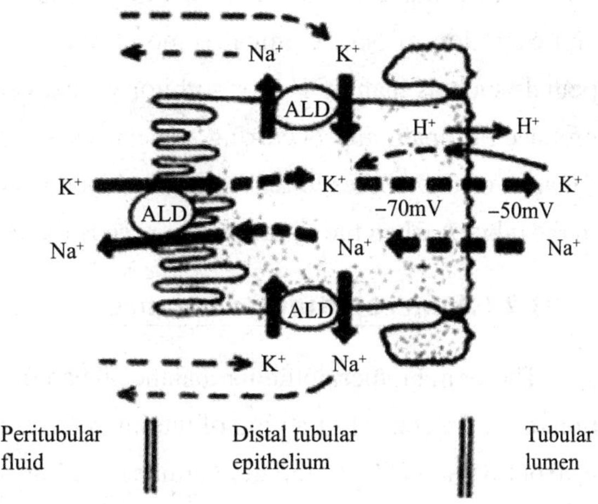

Figure 8–9 Mechanism of Na^+ and K^+ transport through the distal tubular epithelium

---

[1] 形成 NH^+。

[2] 造成更多的 NH_3 扩散。

[3] 小管液中的最多的阴离子主要是 Cl^-。

[4] 小管液的 pH 值。

[5] NH_4Cl 只是弱酸性。

[6] K^+ 同时反向转运进入上皮细胞内。

into the cell is probably caused by the very negative electrical potential created inside the cell[1] when sodium is pumped out into the interstitial fluid. Once the potassium has entered the epithelial cell, it then diffused passively from the cell into the tubular lumen.

Section 4 Regulation of renal tubule and collecting duct

There are many factors that can regulate the urine formation. Factors influencing glomerular filtration have been introduced, and here factors regulating renal tubules and collecting ducts are described.

1 Autoregulation

1.1 Osmotic diuresis[2]

The presence of large quantities of un-reabsorbed solutes in the renal tubules causes an increase in urine volume called osmotic diuresis. Solutes that are not reabsorbed in the proximal tubules exert an appreciable osmotic effect which can hold water in the tubules. Moreover, this fluid has a decreased Na^+ concentration, so the result is a marked increase in urine volume and excretion of Na^+. Clinical osmotic diuresis is produced by the administration of compounds such as mannitol[3] or sorbitol[4] that can be filtered but not be reabsorbed. It is also produced by naturally occurring substances when they are present in amounts exceeding the capacity of the tubules to reabsorb them. In diabetes[5], for example, the glucose that remains in the tubules when the filtrate load exceeds the renal glucose threshold causes polyuria[6].

1.2 Glomerulotubular balance[7]

The term glomerulotubular balance mean that despite variation of GFR (glomerular filtration rate), the constant fraction of the filtered Na^+ and water reabsorbed in the proximal tubular is about 65% ~ 70% of the glomerular filtration rate. Its physiological significance is to maintain the relative stability of urine volume and urine sodium.

[1] 全部或大部分 K^+ 转运进入细胞内可能是由于细胞内产生的负电位。

[2] 渗透性利尿。

[3] 甘露醇。

[4] 山梨醇。

[5] 糖尿病。

[6] 多尿症。

[7] 球管平衡。

2 Humoral regulation

2.1 Antidiuretic hormone[1]

Antidiuretic hormone (ADH) is a 9–peptide neurohormone, and it is synthesized by supraoptic nuclei[2](SON) and paraventricular nuclei[3](PVN) in the hypothalamus[4]. The intracellular synthesis of ADH is transported to the neurohypophysis along the hypothalamus – pituitary bundle[5], and stored in the nerve endings. When these nerve cells are excited, they release ADH and go into the circulation of the blood. ADH can cause vasoconstriction of arterioles by acting on vasopressin V_1 receptors, so ADH can be called vasopressin[6]. In the kidney, after binding to V_2 receptor , ADH increases the intracellular levels of cAMP and then improves the permeability of distal tubules and collecting ducts, thereby promoting the reabsorption of water. ADH also increases the urea permeability of the medullary portion of the collecting duct by activating specific urea transporters in the membrane. This increase in urea permeability contributes to the ability of the kidney to concentrate the urine (Figure 8–10).

There are two factors, the most powerful stimuli, which can affect the production and release of ADH: increase of crystal osmotic pressure[7] and severe loss of blood volume.

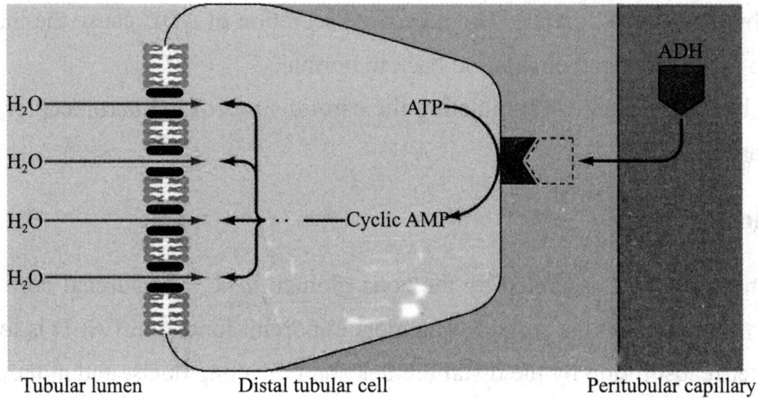

Figure 8–10 The mechanism of ADH

[1] 抗利尿激素。

[2] 视上核。

[3] 室旁核。

[4] 下丘脑。

[5] 下丘脑 – 垂体束。

[6] 血管升压素。

[7] 晶体渗透压。

2.1.1 Crystal osmotic pressure

Crystal osmotic pressure is the most important factor in regulating ADH release under physiological conditions. The osmoreceptors, located in the supraoptic nuclei of the anterior hypothalamus, are sensitive to the changes in plasma osmotic pressure.

When the body lost water, such as profuse sweating[1], severe vomiting or diarrhea, the plasma osmotic pressure increased, and the osmotic pressure receptor stimulation increased, then, ADH release increased, and promote water reabsorption in the distal tubules and collecting ducts. On the other hand, when we drink a large amount of water, the plasma is diluted, and the plasma osmotic pressure is reduced, then, the release of ADH is reduced, and the reabsorption of the distal tubule and the collecting tube is reduced and the urine volume is increased. This increased urine output due to drinking large amount of water is called water diuresis[2]. Water diuresis begins about 15 minutes after ingestion of a water load and reaches its maximum in about 40 minutes. However, when drinking small amounts of isotonic saline, the urine output remains to constant because the plasma osmotic pressure does not change significantly.

2.1.2 Blood volume

The volume receptors exist in the atria (mainly the left atrium) and the thoracic venous. When the circulating blood volume increases, the volume receptors are excited by expansion or stretch stimulation, and then the impulses are transported into the center along the vagus nerve to inhibit the release of ADH. The decreased secretion of ADH cause the increased urine output, which make the blood circulation back to normal.

Arterial blood pressure, by stimulating the carotid sinus of the baroreceptor, can also inhibit the release of ADH.

2.2 Aldosterone

Aldosterone (ALD) is secreted by the zona glomerulosa[3] of adrenal cortex, the outermost and very thin layer on the surface. The most important function of ALD is to increase sodium and water reabsorption by the distal tubules and collecting ducts, and at the same time to increase potassium ion secretion into these tubules. Two factors regulating ALD secretion are explained, rennin–angiotensin–aldosterone system[4] (RAAS) and plasma concentrations of K^+ and Na^+.

2.2.1 RAAS

Renin is an enzyme that is synthesized, stored and secreted by granular cells in the juxta-

---

[1] 大量出汗。

[2] 水利尿。

[3] 球状带。

[4] 肾素－血管紧张素－醛固酮系统。

glomerular apparatus. Renin can catalyze the conversion of angiotensinogen[1] into angiotensin I. Angiotensin I is then converted into the octapeptide angiotensin II by angiotensin–converting enzyme (ACE)[2]. Angiotensinogen is produced by the liver and circulates in the blood. ACE is found in high concentration in vascular endothelium. Therefore, much of the angiotensin II that circulates in the blood is formed in the lungs where there is a large surface area of vascular endothelium. However, angiotensin II can also be produced locally within the kidney itself from intrarenal angiotensinogen[3], without activation of the systemic rennin–angiotensin system[4]. This locally generated angiotensin II is very important in the regulation of GFR and sodium excretion.

Angiotensin II has many effects. It causes vasoconstriction, which can increases arterial blood pressure in the systemic circulation. In the kidney, it can preferentially constrict the efferent arterioles leading to an increase in the glomerular capillary pressure and to maintain GFR constant when renal perfusion pressure is reduced. It stimulates sodium reabsorption by the proximal tubule, and chloride and water follow passively. It stimulates aldosterone secretion by the adrenal cortex. It stimulates ADH secretion from the posterior pituitary gland. It stimulates thirst by an action on the brain. It has a negative–feedback effect on renin secretion.

Angiotensin II is further hydrolyzed by aminopeptidase[5] to produce angiotensin III (7 peptide), which can promote the ALD synthesis and secretion. However, the secretion of angiotensin III is relatively small, so the main component which stimulates aldosterone synthesis and secretion in vivo is angiotensin II. For the secretion connection of rennin, angiotensin and ALD, in physiology they are bound to form a RAAS.

2.2.2 Plasma concentrations of K^+ and Na^+

When plasma K^+ concentration increases or Na^+ concentration decreases, the zona glomerulosa of adrenal cortex can be stimulated to synthesize and secret much more ALD. As a result, plasma K^+ concentration decreases and Na^+ concentration increases. Otherwise, when plasma K^+ concentration decreases or Na^+ concentration increases, ALD concentration is low, and the action of keeping Na^+ and excretion K^+ is weakened. In the end the concentration of K^+ and Na^+ is recovered.

3 Neuroregulation

The renal sympathetic nerve dominates not only the renal blood vessels, but also the

[1] 血管紧张素原。

[2] 血管紧张素转换酶。

[3] 肾脏本身产生的血管紧张素原。

[4] 全身性的肾素 – 血管紧张素系统。

[5] 氨基肽酶。

juxtaglomerular cells and renal tubular epithelial cells. Stimulation of the renal sympathetic nerve increases renin secretion by a direct action of released on β_1-adrenergic receptors on the juxtaglomerular cells. Renal sympathetic nerve stimulation also decreases renal plasma flow by binding α receptors on the vascular smooth muscle. Furthermore, renal sympathetic nerve stimulation promotes the reabsorption of Na^+, Cl^- and water by proximal tubules and medulla loops.

Section 5 Concentration and dilution of urine

One of the most important functions of the kidney is to control the osmolality of the body fluids. When the osmolality falls too low, the kidneys automatically excrete a great excess of water into the urine, a dilute urine [1], to raise the body fluid osmolality. Conversely, when the osmolality of the body fluids is too high, the kidney automatically excrete an excess of solutes into the urine, a concentrated urine [2], thereby reducing the body fluid osmolality. Under normal condition, the final urine osmotic concentration changes between 50 and 1200 mOsm/Kg·H_2O, the concentration and dilution of the kidney to the urine depends largely on the function and structure of the juxtamedullary nephron, the collecting duct, and vasa recta.

1 Formation mechanism of osmotic gradient in the renal medullary

The concentrating mechanism depends on the maintenance of a gradient of increasing osmolality from the outer of medulla to the inner of medulla either in tissue fluid or tubule fluid. This osmotic gradient is produced by the operation of the loops of Henle as countercurrent multipliers [3] and maintained by the operation of the vasa recta [4] as countercurrent exchangers [5]. In physics, the countercurrent system refers to two U-shaped pipe with lower ends connected in parallel, with the opposite direction of the liquid flowing. In the renal medulla, this happened in both the loop of Henle and the vasa recta.

The mechanism of countercurrent multipliers can be explained by using the model in Figure 8-11. In the model, the solute of liquid flows from A pipe to B pipe through the connection part. In the process of liquid flowing, the M_1 film can pump the solute from B to A pipe actively, and the water is impermeable to each other. Therefore, the concentration of solute in A pipe is getting higher and higher, the maximum concentration is appeared in the connection

[1] 稀释尿液。

[2] 浓缩尿液。

[3] 逆流倍增。

[4] 直小血管。

[5] 逆流交换。

part. And then when the liquid flows in the B pipe , the concentration of solute is getting lower and lower. In this way, either in A pipe or in B pipe, the solute concentration is gradually increased from the top to the bottom, that is, the countercurrent multipliers. The M_2 film is permeable to water but impermeable to solute. When the solution with a lower concentration down are flows in C pipe, the water can enter into B pipe continuously, thus, the concentration of solute in C pipe is gradually increased from the top to bottom, finally, the hyperosmotic solution flows out of the C pipe. The arrangement of the loop of Henle and the collecting tube is similar to the countercurrent multiplication modle, so the formation of the medullary osmotic concentration gradient can be explained by the theory of the countercurrent multiplication.

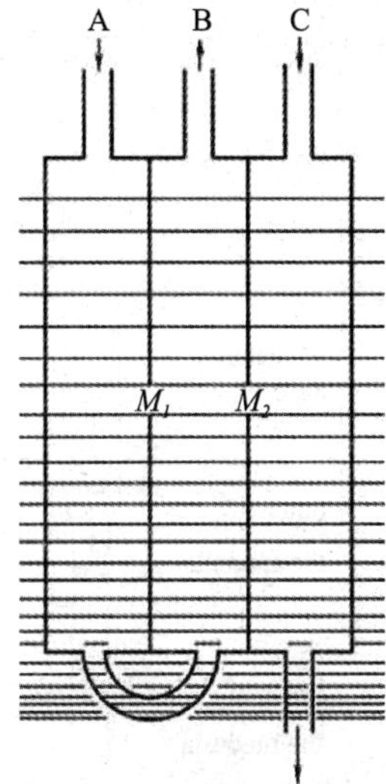

Figure 8–11 The model of countercurrent multipliers

The liquid in A, B and C tubes flows in the direction of the arrow. The M_1 membrane can pump $Na^+$from B into A, and the water is impermeable to each other. The M_2 film is permeable to water

1.1 The formation of osmotic gradient in outer of the medulla

The formation of osmotic gradient in outer of the medulla depends on the active transport of Na^+ and Cl^- in the thick ascending limb. Due to the active reabsorption of NaCl, the osmotic pressure of tube fluid and tissue fluid decreases gradually[1] when the fluid flows from the outer of medulla to the cortex direction (Figure 8–12).

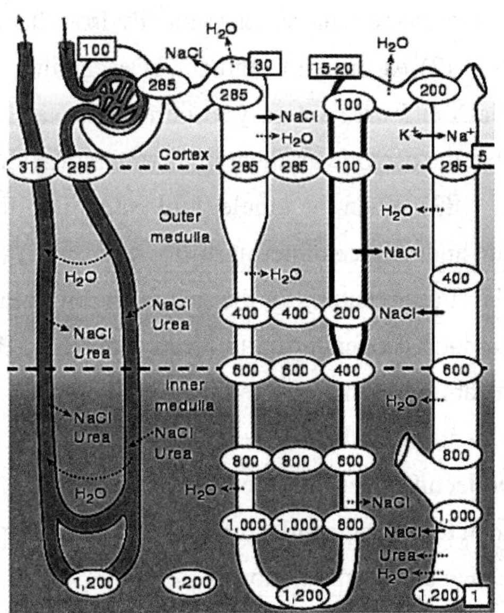

Figure 8–12 The mechanism of the formation of osmotic gradients

1.2 The formation of osmotic gradient in inner of the medulla

The formation of osmotic gradient in inner of the medulla is mainly related to the reabsorption of sodium chloride and recycle of urea (Fig8–13).

[1] 小管液和组织液的渗透压逐渐降低。

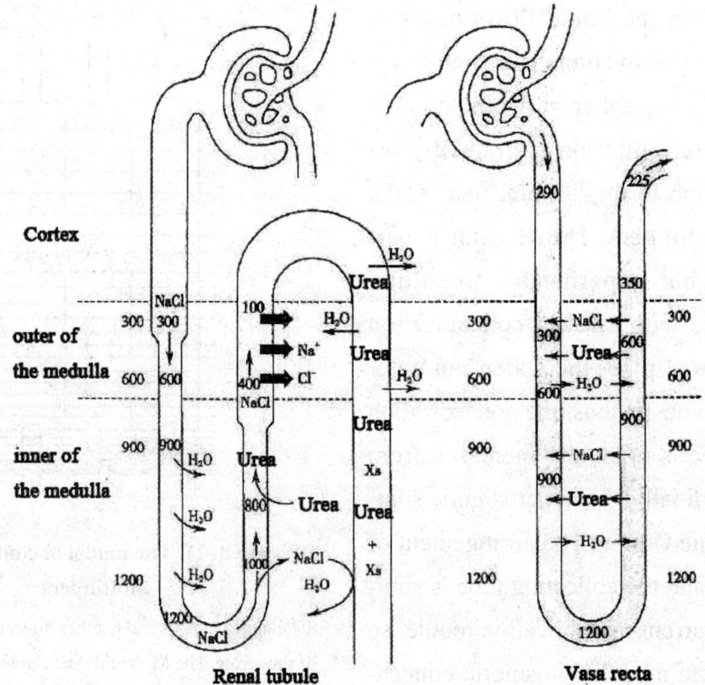

Figure 8–13 The formation of osmotic gradient in renal medulla

(1) At the thin segment of descending limb in the medullary loop, NaCl and urea are not be penetrated[1], and H_2O is easy to be penetrated. While with the reabsorption of H_2O, the osmotic gradient increases gradually from the top to the bottom;

(2) At the thin segment of ascending limb, because the H_2O is impermeable, while the NaCl and urea are easy to permeate, NaCl diffuses into the interstitial fluid continuously, so that the osmotic gradient in the interstitial fluid increases;

(3) When the tubule fluid enters into the collecting duct in the inner medulla, because of the high degree of permeability of urea[2], the urea passes through the tube wall to the interstitial fluid, resulting in the increasing of urea in the interstitial fluid, so that the intramedullary osmotic concentration to further increase. Because the thin ascending limb has moderate permeability to the urea, the urea in the interstitial fluid from the collecting duct can enter the thin ascending limb, and then flows through thick ascending limb, distal convoluted tubule and the collecting duct in the outer where the urea is impermeable or has very low permeability, and then to inner medulla, diffuses into the interstitial fluid from the collecting duct. This process is called urea recirculation[3].

---

[1] NaCl和尿素不具有通透性。

[2] 尿素的高通透性。

[3] 尿素的再循环。

1.3 Countercurrent exchange mechanism in the vasa recta

The medullary blood flow has two characteristics, both exceedingly important for maintaining the high solute concentration in the medullary interstitial fluids. First, the medullary blood flow is very slight in quantity, because of this very sluggish blood flow, removal of solutes is minimal. Second, the vasa recta functions are as a countercurrent exchanger[1] that prevents washout of solutes from the medulla. The slow flow of blood allows diffusion to occur between adjacent segments of descending (incoming) and ascending (outgoing) limbs of the blood vessels while a steep osmotic gradient exists at opposite ends of the system . Thus, in Figure 8–13, as blood flows down the descending limbs of the vasa recta, sodium chloride and urea diffuse into the blood from the interstitium fluid while water diffuses outward into the interstitium, and these two effects cause the osmole concentration in the vasa recta to rise progressively higher, to a maximum concentration of 1200 mOsm/liter at the tips of the vasa recta. Then as the blood flows backup the ascending limbs, all the extra sodium chloride and urea diffuse back out of the blood into the interstitial fluid while water diffuses back into the blood. By the time the blood finally leaves the medulla, its osmole concentration is only slightly greater than that of the blood that had initially entered the vasa recta. As a result, blood flowing through the vasa recta carries only a minute amount of the medullary interstitial solutes away from the medulla, thus the osmotic gradient of the renal medulla can be maintained.

2 The basic process of urine concentration and dilution

The osmotic concentration in renal medullary and ADH are the basic condition for urine concentration. Experiments showed that the tubular fluid is always hypotonic solution after it enters into the distal convoluted tubule. When the hypotonic solution flows into the collecting duct, the H_2O is reabsorbed under the action of ADH, so the H_2O inside the collecting duct is less and the concentration of the tubular fluid is higher, and thus the tubular fluid becomes hypertonic urine. When there is too much H_2O in the body, the plasma osmotic pressure decreases, and less ADH are released, so that the reabsorption of H_2O in the distal convoluted tubule and collecting duct is reduced and the NaCl continues to be reabsorbed actively, resulting in a large amount of hypotonic urine.

Section 6 Urine discharge

Urine discharge (micturition[2]) is the process by which the urinary bladder empties when it becomes filled. Urine is formed continuously at a rate of about 1 ml per minute. Storage and

[1] 逆流交换器。

[2] 排尿。

controlled release is the function of the urinary bladder and its associated sphincters.

1 Innervation of bladder and urethra

The bladder is a distensible hollow organ, the wall of which is made of smooth muscle. The smooth muscle of the bladder is arranged in spiral, longitudinal, and circular bundles. The detrusor muscle [1] is mainly responsible for emptying the bladder during micturition. There is an internal sphincter of urethra [2] at the junction of urethra and bladder. Farther along the urethra is a sphincter of skeletal muscle, which is called external urethral sphincter [3].

The bladder and the internal urethral sphincter are innervated by pelvic nerve [4] (parasympathetic nerve) and hypogastric nerve [5] (sympathetic nerve). The external sphincter is innervated by pudendal nerve [6] (somatic motor nerve [7]). Pelvic, hypogastric and pudendal nerves are both motor and sensory fibers. The postganglionic fibers [8] of motor nerves in pelvic nerves innervate the detrusor muscle. Stimulation of the parasympathetic fibers can cause the constriction of the detrusor muscle. The sensory fibers of the pelvic nerves can detect the stretch degree of the bladder wall and the posterior urethra (Figure 8–14).

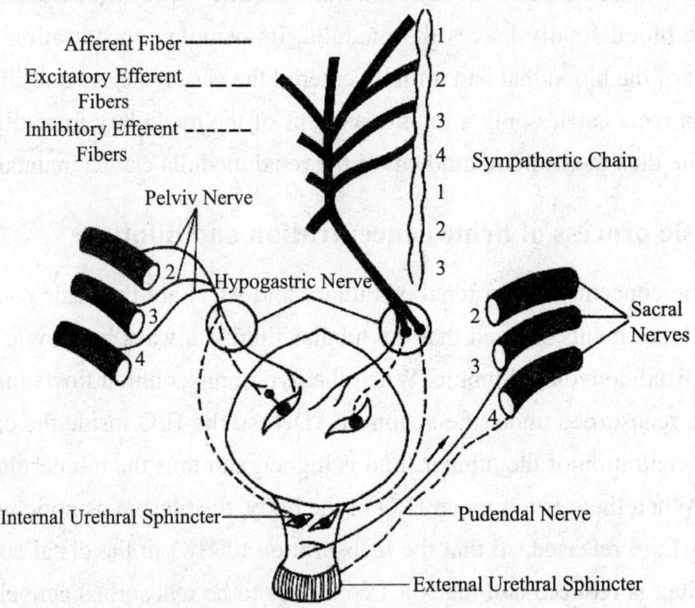

Figure 8–14 Innervation of the bladder and urethra

---

[1] 膀胱逼尿肌。

[2] 膀胱内括约肌。

[3] 尿道外括约肌。

[4] 盆神经。

[5] 腹下神经。

[6] 阴部神经。

[7] 躯体运动神经。

[8] 节后纤维。

2 Micturition reflex [1]

Micturition reflex is a spinal reflex, that is, the reflex can be done at the spinal cord level, but under normal condition, micturition reflex is controlled by the upper center of the brain. When there is no urine in the bladder, the intravesical pressure [2] is about zero. As the bladder contains about 150 to 250 ml of urine, the first desire to void is usually felt. When the volume of bladder is about 400 to 500 ml, an individual will feel uncomfortable. Stimulation of stretch receptors induces reflex contraction of the detrusor muscle and the relaxation of internal urethral sphincter, and urination enters into the posterior urethra. Urine flowing through the urethra stimulates its stretch receptor which reflexly causes further contraction of the detrusor muscle of bladder and relaxation of the external urethral sphincter. This process that urine stimulation of the urethra can further strengthen the activity of micturition center is a positive feedback. In the process of urination, the strong contraction of the abdominal muscles and diaphragm, can increase the intra–abdominal pressure [3], to help urination activity.

[1] 排尿反射。

[2] 膀胱内压。

[3] 腹内压。

Chapter 9 ENDOCRINOLOGY PHYSIOLOGY

Section 1 Introduction

The endocrine system, like the nervous system, adjusts and correlates the activities of the various body systems, making them appropriate to the changing demands of the external and internal environment. Endocrine integration is brought about by hormones[1], chemical messages or signal molecules produced by ductless glands, tissues and cells, and are transported by blood to their target cells. Classically, the endocrine system consists of various endocrine glands, tissues and cells that can produce hormones. The main endocrine glands and hormones of the body are shown in Table 9–1.

1 Chemical classification

There are two general classes of hormones: nitrogenous hormones and steroid hormones[2] according to their chemical structure(Table 9–1). The nitrogenous hormones include peptides, proteins and monoamines[3] (modified amino acids). Peptides and proteins include neuropeptides, pituitary and gastrointestinal hormones. Monoamines comprise catecholamines, histamine, serotonin, and melatonin. Catecholamines (dopamine, noradrenaline and adrenaline) are derived from tyrosine by a series of enzymatic conversions. The steroid hormones are derived from cholesterol. Steroids consist of adrenal, gonadal steroids and 1–25 dihydroxyvitamin D_3[4], which is converted to a hormone. Steroid hormones are highly lipid soluble.

[1] 激素。

[2] 含氮激素和类固醇激素。

[3] 含氮激素包括多肽、蛋白质、单胺类激素。

[4] 类固醇激素包括肾上腺皮质激素、性激素及 1,25（OH）$_2$VitD_3。

Table 9-1 Endocrine Glands, Hormones, and Their Functions and Structure

Gland	Hormones	Major Functions	Structure
Hypothalamus	Thyrotropin-releasing hormone(TRH) [1]	Stimulates secretion of TSH and prolactin	Peptide
	Gonadotropin-releasing hormone(GnRH) [2]	Causes release of LH and FSH	Dopamine
	Growth hormone-releasing hormone(GHRH) [3]	Causes release of growth hormone	Peptide
	Growth hormone inhibitory hormone(GHIH) [4]	Inhibits release of growth hormone	Peptide
	Corticotropin-releasing hormone(CRH) [5]	Causes release of ACTH	Peptide
	Prolactin- releasing factor (PRF) [6]	Causes release of prolactin	Peptide
	Prolactin-inhibiting factor (PIF) [7]	Inhibits release of prolactin	Amine
Anterior pituitary	Growth hormone [8]	Stimulates protein synthesis and overall growth of most cells and tissues	Peptide
	Thyroid-stimulating hormone (TSH) [9]	Stimulates synthesis and secretion of thyroid hormones	Peptide
	Adrenocorticotropic hormone(ACTH) [10]	Stimulates synthesis and secretion of adrenocortical hormone	Peptide
	Prolactin [11]	Promotes development of the female breasts and secretion of milk	Peptide
	Follicle-stimulating hormone (FSH) [12]	Causes growth of follicles in the ovaries and sperm maturation in Sertoli cells of testes	Peptide
	Luteinizing hormone (LH) [13]	Stimulates testosterone synthesis in Leydig cells of testes; stimulates ovulation, formation of corpus luteum, and estrogen and progesterone synthesis in ovaries	Peptide

[1] 促甲状腺激素释放激素。

[2] 促性腺激素释放激素。

[3] 生长激素释放激素。

[4] 生长激素释放抑制激素。

[5] 促肾上腺激素释放抑制激素。

[6] 促乳素释放抑制因子。

[7] 促乳素释放因子。

[8] 生长激素。

[9] 促甲状腺激素。

[10] 促肾上腺皮质激素（ACTH）。

[11] 催乳素。

[12] 促卵泡激素。

[13] 黄体生成素。

续表

Gland	Hormones	Major Functions	Structure
Posterior pituitary	Antidiuretic hormone (ADH) (also called vasopressin)	Increases water reabsorption by the kidneys and causes vasoconstriction and increased blood pressure	Peptide
	Oxytocin	Stimulates milk ejection from breasts and uterine contractions	Peptide
Thyroid	Thyroxine (T_4) and triiodothyronine(T_3)	Increases the rates of chemical reactions in most cells, thus increasing body metabolic rate	Amine
	Calcitonin	Promotes deposition of calcium in the bones and decreases extracellular fluid calcium ion concentration	Peptide
Parathyroid	Parathyroid hormone (PTH)	Controls serum calcium ion concentration by increasing calcium absorption by the gut and kidneys and releasing calcium from bones	Peptide
Adrenal cortex	Cortisol	Has multiple metabolic functions for controlling metabolism of proteins, carbohydrates, and fats; also has anti-inflammatory effects	Steroid
	Aldosterone	Increases renal sodium reabsorption, potassium secretion, and hydrogen ion secretion	Steroid
Adrenal medulla	Norepinephrine, epinephrine	Same effects as sympathetic stimulation	Amine
Pancreas	Insulin (B-cells)	Promotes glucose entry in many cells, and in this way controls carbohydrate metabolism	Peptide
	Glucagon (A-cells)	Increases synthesis and release of glucose from the liver into the body fluids	Peptide

2 The way of hormone action

Generally, there are four methods of hormone action forms. Most hormones are transported to the distal organs via blood stream, which is called telecrine[1]. Some hormones diffuse into the extracellular fluid and act on target cells that are situated very close to the producer cell, which is called paracrine[2]. And some neurons can secret chemical substances (neurohormones) that reach the circulating blood and influence the function of cells at another location

[1] 远距分泌。

[2] 旁分泌。

in the body, which is called neurocrine[1]. While autocrine[2] is that a cell secretes chemical substances that affect the function of the same cell by binding to the cell surface receptors. By these four forms hormones can regulate extensive functions of the body.

3 Physiological functions and characteristics

3.1 Physiological functions of hormones

The functions of hormones are multiple and complex, and they can be classified as follows: ① regulate the metabolism; ② promote the cell proliferation and differentiation; ③ regulate the growth and activity of nervous system; ④ regulate reproduction, maintain normal sex function; ⑤ regulate the activity of cardiovascular system and functions of kidney, etc.

3.2 Characteristics of hormones

Regardless of their chemical structures, all hormones have several characteristics:

3.2.1 Specificity[3] Classical endocrine hormones are secreted into the blood and transported to their distant target cells, which are equipped with receptors that recognize each hormone. The first step of a hormone's action is to bind to specific receptors at the target cell, then the hormone can activate the physiological process inside the cells.

3.2.2 High efficiency[4] Hormones are present in the circulation in low concentrations. The plasma concentrations of hormones range between nmol/L and pmol/L. When the hormone combines with its receptor, it usually initiates a cascade of reactions[5] in the cell, with each stage becoming more powerfully activated so that even small concentrations of the hormone can have a large effect. One molecule hormone bound to a cell receptor may release 10,000 times more cAMP in the cell. cAMP works as an amplifier of the hormone signal, so the action of the hormone can be amplified.

3.2.3 Interactions of hormones[6] The hormones can interact with each other. Some are strengthened by others, but some are antagonists to others. There are also some kinds of hormones who do not act directly on the cells, but they can enlarge the effect of other hormones. This is called the permissive action of the hormone, e. g. corticosteroid can enhance the vasoconstrictive effect of noradrenaline.

---

[1] 神经分泌。

[2] 自分泌。

[3] 特异性。

[4] 高效性。

[5] 级联反应。

[6] 激素的相互作用。

4 Mechanism of hormones

4.1 The second messenger hypothesis

For the nitrogenous hormone, like peptides and amino acid hormones, the second messenger hypothesis[1] is the main mechanism of action (Figure 9–1). According to the second messenger hypothesis, in many cases, the binding of polypeptide to the receptors promotes synthesis of cAMP by activating adenylatecyclase (AC), which is an enzyme locating in the plasma membrane. cAMP serves as an intracellular mediator or second messenger to activate or inhibit intracellular enzymes by activating a cAMP–dependent protein kinase (i. e. , PKA), which in turn phosphorylates specific proteins in the cell, triggering biochemical reactions that ultimately lead to the cell's response to the hormone.

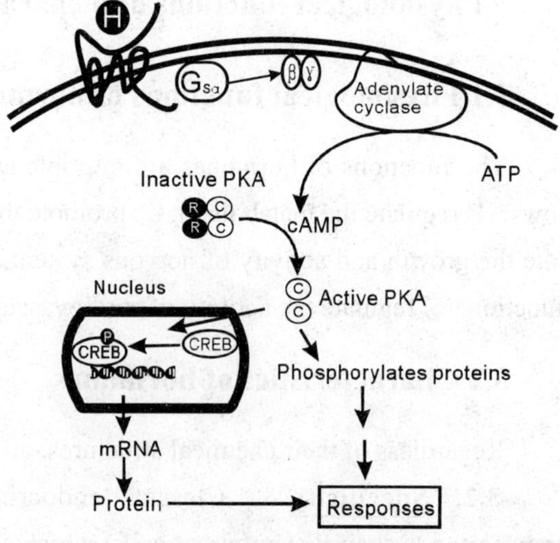

Figure 9–1 The second messenger hypothesis

There is another action path of hormones. The binding of the hormone to the surface receptors causes an activation of a membrane–associated enzyme, phospholipase C, which generates two potent intracellular signals from membrane phospholipids– inositol 1, 4, 5–triphosphate (IP_3) and diacylglycerol (DG). These enzymes cause releas of Ca^{2+}or the phosphorylation of specific proteins, leading to the cell's response.

In many target cells a hormone may trigger production of more than one of these second messengers.

4.2 The genetic expression hypothesis[2]

Receptors for steroid hormones are soluble intracellular proteins. The lipid–soluble steroid hormone diffuses across the cell membrane and enters the cytoplasm of the cell, where it binds with a specific receptor protein. Some receptors normally also exist in the nucleus. The combined receptor protein–hormone then diffuses into or is transported into the nucleus, where the combination binds at specific points on the DNA strands in the chromosomes, which acti-

[1] 第二信使学说。

[2] 基因表达学说。

vates the transcription process of specific genes to form mRNA. Eventually, the mRNA diffuses into the cytoplasm, where increase the synthesis of certain cellular proteins. Larger amounts of specific mRNA have been found in steroid treated target cells(Figure 9–2).

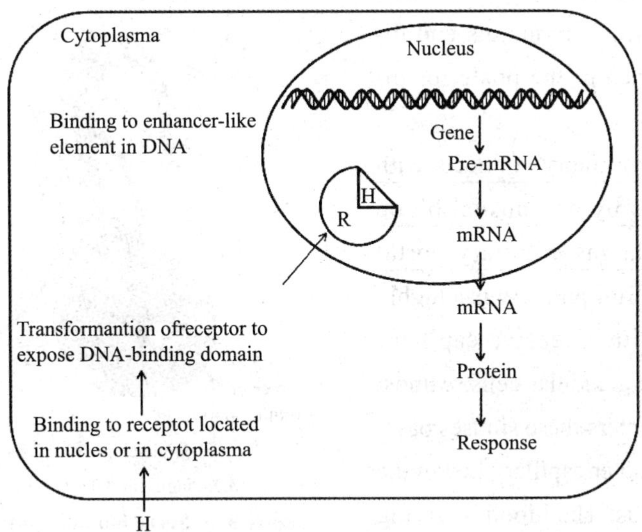

Figure 9–2 The genetic expression hypothesis

Section 2 Hypothalamus and pituitary hormones

In central nervous system, some neurons not only can initiate and conduct stimulation, but also can synthesize and release hormones. These neurons are called endocrine neurons[1]. It has been identified that endocrine neurons are major in hypothalamus. The hypothalamus is the portion of the anterior end of the diencephalon that lies below the hypothalamic sulcus and in front of the interpeduncular nuclei. It is divided into a variety of nuclei and nuclear areas. The supraoptic nucleus (SON) and the paraventricular nucleus (PVN) in the hypothalamus are the major sites for nervous endocrine system.

The pituitary gland is composed of two adjacent lobes—the anterior pituitary and the posterior pituitary. The anterior pituitary is also called adenohypophysis, and the posterior pituitary is also known as neurohypophysis. There are neural connections, between the hypothalamus and the posterior lobe of the pituitary gland[2]. Actually, the posterior pituitary is an extension of the neural components of the hypothalamus[3]. The axons of SON and PVN pass

[1] 在中枢神经系统中，一些神经元不仅能产生和传导兴奋，而且能够合成和释放激素，这些神经元称为内分泌神经元。

[2] 下丘脑和垂体后叶之间有神经联系。

[3] 神经垂体为下丘脑的延伸结构。

down the infundibulum and end within the posterior pituitary in close proximity to capillaries (Figure 9–3). Thus, these neurons do not form a synapse with other neurons. Instead, their terminals end directly on capillaries in the posterior pituitary.

The anterior pituitary connects with the hypothalamus by an unusual blood vessel—hypothalamus–pituitary portal system[1]. The anterior pituitary is a highly vascular gland with extensive capillary sinuses among the glandular cells. Almost all the blood that enters these sinuses passes first through another capillary bed in the lower hypothalamus. The blood, carrying hypothalamic, flows through hypothalamus–pituitary portal system directly into the anterior pituitary (Figure 9–3).

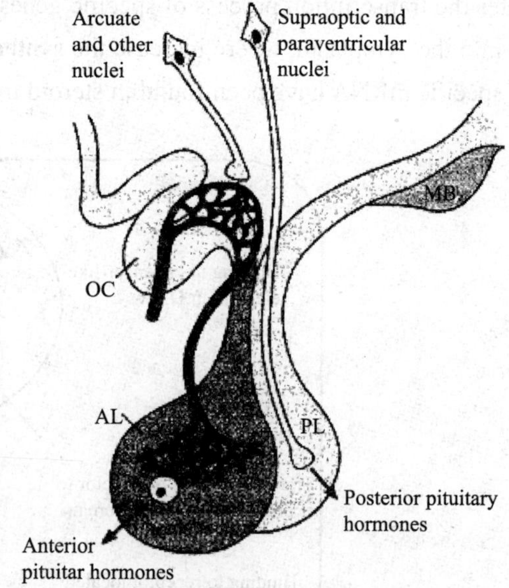

Figure 9–3 Secretion of hypothalamic hormones

1 Hypothalamic–neurohypophysis system

The SON and PVN in the hypothalamus terminate in neurohypophysis. These are called hypothalamic–neurohypophyseal system. Antidiuretic hormone (ADH) or vasopressin (VP) is synthesized in the cell bodies of the SON, and the oxytocin in the PVN[2].

1.1 Antidiuretic hormone[3]

ADH plays an important regulatory role in water excretion into the urine from kidney and maintenance of fluid osmolarity, blood volume and blood pressure[4]. This antidiuretic effect and its regulation have been discussed in detail in Chapter 8. ADH is also called VP because its vasoconstrictive function. 5 pg/mL of ADH is sufficient for maximal antidiuresis but inadequate to produce a widespread pressure response. Hemorrhage, on the other hand, can result in levels of ADH 10 ~ 100 times as high. At these concentrations, ADH may indeed exert a vaso-

[1] 垂体前叶与下丘脑之间通过垂体－门脉系统相联系。

[2] 抗利尿激素由主要由视上核合成，而缩宫素主要由室旁核合成。

[3] 抗利尿激素。

[4] 抗利尿激素在肾对水的重吸收、尿的浓缩与稀释、血容量及血压的调节中发挥重要作用。

constrictor effect.

1.2 Oxytocin [1]

Oxytocin has two main actions: milk ejection and uterine contraction [2]. This peptide is released in response to neural signals that arise in the nipple stimulated by suckling. It is also released when a mother hears her baby cry [3]. The oxytocin is then carried by the blood to the breasts, where it causes contraction of myoepithelial cells that lie outside of and form a lattice-work surrounding the alveoli of the mammary glands. In less than a minute after the beginning of suckling, milk begins to flow. In addition, Oxytocin powerfully stimulates contraction of the pregnant uterus, especially toward the end of gestation. Generally, estrogen sensitizes the myometrium to stimulation by oxytocin, and progesterone makes it more resistant to such stimulation. It is possible that the peptide could play a significant role during the process called labor. Mechanical stimulation of various regions of the female genital tract can elicit oxytocin release reflex.

2 Hypothalamic–adenohypophysissystem

It is now clear that specialized classes of hypothalamic neurons (hypophysiotrophic neurons) terminate in the capillary loops found in the median eminence at the start of the portal system. These neurons secrets neuropeptides (hypothalamic regulatory peptides) into the portal blood that act on the anterior pituitary cells to control the synthesis and secretion of the anterior pituitary hormones[4]. Because of the short distance traveled by these blood–born hormones, their leftover concentration in the general circulation are especially small.

2.1 Hypothalamic regulatory peptides

Hypophysiotrophic neurons in the hypothalamus synthesize and secrete the hypothalamic releasing and inhibitory hormones that control secretion of the anterior pituitary hormones. The major hypothalamic releasing and inhibitory hormones are summarized in Table 9–1 and are the following:

(1) Thyrotropin–releasing hormone (TRH) Being the first hypothalamic hormone isolated, it is a tripeptide with a N–terminal pyroglutamic acid residue that stimulates the secretion of both TSH and prolactin.

---

[1] 缩宫素。

[2] 缩宫素有两个主要作用：一是引起射乳反射，二是引起子宫平滑肌收缩。

[3] 吸吮乳头或婴儿的啼哭声通过神经传递引起缩宫素的分泌。

[4] 下丘脑促垂体区神经元分泌的肽类物质，经垂体门脉系统运输到垂体前叶，调节垂体前叶激素的分泌。

(2) Gonadotropin-releasing hormone (GnRH) It is a decapeptide that promotes the synthesis and secretion of both LH and FSH.

(3) Corticotrophin-releasing hormone (CRH) This is a 41 amino acids (a. a.) polypeptide that stimulates the release of adrenocorticotropic hormone (ACTH).

(4) Growth hormone releasing hormone (GHRH) It is a 40 ~ 44 a. a. polypeptide that promotes GH release.

(5) Growth hormone inhibiting hormone (GHIH) It is a 14 or 28 a. a. polypeptide that slows the secretion of two pituitary hormones, GH and TSH. It depresses the secretion of several others systemic hormones and peptides produced in peripheral endocrine and non-endocrine glands.

(6) Prolactin releasing factor (PRF) This is a 31 amino acids (a. a.) polypeptide that is present in hypophyseoportal vessel blood in sufficient concentration to promotes PRL release.

(7) Prolactin inhibitory factor (PIF) It inhibits PRL secretion. Dopamine is the most important PIF that is present in hypophyseoportal vessel blood in sufficient concentration to inhibit PRL release.

As it is clear from this list that most of the releasing hormones act on one or two classes of anterior pituitary cells. This permits higher central nervous system centers to directly influence the synthesis and release of pituitary hormones by modulating the activity of hypothalamic neurosecretory neurons. Several monoaminergic neuronal pathways that regulate the secretion of neurosecretory neurons have been described to act as the link between various brain center and hypothalamic control of the pituitary. It is through these neuronal connections that such stimuli as stress, environmental factors and certain drugs that act on the central nervous system can modulate the secretion of prolactin.

2.2 Anterior pituitary hormones

The anterior pituitary gland can secrete growth hormone (GH), adrenocorticotropic (ACTH), thyroid-stimulating hormone (TSH), luteinizing hormone (LH), follicle-stimulating hormone (FSH), lactotropes-prolactin (PRL) and melanophore stimulating hormone(MSH). Among them, TSH, ACTH, LH and FSH exert their principal effects by stimulating target glands, including thyroid gland, adrenal cortex, ovaries, testicles, and mammary glands, whose functions will be discussed in subsequent sections along with the target glands. In this section, GH and PRL will be introduced in details.

2.2.1 Growth hormone

Growth hormone is produced and released by the acidophil cells in anterior pituitary. It is a small protein molecule that contains 191 amino acids in a single chain and has a molecular weight of 22,005. Growth hormones from various species are different and show species specificity[1]. Growth hormone, in contrast to other hormones, does not function through a target gland but exerts its effects directly on all or almost all tissues of the body.

2.2.1.1 Physiological effects of growth hormone

(1) Effects on growth[2] In young animals in which the epiphyses of the long bones have not yet united with the shafts, further growth is inhibited by hypophysectomy but can still be enhanced by daily injections of growth hormone. Growth hormone accelerates chondrogenesis, and as the cartilaginous epiphysial plates widen, they lay down more bone matrix at the ends of long bones. In this way, stature is increased, and prolonged treatment with growth hormone leads to gigantism. When growth hormone secretion is low in young child, dwarfism is produced[3]. When the bony fusion occurs between the shaft and the epiphysis at each end, linear growth is no longer possible, and growth hormone produces the pattern of bone and soft tissue deformities known in humans as acromegaly[4].

(2) Effects on metabolism[5] Aside from its general effect in causing growth, growth hormone has multiple specific metabolic effects. ① Growth hormone promotes protein deposition in tissues[6] The precise mechanisms by which growth hormone increases protein deposition are not known. ② Growth hormone enhances fat utilization for energy[7]. Growth hormone can cause the release of fatty acids from adipose tissue and enhance the conversion of fatty acids to acetyl coenzyme A (acetyl–CoA) and its subsequent utilization for energy. ③ Growth hormone decreases carbohydrate utilization[8] Growth hormone causes multiple effects that influence carbohydrate metabolism, including decreased glucose uptake in tissues such as skeletal muscle and fat, increased glucose production by the liver and increased insulin secretion[9].

2.2.1.2 Regulation of growth hormone secretion

(1) Hypothalamic control of growth hormone secretion[10]. The secretion of growth hormone is controlled via the hypothalamus. The hypothalamus secretes growth hormone releas-

---

[1] 生长激素由垂体前叶的嗜酸细胞分泌，具有显著的种属差异性。人生长激素由 191 个氨基酸残基组成，分子量约为 22KD。

[2] 促进生长。

[3] 幼儿期生长激素应用过多导致巨人症，而生长激素分泌过少患侏儒症。

[4] 骺发生骨性融合，长骨不再生长，而短骨及其软组织异常生长，出现肢端肥大症。

[5] 对代谢的影响。

[6] 生长激素促进蛋白质在组织沉积。

[7] 生长激素促进脂肪转变成能量。

[8] 生长激素降低了碳水化合物的代谢。

[9] 生长激素引起碳水化合代谢改变主要包括以下机制：①降低骨骼肌及脂肪组织对葡萄糖的吸收；②增强了肝脏的糖异生；③促进胰岛素的分泌。

[10] 下丘脑调控生长激素的分泌。

ing hormone (GHRH) and the growth hormone inhibiting hormone (GHIH), into the portal hypophysial blood, and control growth hormone secretion [1]. Growth hormone secretion is subject to negative feedback control. Growth hormone increases circulating IGF-Ⅰ, and IGF-Ⅰ in turn exerts a direct inhibitory action on growth hormone secretion from the pituitary [2].

(2) Stimuli affecting growth hormone secretion [3] The stimuli that increase growth hormone secretion fall into three general categories: conditions such as hypoglycemia and fasting in which there is an actual or threatened decrease in the substrate for energy production in the cells; conditions in which there are increased amounts of certain amino acids in the plasma; and stressful stimuli [4]. Although the growth hormone responses to the other stimuli are relatively reproducible, they may vary from individual to individual. A spike in growth hormone secretion occurs with considerable regularity upon going to sleep, but the significance of the association between growth hormone and sleep is an enigma [5]. Growth hormone secretion is increased in subjects during normal REM sleep.

Glucose infusions lower plasma growth hormone levels and inhibit the response to exercise. The increase produced by 2-deoxyglucose is presumably due to intracellular glucose deficiency, since this compound blocks the catabolism of glucose 6-phosphate. Sex hormones, particularly estrogens, increase growth hormone responses to provocative stimuli such as arginine and insulin. Growth hormone secretion can also be increased by L-dopa. GH secretion is inhibited by cortisol, FFA, and medroxyprogesterone.

2.2.2 Prolactin

Prolactin (PRL) contains 199 amino acids with molecular weight about 22,000. The normal plasma prolactin concentration is approximately 5 ng/mL in men and 8 ng/mL in women.

2.2.2.1 Physiological effects of prolactin

Prolactin causes milk secretion from the breast after estrogen and progesterone priming [6]. Its effect on the breast involves increased action of mRNA and increased production of casein and lactalbumin. However, the action of the hormone is not exerted on the cell nucleus and is prevented by inhibitors of microtubules.

Prolactin also inhibits the effects of gonadotropins, possibly by an action at the level of the ovary, It prevents ovulation in lactating women [7]. The function of prolactin in normal

[1] 生长激素的分泌受下丘脑生长激素释放激素及生长激素释放抑制激素的双重调控。

[2] 生长激素的分泌受到负反馈调节。生长激素促进血液胰岛素样生长因子释放，而胰岛素样生长因子直接抑制腺垂体分泌生长激素。

[3] 刺激引起生长激素的分泌。

[4] 低血糖、血液中氨基酸增多、应激刺激等均能促进生长激素的分泌。

[5] 生长激素分泌的峰值出现在睡眠期，但是生长激素与睡眠关联的意义仍然不清楚。

[6] 催乳素在雌激素与孕激素共同作用下，促进乳腺分泌乳汁。

[7] 催促乳素抑制促性腺激素的对卵巢的作用，从而防止哺乳期女性排卵。

males is unsettled, but excess prolactin secreted by tumors causes impotence.

2.2.2.2 Regulation of prolactin secretion

Prolactin secretion is regulated by the hypothalamus. The effect of the hypothalamic prolactin–inhibitory hormone (PIH) dopamine is normally greater than the effects of the various hypothalamic peptides with prolactin–releasing activity[1]. In human prolactin secretion is increased by exercise, surgical and psychologic stresses, and stimulation of the nipple. Secretion is increased during pregnancy, reaching a peak at the time of parturition. After delivery, the plasma concentration falls to nonpregnant levels in about 8 days. Suckling produces a prompt increase in secretion. L–Dopa decreases prolactin secretion by increasing the formation of dopamine. TRH stimulates the secretion of prolactin in addition to TSH, and there are additional prolactin–releasing polypeptides in hypothalamic tissue. Estrogens produce a slowly developing increase in prolactin secretion as a result of a direct action on the lactotropes.

2.2.3 Melanophore stimulating hormone

Melanophore stimulating hormone (MSH) is formed in the intermediate–lobe cells, including α–MSH, β–MSH and γ–MSH.

In mammals, there are melanocytes, which contain melanosomes and synthesize melanins. The melanocytes then transfer the melanosomes to skin cells (keratinocytes) in hair follicles and other portions of the skin. This accounts for the pigmentation of hair and skin. The melanocytes contain melanotropin receptors that have been cloned, and treatment with MSHs accelerates melanin synthesis, causing readily detectable darkening of the skin in humans in 24 hours.

MRF and MIF secreted by hypothalamus control the secretion of MSH, and normally the action of MIF is prior to that of MRF.

Section 3 Thyroid Hormones

The thyroid gland is one of the largest of the endocrine glands, normally weighing 15 to 20 grams in adults. The thyroid gland maintains the level of metabolism in the tissues that is optimal for their normal function by producing, in its follicular cells, two major thyroid hormones: triiodothyronine (T_3)[2], and tetraiodothyronine (T_4)[3]. Thyroid hormones are essential for normal neural development, linear bone growth, and proper sexual maturation[4].

[1] 催乳素的分泌受下丘脑调节，正常情况下，下丘脑催乳素抑制因子的抑制调控作用明显强于催乳素释放因子的作用。

[2] 三碘甲腺原氨酸。

[3] 四碘甲腺原氨酸。

[4] 甲状腺激素对神经系统发育、骨骼生长及性成熟发挥重要作用。

1 Synthesis and metabolism of thyroid hormones

To form normal quantities of thyroxine, about 50 milligrams of ingested iodine in the form of iodides are required each year, or about 1 mg/week.

1.1 Synthesis of thyroid hormones

The synthesis in the thyroid gland takes place in the following way (Figure 9–4):

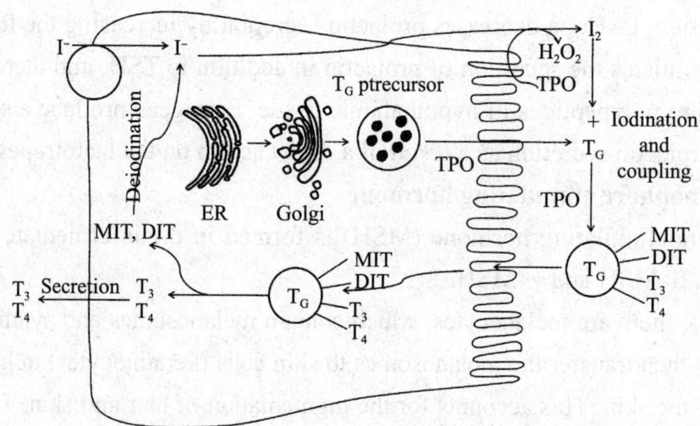

MIT, monoiodotyrosine; DIT, diiodotyrosine; T_3, triiodothyronine;

T_4, thyroxine; TG, thyroglobulin; TPO: thyroid peroxidase.

Figure 9–4 Thyroid hormones formation and thyroid hormones secretion

1.1.1 Iodide trapping of follicular cells [1]

Dietary iodine (I_2) is reduced to iodide (I^-) in the gastrointestinal tract, then it is rapidly absorbed and circulates in the form of iodide. The basal membrane of the follicular cells in the thyroid gland has the specific ability to pump the iodide actively to the interior of the cell. This is called iodide trapping. Iodide is transported into the cell against an electrochemical gradient-by Na^+–I^- symporter. The Na^+–I^-symporter is linked to a Na^+–K^+ pump, which requires energy in the form of oxidative phosphorylation (ATP). The rate of iodide trapping by the thyroid is influenced by several factors, the most important being the concentration of TSH.

1.1.2 Oxidation of the iodide ion [2]

Iodide is instantly activated with hydrogen peroxide as oxidant by a thyroid peroxidase (TPO) [3] to an oxidized form of iodine, either nascent iodine (I^0) or I_3^-, that is then capable of combining directly with the amino acid tyrosine at the colloid surface of the apical membrane.

---

[1] 甲状腺滤泡摄碘。

[2] 碘离子的氧化。

[3] 甲状腺过氧化物酶。

The TPO is either located in the apical membrane of the cell or attached to it.

1.1.3 Iodination of tyrosine [1]

The rough endoplasmic reticulum synthesizes a large storage molecule called thyroglobulin. Iodide–free thyroglobulin is transported in vesicles to the apical membrane, where they fuse with the membrane and finally release thyroglobulin at the apical membrane. At the apical membrane the oxidised iodide is attached to the tyrosine units in thyroglobulin at one or two positions, forming the hormone precursors mono–iodotyrosine (MIT), and di–iodotyrosine (DIT), respectively. This and the following reactions are dependent on TPO in the presence of hydrogen peroxide both located at the apical membrane.

1.1.4 Coupling [2]

As MIT couples to DIT, it produces tri–iodothyronine (3,5, 3'–T_3), whereas two DIT molecules form tetra–iodothyronine (T_4). These two molecules are the two thyroid hormones. Small amounts of the inactive reverse T3 (3, 3', 5'– T_3) is also synthesized.

1.2 Metabolism of thyroid hormones

1.2.1 Secretion

The human thyroid secretes about 80 μg (103 nmol) of T_4, 4μg (7 nmol) of T_3, however, MIT and DIT are not secreted. The thyroid cells ingest colloid by endocytosis. This chewing up at the edge of the colloid produces the reabsorption lacunae seen in active glands. In the cells, the globules of colloid merge with lysosomes. The peptide bonds between the iodinated residues and the thyroglobulin are broken by proteases in the lysosomes, and T_4, T_3, DIT, and MIT are liberated into the cytoplasm. The iodinated tyrosines are deiodinated by a microsomal iodotyrosine deiodinase enzyme. This enzyme does not attack iodinated thyronines, and T_4 and T_3 pass into the circulation. The iodine liberated by deiodination of MIT and DIT is reutilized in the gland and normally provides about twice as much iodide for hormone synthesis as the iodide pump does.

1.2.2 Transportation

On entering the blood, over 99 % of the T_4 and T_3 combines immediately with several of the plasma proteins, they combine mainly with thyroxine–binding globulin and much less so with thyroxine–binding prealbumin and albumin [3]. The free thyroid hormones in plasma are in equilibrium with the protein–bound thyroid hormones in plasma and in tissues. Free thyroid hormones are added to the circulating pool by the thyroid. It is the free thyroid hormones in

---

[1] 酪氨酸的碘化。

[2] 缩合。

[3] T_3、T_4 释放入血之后，99% 以上与血浆中的转运蛋白结合。其中，最重要转运蛋白是甲状腺转运蛋白，其次为甲状腺结合球蛋白与白蛋白。

plasma that are physiologically active.

1.2.3 Elimination

The T_3 is eliminated quickly (half-life: 24 hours), because it has the lowest affinity of plasma-binding protein. The T_4 molecule has a biological half-life of 7 days[1]. T_4 is likely to be a prohormone, which is deiodinased by monodeiodinase to the more potent T_3 just before it is used in the cells. Thus T_3 is probably the final active hormone, although it is present only in a very low concentration. Most of the daily T_4 released from the thyroid gland undergoes deiodination, with subsequent deamination and decarboxylation. Some of the hormone molecules are coupled to sulphate and glucuronic acid in the liver and are excreted in the bile. In the intestine most of the coupled molecules are hydrolysed, and the hormones are reabsorbed by the blood, whereby they reach hepar again (the enterohepatic circuit).

2 Physiological functions of the thyroid hormones

2.1 Physiological functions

2.1.1 Calorigenic action[2]

The thyroid hormones increase the metabolic activities of almost all the tissues of the body. The basal metabolic rate can increase to 60% to 100% above normal, when large quantities of the hormones are secreted.

Some of the calorigenic effect of thyroid hormone is due to metabolism of the fatty acids they mobilize. In addition, thyroid hormones increase the activity of the membrane-bound Na^+-K^+ ATPase in many tissues. Large doses of thyroid hormones cause enough extra heat production to lead to a slight rise in body temperature, which in turn activates heat-dissipating mechanisms. And deficiency of thyroid hormone secretion caused decreased heat production, leading to temperature decrease.

2.1.2 Effects of substance metabolism

2.1.2.1 Effects on protein metabolism

The physiological dose of thyroid hormones are to activate nuclear transcription of large numbers of genes. Therefore, in virtually all cells of the body, great numbers of protein enzymes, structural proteins, transport proteins, and other substances are synthesized. The net result is generalized increase in functional activity throughout the body[3].

In hypothyroidism, insufficient secretion of T_3 and T_4 leads to reduced protein synthesis. The skin normally contains a variety of proteins combined with polysaccharides, hyaluronic

[1] 血浆中 T_3 的半衰期约为 1 天，T_4 的半衰期约为 7 天。

[2] 产热效应。

[3] 生理水平的甲状腺激素激活基因的转录，从而合成大量的酶、结构蛋白、运输蛋白等其他物质，最终效应促进机体的功能活动。

acid, and chondroitin sulfuric acid. These complexes accumulate, promoting water retention and the characteristic puffiness of the skin (myxedema) [1].

2.1.2.2 Stimulation of carbohydrate metabolism

Thyroid hormone increases the rate of absorption of glucose from the gastrointestinal tract [2]. In a patient with hyperthyroidism, therefore, the plasma glucose level rises rapidly after a carbohydrate meal, sometimes exceeding the renal threshold. However, it falls again at a rapid rate.

2.1.2.3 Effects on cholesterol metabolism

Thyroid hormones lower circulating cholesterol levels [3]. The plasma cholesterol level drops before the metabolic rate rises, which indicates that this action is independent of the stimulation of O_2 consumption. The decrease in plasma cholesterol concentration is due to increased formation of LDL receptors in the liver, resulting in increased hepatic removal of cholesterol from the circulation.

2.1.3 Effects on growth

Thyroid hormones are essential for normal growth and skeletal maturation[4]. In hypothyroid children, bone growth is slowed and epiphysial closure delayed. In the absence of thyroid hormone, growth hormone secretion is also depressed, and thyroid hormones potentiate the effect of growth hormone on the tissues.

Cretinism refers to a clinical condition caused by congenital hypothyroidism or infantile iodide deficiency [5]. And supply enough iodine in pregnancy can prevent cretinism. Supplement of thyroid hormones as soon as possible is therapy for cretinism.

2.1.4 Effects on the nervous system

Thyroid hormones can promote the proliferation and differentiation in the immature brain tissues, so intelligence in cretinism is low [6]. Thyroid hormones can also increase the rapidity of cerebration; conversely, lack of thyroid hormones decrease this function [7]. The hyperthyroid individual is likely to have extreme nervousness and many psychoneurotic tendencies, such as anxiety complexes, extreme worry, and paranoia.

2.1.5 Effects on the cardiovascular system

Thyroid hormones increase the number and affinity of β-adrenergic receptors in the heart

[1] 皮肤中含有多聚糖、透明质酸、软骨素硫酸等大量蛋白质，甲状腺功能低下时，这些蛋白质在组织中沉积，形成黏液性水肿。

[2] 甲状腺激素促进小肠黏膜对葡萄糖的吸收。

[3] 甲状腺激素能够降低血浆中胆固醇浓度。

[4] 甲状腺激素是维持正常生长发育和骨成熟不可缺少的激素。

[5] 先天性甲状腺功能低下或婴幼儿碘缺乏会导致克汀病。

[6] 甲状腺激素促进神经系统的生长和分化，所以克汀病表现为智力发育障碍。

[7] 甲状腺激素能够提高大脑的兴奋性，相反，甲状腺激素功能低下大脑的兴奋性降低。

and consequently increase its sensitivity to the inotropic and chronotropic effects of catecholamines.

3 Control of thyroid hormone secretion

3.1 Hypothalamic–pituitary–thyroid axis

Thyroid hormone secretion is controlled by hypothalamic–pituitary–thyroid axis (Figure 9–5).

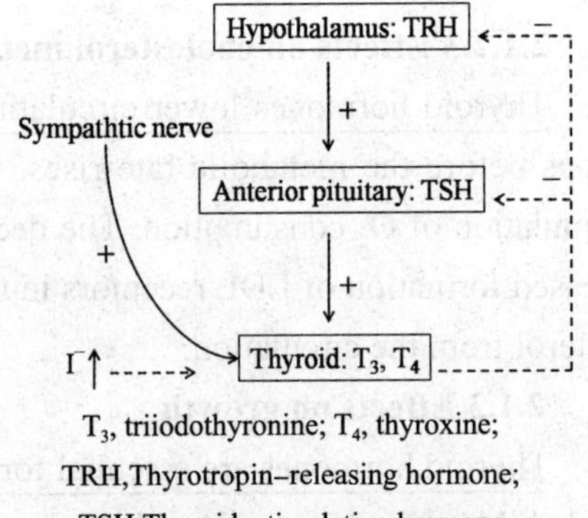

T_3, triiodothyronine; T_4, thyroxine;
TRH,Thyrotropin–releasing hormone;
TSH,Thyroid–stimulating hormone

Figure 9–5 Regulation of thyroid secretion

3.1.1 Control by TSH

TSH is the major hormone for the regulation of thyroid: ① The TSH stimulates not only the release of performed thyroid hormone, but also the synthesis of thyroid hormone[1]. The effect on synthesis includes increasing in iodide pump activity, in peroxidase activity and organification, and in coupling of iodotyrosine to form T_4 and T_3; ② It can also increase the growth of the entire gland[2].

The synthesis and secretion of TSH is under positive control of the hypothalamic hormone TRH[3]. This tripeptide binds to specific receptors on the thyrotrophic cells and stimulates both synthesis and secretion of TSH. TRH neurons is controlled by other part of central nervous system, environment factors can affect on the TRH neurons, e. g. , cold stimulus can greatly increase the secretion of TRH, thus increasing the secretion of TSH and thyroid hormone.

3.1.2 Negative effect of thyroid hormone on TSH

Thyroid hormone has a negative effect on TSH secretion[4]. Increased thyroid hormone in the body fluids decreases secretion of TSH by the anterior pituitary. When the rate of thyroid hormone secretion rises to about 1.75 times normal, the rate of TSH secretion falls essentially to zero. in In contrast to, decreased thyroid hormone in the body fluids increases secretion of TSH by the anterior pituitary.

3.2 Autoregulation

Autoregulatory response is demonstrable when the level of TSH is constant or insuffi-

[1] 促甲状腺激素是调节甲状腺功能的主要激素，不仅能促进甲状腺激素的释放，也能促进甲状腺激素的合成。

[2] TSH 能促进甲状腺的增生。

[3] 下丘脑促甲状腺激素释放激素调节着腺垂体促甲状腺激素的合成和分泌。

[4] 甲状腺激素对促甲状腺激素具有负反馈调节作用。

cient. The iodide transport is associated with iodine intake. When intake is too more, the inhibition of iodide transport occur, if intake insufficient the inhibition is abolished. It appears that the autoregulatory mechanisms seek to maintain constancy of thyroid hormone store, in contrast to the classic feedback control via TSH, which seeks to maintain the level of the plasma or tissue concentration of thyroid hormone [1].

3.3 Automatic nervous system

When sympathetic nerve excited, the synthesis and secretion of thyroid hormone increase and parasympathetic nerve inhibit the thyroid hormones [2]. Besides, estrogen, GH and adrenocorticoids can all affect the secretion of T_3, T_4.

Section 4 Hormones regulating calcium and phosphorus metabolism

1 Parathyroid hormone

Parathyroid hormone (PTH) is a polypeptide composed of 84 amino acids that is secreted by the chief cell of the parathyroid gland. Two primary target tissues for PTH are the bone and the kidneys, where PTH acts to increase the plasma calcium concentration. The actions of PTH are mediated by the binding of PTH to specific receptors on the target cells and the subsequent stimulation of adenylatecyclase activity and cAMP production.

1.1 Physiological functions of Parathyroid hormone

1.1.1 Actions on the bone

PTH accelerates osteolysis thereby mobilizing calcium and phosphate. The effect of PTH on bone develops in two phases. The earlier phase is more rapid, and a significant plasma calcium increase is seen in minutes; the later phase is slower and requires at least 12 ~ 14 hours of exposure to PTH, but the increase in plasma calcium is sustained for a longer time [3]. The osteocyte, through its cytoplasmic processes in the canalicular system, has a larger surface area in contact with fluid that bathe calcium crystals and it may function as a calcium pump, transporting calcium from the periosteocytic space of the bone into blood in response to PTH. Osteoclast, on the other hand, may mediate the slower but sustained mobilization of calcium

[1] 自身调节主要维持甲状腺激素储存量的相对稳定，而反馈调节主要维持血浆或组织中甲状腺激素浓度的相对稳定。

[2] 当交感神经兴奋，甲状腺激素的合成和分泌增加，副交感神经兴奋，甲状腺激素的合成和分泌减少。

[3] 甲状旁腺激素升高血钙的快速效应在数分钟内发生，延迟效应在 12 ~ 14 小时产生，但升高血钙的持续时间长。

through active resorption.

1.1.2 Actions on the kidneys

PTH acts on the kidneys to increase resorption of calcium in the distal tubules and the collecting tubes. PTH also increases phosphate excretion by inhibiting their resorption in the proximal tubules [1]. The consequences of this action have several indirect effects on calcium homeostasis. The most important effect of phosphaturia is stimulation of enzymes in the renal tubular cells that convert vitamin D to the biologically active form $1,25(OH)_2D_3$. This results in the $1,25(OH)_2D_3$ mediated increase in intestinal absorption of calcium and further increase in bone resorption.

1.1.3 Actions on the gut

The PTH action on the gut is indirect. PTH stimulates the renal production of biologically active vitamin D (1,25–dihydroxy–vitamin D, calcitriol), which stimulates the active absorption of Ca^{2+} and phosphate across the gut mucosa, and potentiates the action of PTH on bone resorption [2].

1.2 Regulation of PTH

PTH is regulated by plasma calcium concentration. When the circulating Ca^{2+} level falls, the parathyroid cells are stimulated to release PTH; when Ca^{2+} rises above the equilibrium level, the parathyroid cells are inhibited. Besides, the increase of plasma phosphorus or the secretion of calcitonin, can all decrease the calcium level thus increasing the secretion of PTH.

2 Calcitonin

Calcitonin (CT) is a 32 amino acids polypeptide. It is synthesized and secreted by the parafollicular cells (C cells) found interspersed between individual follicles of the mammalian thyroid gland.

2.1 Physiological functions of calcitonin

The most obvious effect of calcitonin is inhibition of the absorptive activities of the osteoclasts, and thereby lowers the circulatory calcium and phosphate level [3]. This action is direct and is apparently due to inhibition of the calcium permeability of osteoblasts and osteoclasts. Calcitonin also decreases osteoclast activity and number. In adults, the hormone is relatively inactive, and its regulatory importance in maintenance of calcium homeostasis has been questioned. However, it is more active in young individuals and may play a role in skeletal de-

---

[1] 甲状旁腺激素促进远端小管和集合管对钙的重吸收，通过抑制近端小管对磷的重吸收而增加磷的排泄。

[2] 甲状旁腺激素促进 1,25（OH）$_2$VitD$_3$ 的生成，而 1,25（OH）$_2$VitD$_3$ 促进小肠对钙的吸收。

[3] 降钙素主要通过抑制破骨细胞骨吸收，降低血钙和血磷水平。

velopment.

Additional actions include increasing sodium, calcium and phosphate excretion in the urine and decreasing gastric acid secretion. Since gastrointestinal hormones stimulate calcitonin secretion and calcitonin inhibits gastric acid secretion, it has been suggested that it protects against postprandial hypercalcemia.

2.2 Regulation of calcitonin

The primary stimulus for calcitonin secretion is increased plasma calcium ion concentration [1]. When plasma Ca^{2+} is higher than 45 mmol/L, secretion increases along with the increase of plasma calcium; if lower than 45 mmol/l, calcitonin decreases. Besides, Vitamin D_3 can be hydroxylated in liver and kidney to form $1,25(OH)_2D_3$. This substance also participates in the metabolism of calcium and phosphours.

3 Vitamin D_3

Several compounds derived from sterols belong to the vitamin D family, and they all perform more or less the same functions. Vitamin D_3 (also called cholecalciferol) is the most important of these and is formed in the skin as a result of irradiation of 7–dehydrocholesterol, a substance normally in the skin, by ultraviolet rays from the sun. Therefore, appropriate exposure to the sun prevents vitamin D deficiency.

The first step in the activation of cholecalciferol is to convert it to 25–hydroxycholecalciferol (25–OH–D) by 25–hydroxylase in the liver. The process is a limited one, because the 25–hydroxycholecalciferol has a feedback inhibitory effect on the conversion reactions.

The second step in the activation of cholecalciferol is to convert 25–hydroxy– cholecalciferol to 1,25–dihydroxycholecalciferol by 1α–hydroxylase in the proximal tubules of the kidneys. 1,25–dihydroxycholecalciferol is by far the most active form of vitamin D. Therefore, in the absence of the kidneys, vitamin D loses almost all its effectiveness.

3.1 Physiological functions of vitamin D

The active form of vitamin D, 1,25–dihydroxycholecalciferol, has several effects on the intestines, kidneys, and bones that increase absorption of calcium and phosphate into the extracellular fluid and contribute to feedback regulation of these substances.

(1)1,25–dihydroxycholecalciferol itself functions as a type of 'hormone' to promote intestinal absorption of calcium and phosphate flux through the gastrointestinal epithelium [2]. It does this principally by increasing formations of calcium–binding proteins in the intestinal epithelial cells, calcium–stimulated ATPases in the brush border and alkaline phosphatases in the

[1] 血钙浓度增加是刺激降钙素分泌的主要因素。

[2] 1,25（OH）$_2$VitD$_3$ 促进小肠黏膜上皮对钙、磷的吸收。

epithelial cells.

(2)Vitamin D also increases calcium and phosphate absorption by the epithelial cells of the renal tubules, thereby tending to decrease excretion of these substances in the urine [1]. However, this is a weak effect and probably not the major importance in regulating the extracellular fluid concentration of these substance.

(3)Vitamin D plays important roles in both absorption and bone deposition [2]. The administration of extreme quantities of vitamin D causes absorption of bone. In the absence of vitamin D, the effect of PTH in causing bone absorption is greatly reduced or even prevented, and the mechanism of this action of vitamin D is not known. Vitamin D in smaller quantities promotes bone calcification. One of the ways in which it does this is to increase calcium and phosphate absorption from the intestine. However, even in the absence of such increase, it enhances the mineralization of bone and again, the mechanism of the effect is unknown.

Vitamin D deficiency causes rickets in children and osteomalacia in adults [3]. The deficiency is caused by insufficient diet, inadequate absorption as in fat malabsorption, insufficient synthesis in the skin, or abnormal conversion to its potent form in the liver and kidneys.

3.2 Regulation of vitamin D

The formation of 25–dihydroxycholecalciferol does not appear to be stringently regulated. However, the formation of 1,25–dihydroxycholecalciferol in the kidneys, which is catalyzed by 1α–hydroxylase, is regulated in a feedback fashion by plasma Ca^{2+} and PO_4^{3-}. The formation is facilitated by PTH, and when the plasma Ca^{2+} level is low, PTH secretion is increased. When the plasma Ca^{2+} level is high, little 1,25–dihydroxycholccalciferol is produced, and the kidneys produce the relatively inactive metabolite 24,25–dihydroxycholecalciferol instead. This effect of Ca^{2+} on production of 1,25–dihydroxycholecalciferol is the mechanism that brings about adaptation of Ca^{2+} absorption from the intestine. The production of 1,25–dihydroxycholecalciferol is also increased by low and inhibited by high plasma PO_4^{3-} level, by a direct inhibitory effect of PO_4^{3-} on 1α–hydroxylase.

Section 5 Hormones secreted by the adrenal gland

The two adrenal glands lie at the superior poles of the two kidneys. Each gland is composed of an outer layer of striated cells (the cortex) and inner core (the medulla). Adrenal cortex secretes an entirely different group of hormones, called corticosteroids. (Mineral corticoids, glucocorticoids, and sex hormones) . The adrenal medulla is a part of the automatic nervous system and is a primary source of circulating catecholamines (adrenaline and noradrenaline)

---

[1] 1,25（OH）$_2$VitD$_3$ 促进肾小管上皮细胞对钙、磷的重吸收，从而使尿中的钙、磷排泄减少。

[2] 1,25（OH）$_2$VitD$_3$ 对骨吸收和骨沉积两方面都具有重要的作用。

[3] VitD 缺乏在儿童导致佝偻病，而在成人引起骨软化症。

1 Adrenocortical hormones

The adrenal cortex is composed of 3 distinct layers of cells: the outer layer (the zone glomerulosa), the middle layer (the zone fasciculata), and the inner layer (the zone reticularis). Each layer synthesizes and secrets a different steroid hormone and this is accomplished by differences in the enzymatic machinery that catalyzes the individual steps in steroid biosynthesis. The outer layer produces aldosterone, which acts on salt–transporting epithelia to lead to Nacl retention, K^+ loss, H^+ excretion and indirectly to water retention. It helps maintain extracellular volume and is regulated by the plasma K^+ levels and the renin–angiotensin system. The middle layer produces mainly cortisol in man. Cortisol helps to sustain blood sugar, blood pressure and products from stress. The inner layer produces androgen, which have minimal intrinsic biologic activity and must be converted to more potent compounds by peripheral tissues.

Aldosterone is called a 'mineralocorticoid' and cortisol called a 'glucocorticoid'. These terms are not precise, but they are continuous. A general term for both kinds of hormone is corticosteroid. Since aldosterone has been discussed and sex steroids will be discussed in chapter 10, only the glucocorticoids will be discussed here.

1.1 Physiological functions of glucocorticoid

At least 95% of the glucocorticoid activity of the adrenocortical secretions results from the secretion of cortisol, known also as hydrocortisone. In addition to this, a small but significant amount of glucocorticoid activity is provided by corticosterone.

1.1.1 Effect of glucocorticoid on carbohydrate metabolism

Glucocorticoid was discovered to increase the concentration of glucose in the blood[1]. This is caused by two different functions of glucocorticoid: glucocorticoid depresses utilization of glucose by the tissue cells, consequently, the glucose accumulates in the extracellular fluid instead of being utilized fully by the tissue cells[2]; glucocorticoid causes the liver cells to convert proteins and the glycerol portion of fats into glucose, a process called gluconeogenesis[3]. It is very important during starvation because it supplies a continual source of glucose in the blood even when the person is not ingesting glucose.

1.1.2 Effect of glucocorticoid on protein metabolism

One of the principal effects of glucocorticoid on the metabolic systems of the body is reduction of protein stores in essentially all body cells except those of the liver[4]. It does this by both decreased protein synthesis and increased catabolism of protein already in the cells. Both

[1] 糖皮质激素能够升高血液中葡萄糖的水平。

[2] 糖皮质激素使组织对葡萄糖的利用减少，导致血糖升高。

[3] 糖皮质激素诱导肝脏糖异生增强，使糖原增多，血糖升高。

[4] 糖皮质激素能促进除肝脏以外的全身其他组织细胞内蛋白质减少。

these effects may result from decreased amino acids transport into extrahepatic tissues. It also depresses the formation of RNA and subsequent protein synthesis in many extrahepatic tissues, especially in muscle and lymphoid tissue.

1.1.3 Effect of glucocorticoid on fat

It mobilizes fat from the fat depots in much the same manner that it mobilizes amino acids from the cells. This increases the concentration of free fatty acids in the plasma, which also increases their utilization for energy. Cortisol also seems to have a direct effect to enhance the oxidation of fatty acids in the cells[1]. It can also affect the distribution of fat, making fat accumulate on the face, shoulder and back but less in limbs[2], therefore, many people with excess cortisol secretion develop a peculiar type of obesity, with excess deposition of fat in the chest and head regions of the body, giving a buffalo–like torso and a rounded 'moon face'[3].

1.1.4 Effect of glucocorticoid on water metabolism

Glucocorticoid has a slight function of promoting the renal tubule to reabsorb Na^+ and excrete K^+, and it is helpful in water excretion by increasing glomerular plasma flow[4]. Adrenal insufficiency is characterized by inability to excrete a water load. The load is eventually excreted, but the excretion is so slow that there is danger of water intoxication. Only glucocorticoids repair this deficit.

1.1.5 Resistance to stress

Almost any type of stress, whether physical or neurogenic, causes an immediate and marked increase in ACTH secretion by the anterior pituitary gland, followed within minutes by greatly increased adrenocortical secretion of cortisol[5]. The rise is essential for survival. The reason that an elevated circulatory glucocorticoid level is essential for resisting stress remains for the most part unknown. The physiological benefit of increased glucocorticoid secretion may derive from its permissive action that allows other hormones to act more effectively. Most of the stressful stimuli that increase ACTH secretion also activate the sympathoadrenal medullary system, and part of the functions of the circulatory glucocorticoid may be the maintenance of vascular reactivity to catecholamines.

1.1.6 Effects on blood cells

Glucocorticoids increase the number neutrophils, platelets, and red blood cells[6]; Glu-

[1] 糖皮质激素导致血浆中游离脂肪酸的浓度增加，并增强游离脂肪酸的氧化供能，同时，它也加强了细胞内脂肪酸氧化功能。

[2] 糖皮质激素使体内脂肪重新分布，主要沉积在面部、肩部和背部，而四肢分解较强，储存较少。

[3] 满月脸。

[4] 糖皮质激素有较弱促进肾小管排钠保钾作用，此外，糖皮质激素还可增加肾小球血浆流量，有利于水的排出。

[5] 无论人体受到身体还是精神上的各种应激，腺垂体分泌的促肾上腺皮质激素的浓度增加，几分钟内糖皮质激素的分泌也大大增加。

[6] 糖皮质激素可增加血中红细胞、血小板和中性粒细胞的数量。

cocorticoids also lower the number of eosinophils and lymphocytes in the blood[1], this effect begins within a few minutes after the injection of cortisol and becomes marked within a few hours. Glucocorticoids decrease the circulating lymphocyte count and the size of the lymph nodes and thymus by inhibiting lymphocyte mitotic activity. They can reduce secretion of cytokines. The reduced secretion of cytokine leukin–2 (IL–2) leads to reduced proliferation of lymphocytes, and these cells undergo apoptosis.

1.1.7 Effect on cardiovascular system

Glucocorticoids can strengthen the effect of catecholamines on vascular muscles[2]. Catecholamines are much less active on vascular smooth muscle in the absence of glucocorticoids. This is the permissive reaction for glucocorticoid. It can also increase the contractility of cardiac muscles.

1.1.8 Other effects

Increase the sensitivity of parietal cells to vagus nerves and gastrin, increase the HCl and pepsinogen secretion, and inhibit the protein synthesis and connective tissue proliferation, so large dose of glucocorticoid can initiate an ulcer. Besides, it can increase the excitability, maintain the normal functions of central nervous system. It has anti–inflammation, anti–allergic, anti– intoxicant and anti–shock functions with large dose[3].

1.2 Regulation of glucocorticoid secretion

The glucocorticoid secretion is regulated by feedback mechanisms (Figure 9–6).

Secretion of glucocorticoid is controlled almost entirely by ACTH secreted by the anterior pituitary gland[4]. This hormone, also called corticotrophin or adrenocorticotropin, is derived from a larger precursor polypeptide synthesized in corticotroph cells of the anterior pituitary. The major hypothalamic compound that stimulates synthesis and secretion of ATCH is CRH[5], which is produced by hypophysiotrophic neurons located in anterior portions of the paraventricular nucleus of the hypothalamus. These neurosecretory neurons receive multiple inputs from higher centers of the brain that can stimulate the release of CRH into the hypophyseal portal vessels. Other hy-

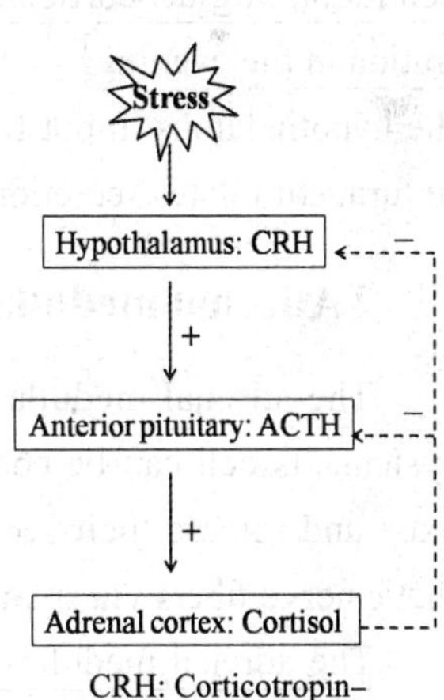

CRH: Corticotropin–releasing hormone; ACTH: Adrenocorticotropic hormone

Figure 9–6 Feedback control of the secretion of cortisol

[1] 糖皮质激素可减少淋巴细胞和嗜酸性粒细胞的数量。

[2] 糖皮质激素能够增加儿茶酚胺类物质对血管平滑肌的收缩功能。

[3] 大剂量应用糖皮质激素产生抗炎、抗过敏、抗病毒、抗休克的药理作用。

[4] 糖皮质激素的分泌主要受 ACTH 的调控。

[5] ACTH 的分泌受下丘脑 CRH 的调控。

pothalamic hormones that have been shown to stimulate ACTH secretion include vasopressin and angiotensin II. The role of these compounds in the normal regulation of ACTH secretion remains to be established.

Glucocorticoids have direct negative feedback effects on hypothalamus to decrease the formation of CRF and the anterior pituitary gland to decrease the formation of ACTH[1]. Both of these feedbacks help regulate the plasma concentration of glucocorticoids.

Glucocorticoids suppress pituitary ACTH synthesis and secretion through long–loop feedback. The mechanism by which glucocorticoid suppresses ACTH secretion appears to involve glucocorticoid receptors located within the corticotroph since glucocorticoid has been shown to suppress ACTH secretion in dispersed pituitary cells in culture. Glucocorticoid has also been reported to inhibit CRH secretion by the hypothalamus, although this is still a subject of controversy. Lastly ACTH directly inhibits the release of CRH through a short–loop feedback probably as a result of retrograde flow of blood in the hypophyseal portal system.

Secretion of the ACTH is episodic and this pulsatile release is also in other pituitary hormones. The half–life of the circulating ACTH is 20 minutes[2], pulses of ACTH secretion occur every 20 to 30 minutes and these smaller secretary pulses are superimposed on the larger fluctuations in serum ACTH levels that are due to circadian rhythms. In man the maximal concentration of glucocorticoid in the blood occurs in the early morning, with the minimal concentration in the evening[3]. The source of the rhythm appears to be in suprachiasmatic nucleus of the hypothalamus. Input from hypothalamus is responsible for cyclic increase in CRH, which, in turn, stimulates secretion of ACTH and glucocorticoid.

2 Adrenal medulla hormones

The adrenal medulla is functional and embryological part of the sympathetic–nervous system. Its cell can be considered as postganglionic sympathetic cells, which have lost their axon and release their secretions into the blood. They are supplied by preganglionic sympathetic nerve fibers via splanchnic nerves.

The adrenal medulla secretes two physiologically active catecholamines–adrenaline (epinephrine) and noradrenaline (norepinephrine)[4].

2.1 Actions of adrenaline and noradrenaline

The physiological actions of adrenaline and noradrenaline cannot be considered in isolation because their release is invariably associated with activity in the sympathetic nervous

[1] 糖皮质激素对下丘脑 CRH 和腺垂体 ACTH 分泌具有反馈调控作用。

[2] ACTH 的半衰期是 20 分钟。

[3] 糖皮质激素的分泌呈日夜节律性，清晨进入分泌高峰，入睡后分泌逐渐减少。

[4] 肾上腺髓质分泌儿茶酚胺，即肾上腺素和去甲肾上腺素。

system as a whole. Adrenaline and noradrenaline are almost always released by the adrenal medullae at the same time that the different organs are stimulated directly by generalized sympathetic activation. Thus, they are called sympathoadrenomedullary system [1].

The metabolic effects include breakdown of hepatic glycogen (glycogenolysis), breakdown of fat store (lipolysis) and increased heat production and oxygen consumption by many tissues. They can augment the cardiac output, constrict the vessels and increase myocardial contractility. Besides, catecholamine has a number of actions on motility and secretion of the alimentary tract. Insulin release is inhibited by an effect of catecholamines. Furthermore, they have a number of important effects on the CNS to increase its excitability.

Emergency reaction [2] hypothesis of Cannon: The concerted discharge of the sympathetic system and the associated stimulation of adrenomedullary secretion serve to produce in an animal a complex emergency response which is well suited to prepare it for fight or flight. Thus the blood pressure and cardiac output increase and blood is diverted to skeletal muscle. Glycogenolysis and lipolysis help provide substrate for muscle metabolism. Brochodilaltion and respiratory stimulation increase respiratory gas exchange. The spleen contracts and effectively transfuses RBC -rich additional blood into the general circulation. It should be noted that the sympathetic discharge is associated with stimulation of the pituitary adrenocortical axis.

2.2 Control of adrenomedullary secretion

The adrenal medulla probably has no resting secretion but can be provoked to release catecholamines by sympathetic nerve in response to a variety of stressful circumstances. Released adrenaline and noradrenaline are inactivated extremely rapidly and their half-life is only 20 seconds. Either the hormones are removed from the circulation by uptake into sympathetic nerve terminals or they are broken down within the blood and tissues.

Section 6 Insulin and glucagon

Pancreatic islets are the cell mass distributed in the pancreas. The pancreatic islets contain three major types of cells, A, B, and D cells, which are distinguished from one another by their morphological and staining characteristics. The B cells, constituting about 60% of all the cells of the islets, lie mainly in the middle of each islet and secrete insulin. The A cells, about 25% of the total, secrete glucagon. And the D cells, about 10% of the total, secrete somatostatin [3]. In addition, at least one other type of cell, the PP cell, is present in small numbers in the islets and secretes a hormone of uncertain function called pancreatic polypeptide. Among them, insulin and glucagon are more important.

---

[1] 肾上腺髓质激素的作用与交感神经密切联系，难以分开，两者组成交感 - 肾上腺髓质系统。

[2] 应急反应。

[3] 胰岛 B 细胞分泌胰岛素、A 细胞分泌胰高血糖素、D 细胞分泌生长抑素。

1 Insulin

Insulin is the major factor stimulating energy storage and anabolic reactions in the body[1]. Pre–proinsulin is the precursor of insulin. When pre–proinsulin reaches the endoplasmic reticulum, enzymes separate the molecule from the signal molecule to form proinsulin. In the Golgi apparatus enzymes cleave proinsulin to insulin (51 amino acids in two chains: A and B) and the C peptide (Connecting peptide). They are wrapped in the same secretion granule, and expelled from the cell by exocytosis. When the secretory granules release proinsulin to the portal blood and later the extracellular fluid volume, connecting peptide (C–peptide) and two amino acids breaks off. The split products are carried to the liver, where half of the insulin molecules are degraded and extracted. The degradation products are broken down and eliminated by the kidney. The kidneys only eliminate C–peptide and its rate of production reflects the rate of insulin secretion.

1.1 Action mechanism of insulin

To initiate its effects on target cells, insulin first binds with and activates a membrane receptor protein[2]. It is the activated receptor, not the insulin, that causes the subsequent effects.

The insulin receptor is a tetrameric protein complex with two α–subunits extracellularly, and two β–subunits traversing the membrane of target cells. The insulin binds with the α–subunits on the outside of the cell, but because of the linkages with the β–subunits, the portions of the protruding into cell become auto–phosphorylated. This makes them become an activated enzyme, a local tyrosine kinase, which in turn causes phosphorylation of multiple other intracellular enzymes. The net effect is to activate some of these enzymes while inactivating others. In this way, insulin directs the intracellular metabolic machinery to produce the desired effects on carbohydrate, fat, and protein metabolism. Finally, the insulin–receptor complex is internalized by the cell, insulin is broken down and the insulin–receptor recycles to the cell surface for further use.

1.2 Physiological functions of insulin

1.2.1 Effect of insulin on carbohydrate metabolism

Insulin can reduce the blood glucose concentration because it can cause rapid uptake and use of glucose by almost all tissues of the body, but especially by the muscles, adipose tissue, and liver[3]. And insulin inhibits the gluconeogenesis from glycogenic amino acids in the liv-

[1] 胰岛素是体内能量储存和合成代谢反应的主要因素。

[2] 胰岛素对靶细胞的调节效应主要通过与靶细胞膜上胰岛素受体结合而发挥作用。

[3] 胰岛素可促进各组织细胞（尤其是肌肉、脂肪组织以及肝脏）摄取血液中的葡萄糖，并加速葡萄糖在细胞内的氧化，从而降低血糖浓度。

er[1]. If insulin secretes greatly, it leads to coma or shock. And insulin lacking leads to diabetes.

1.2.2 Effect of insulin on proteins metabolism

Insulin promotes the accumulation of protein in muscle, liver and other cells, by stimulating the uphill transport of many amino acids into cells, by stimulating the incorporation of amino acids into protein through an effect at the translational level and by retarding the degradation of tissue proteins[2].

Because insulin is required for the synthesis of proteins, it is as essential for growth of a human being as growth hormone is. Combination of growth hormone and insulin cause dramatic growth. Thus, it appears that the two hormones function synergistically to promote growth, each performing a specific function that is separate from that of the other.

1.2.3 Effect of insulin on fat metabolism

Insulin promotes lipogenesis in the fat stores; however, it inhibits lipolysis. And it increases the synthesis of cholesterol in the liver, in particular the rate of very low density lipoprotein (VLDL) formation[3].

1.3 Regulation of insulin release

1.3.1 Plasma glucose

The most important stimulant for insulin release is blood glucose concentration[4]. Glucose can act directly on B cells to promote the secretion of insulin. Insulin is released greatly in 30 s, and in 5 ~ 10 min, it decreases by 50%, then the 2nd peak appears in 2 ~ 3 hours and lasts for a link time. That is, any rise in blood glucose increases insulin secretion, and the insulin in turn reduces the blood glucose concentration back toward the normal value.

1.3.2 Amino acids and fatty acids

If amino acids, fatty acids, ketone body increase, B cell secretes insulin[5]. And the amino acids strongly potentiate the glucose stimulus for insulin secretion, whereas fatty acid attenuates the effect.

1.3.3 Other hormones

Gastrin, secretin, cholecystokinin stimulate the secretion of insulin. Growth hormone, estrogen and corticosteroid can also increase the secretion. Parasympathetic hormone can increase the secretion and inhibition of release is induced by adrenaline and sympathetic nervous system.

---

[1] 胰岛素可抑制生糖氨基酸在肝的糖异生过程。

[2] 胰岛素促进肌肉、肝脏和其他组织细胞蛋白质的合成，主要作用的环节是：促进氨基酸通过膜的转运进入细胞；促进蛋白质的合成过程；延缓组织蛋白质的降解。

[3] 胰岛素可促进脂肪的合成与储存，抑制脂肪的分解，促进肝脏合成胆固醇和低密度脂蛋白。

[4] 血糖浓度是调节胰岛素分泌的最重要因素。

[5] 氨基酸、脂肪酸和酮体促进胰岛素的分泌。

2 Glucagon

The glucagon from the A cells of the pancreatic islets only contains 29 of the 160 amino acid residues in pro-glucagon.

2.1 Actions of glucagon

Glucagon has several functions that are diametrically opposed to those of insulin. Most important of these functions is to increase the blood glucose concentration, an effect that is exactly the opposite that of insulin [1]. Glucagon stimulates adenylcyclase in the hepatocytes. Then adenylcyclase activates phosphorylase that breaks down glycogen. Actually, glucagon triggers a glycogenolytic cascade, so those considerable amounts of glucose are released in response to the fall in blood glucose. In addition, glucagon stimulates the hepatic production of glucose from glycerol, alanine and lactate. Glucagon is a direct antagonist to insulin, being catabolic in its actions (gluconeogenetic, glycogenolytic, lipolytic and ketogenic, and deaminating amino acids).

Glucagon also stimulates gluconeogenesis from glycogenic amino acids in the liver and thus increases urea-genesis. Glucagon stimulates ketogenesis. In addition to the ketogenic effect, intestinal glucagon is a potent stimulator of insulin secretion – as are other members of the incretin family. Incretins act by increasing cAMP in the B cells.

2.2 Release of glucagon

The blood glucose concentration is by far the most potent factor that controls glucagon secretion. Conditions where there is intracellular lack of glucose, for example, hunger, insulin deficiency, protein rich meals and amino acid infusion, liberate glucagon from the A cells of the pancreatic islets to the pancreatic vein and then to the portal vein. High blood glucose concentration and free fatty acid concentration inhibit glucagon secretion.

Section 7 Other hormones

1 Prostaglandin

Prostaglandins(PG) are a group of tissue hormones widely found in humans and animals. PG does not belong to circulating hormones, but is produced and released locally, and regulates the function of local tissues and organs. PG is converted from peanut four acid into various forms of PG.

The structure of PG is a 20 carbon unsaturated fatty acid composed of a five ring and two

[1] 胰高血糖素最重要的作用是升高血糖，这与胰岛素的作用相反。

side chains. According to the difference of substituents (mainly hydroxyl and hydrogen) in the five element fat ring of the molecule, PG is divided into A, B, C, D, E, F and so on. They are expressed by PGA, PGB, PGC, PGD, PGE, PGF and so on;

The number of double bonds in the molecular side chain is marked in the lower right corner of each letter, such as PGE_2 or PGF_2. Different type of PG has different functions. For example, PGE_2 can relax bronchial smooth muscle and reduce ventilation resistance, while PGF_2 acts on the contrary.

2 Melatonin

The pineal gland (epiphysis) is known to secrete melatonin[1]. The amphibian pineal contains an indole, N–acetyl–5–methoxy tryptamine, named melatonin because it lightens the skin of tadpoles. However, it does not appear to play a physiologic role in the regulation of skin color. Melatonin may function as a timing device to keep internal events synchronized with the light–dark cycle in the environment[2]. In humans and all other species studied to date, melatonin synthesis and secretion are increased during the dark period of the day and maintained at a low level during the daylight hours.

3 Leptin

LP (Leptin) is a protein secreted by adipose tissue, mainly composed of white adipose tissue and consists of 146 amino acid residues. Leptin has a wide range of biological effects, of which the most important is the metabolic regulation center in the hypothalamus, which plays an important role in inhibiting appetite, reducing energy intake, increasing energy consumption and inhibiting fat synthesis.

---

[1] 褪黑素由松果体分泌。

[2] 褪黑素可使生物体的内源性节律与环境周期保持一致。

Chapter 10 REPRODUCTION

Section 1 Male reproduction

The male reproductive system includes the two testes[1], the system of ducts that store and transport sperms[2] to the exterior, the glands (seminal vesicle, prostate, and urethral gland), and the penis[3]. The duct system, glands, and penis constitute the male accessory reproductive organs[4]. The testis is male gonad, which is the source of spermatozoa and produce the male sex hormone testosterone[5]. The function depends on two structures in the testis. One is seminiferous tubule where spermatogenesis[6] occurred. The other is Leydig cells (interstitial cells)[7] between these tubules which secrete testosterone.

1 Function of testis

1.1 Spermatogenesis

Spermatogenesis indicates that the development of spermatozoa[8] from spermatogonia[9] which distributed around the periphery of the seminiferous tubules[10]. Spermatogonia is firstly divided into primary spermatocytes[11]. Then the primary spermatocytes undergo meiosis, producing two secondary spermatocytes. Secondary spermatocytes undergo meiosis and turn into

[1] 睾丸：男性的主性器官。

[2] 精子。

[3] 阴茎。

[4] 附性器官。

[5] 睾酮。

[6] 精子发生。

[7] 间质细胞。

[8] 精子。

[9] 精原细胞。

[10] 曲细精管。

[11] 精母细胞。

round spermatids and produce spermatozoa which have the structures of head, midpiece and tails. At each stage of spermatogenesis, the Sertoli cells[1] secrete the protein hormone (inhibin) and nutrition to support germs development.

1.2 Secreting testosterone and inhibin

1.2.1 Testosterone

Testosterone is the dominant sex hormone whose functions include:

(1) Maintain spermatogenesis.

(2) Stimulate differentiation and growth of male reproductive system.

(3) Develop the secondary sex characteristics.

(4) Affect metabolism: Increase the synthesis and decrease the breakdown of protein; increase erythrocyte production; promote bone growth by increasing Ca^{2+} and phosphate absorption.

1.2.2 Inhibin

Inhibin, a peptide hormone secreted by Sertoli cells, has a molecular weight of 31000 ~ 32000. In addition to its supporting spermatogenesis, inhibin has a strong inhibitory effect on pituitary secretion and synthesis of FSH, while the physiological dose of inhibin has no significant effect on the secretion of LH.

2 Hormonal control of male reproduction

GnRH produced by the hypothalamus is carried in the hypophyseal portal system to the anterior pituitary(Figure10–1). This stimulates the release of gonadotrophins, FSH and LH, which are carried by circulation to testis and other target cells. FSH stimulates sertoli cells to support spermatogenesis. LH promotes testosterone secretion from Leydig cells. Testosterone exerts a negative feedback factor on inhibiting hypothalamic and anterior pituitary secretion.

The negative feedback regulation of inhibin on FSH secretion of pituitary gland is coordinated with the negative

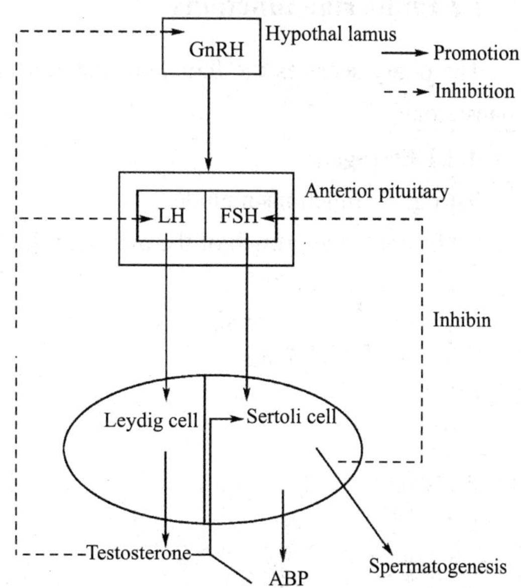

Figure 10–1 Hormonal control of testicular function

[1] 支持细胞。

feedback regulation of testosterone on hypothalamus and pituitary gland, ensuring the normal generation of sperm.

Section 2 Female reproduction

The female reproductive system includes the two ovaries[1] and the female reproductive tract–two fallopian tubes[2], the uterus[3], the cervix, and the vagina. These structures are termed the female internal genitalia.

1 Functions of ovary

1.1 Oogenesis

Oogenia[4] is proliferated by mitotic division and undergoes a maturation process to form the primary oocytes before birth. Primary oocyte[5] is surrounded by the basal lamina and a single layer of granulosa cells[6] to form primary follicle which can further be developed into the second follicle[7]. The second follicle contains a primary oocyte surrounded by several layers granulosa cells which form zonapellucida[8]. The theca cell which differentiated from stromal cell also multiplies and differentiates to form the theca interna[9] surrounded by the theca externa. One follicle becomes dominant and enlarges further. The mature follicle will discharge the secondary oocyte with zonapellucida and adherent granulosa cells.

1.2 Endocrine functions

The ovary secretes the female sex steroid hormones: estrogen[10] (mainly estradiol) and progesterone[11].

1.2.1 Estrogen

Estrogen's functions include:

(1) Promote the growth of the ovarian follicles.

---

[1] 卵巢：女性的主性器官。

[2] 输卵管。

[3] 子宫。

[4] 卵原细胞。

[5] 卵子。

[6] 颗粒细胞。

[7] 卵泡。

[8] 放射冠：柱状颗粒细胞呈放射状排列。

[9] 卵泡内膜。

[10] 雌激素。

[11] 孕激素。

(2) Develop the secondary sex characteristics.

(3) Affect metabolism: Increase the synthesis of protein; promote bone growth by increasing Ca^{2+} and phosphate absorption; decrease the cholesterol level.

1.2.2 Progesterone

Progesterone's functions include:

(1)Promote necessary conditions for the maintenance of pregnancy after implantation. ① On the basis of estrogen, progesterone can thicken the endometrium. ② During the pregnancy, progesterone can decrease uterine smooth muscle excitability, so having tocolysis effect. ③ Progesterone can reduce the maternal immune rejection of the fetus.

(2) Promote breast development and growth.

(3) Thermogenesis: progesterone can cause basal body temperature to rise by about 0.5℃ after ovulation, and maintain this level in luteal phase. The body temperature performances a brief decline before ovulation, then rises after ovulation, so clinically the biphasic changes in body temperature often are selected as one of the signs of ovulation.

(4) The effect on smooth muscle: Progesterone reduces the tension of blood vessel and digestive tract smooth muscle. Some people think that this is one of the reasons why pregnant women are prone to constipation and hemorrhoids.

2 Menstrual cycleand the hormonal control

Each menstrual cycle[1] lasts 28 days approximately(Figure10–2). This includes changes in the ovary known as ovarian cycle[2] and uterus known as uterine cycle[3].

The reproductive system of woman shows regular cyclic changes that may be regarded as periodic preparations for fertilization and pregnancy. In human, the cycle is a menstrual cycle, and its most conspicuous feature is the periodic vaginal bleeding[4] that occurs with the shedding of the uterine mucosa[5] (menstruation).

2.1 Ovarian cycle

Ovarian cycle consists of a 14–day follicular phase[6] followed by ovulation[7] and a 14–day luteal phase[8].

[1] 月经周期。

[2] 卵巢周期。

[3] 子宫周期。

[4] 阴道出血。

[5] 子宫内膜脱落。

[6] 卵泡期。

[7] 排卵。

[8] 黄体期。

2.1.1 Follicular phase

In follicular phase, several of these follicles enlarge, and a cavity forms around the ovum[1] (antrum[2] formation). This cavity is filled with follicular fluid. In humans, one of the follicles in one ovary becomes the dominant follicle[3], while the others regress, forming atretic follicles[4].

2.1.2 Ovulation

At about the 14th day of the cycle, the distended follicle ruptures, and the ovum is extruded into the abdominal cavity. This is the process of ovulation. The ovum is picked up by the fimbriated ends of the uterine tubes (oviducts).

2.1.3 Luteal phase

After ovulation, the granulosa and theca cells of the follicle lining promptly begin to proliferate into yellowish, lipid-rich luteal cells, forming the corpus luteum[5]. This initiates the luteal phase of the menstrual cycle, during which the luteal cells secrete estrogens and progesterone. If pregnancy occurs, the corpus luteum persists. If there is no pregnancy, the corpus luteum begins to degenerate and is eventually replaced by scar tissue, forming a corpus albicans[6] (Figure 10-2).

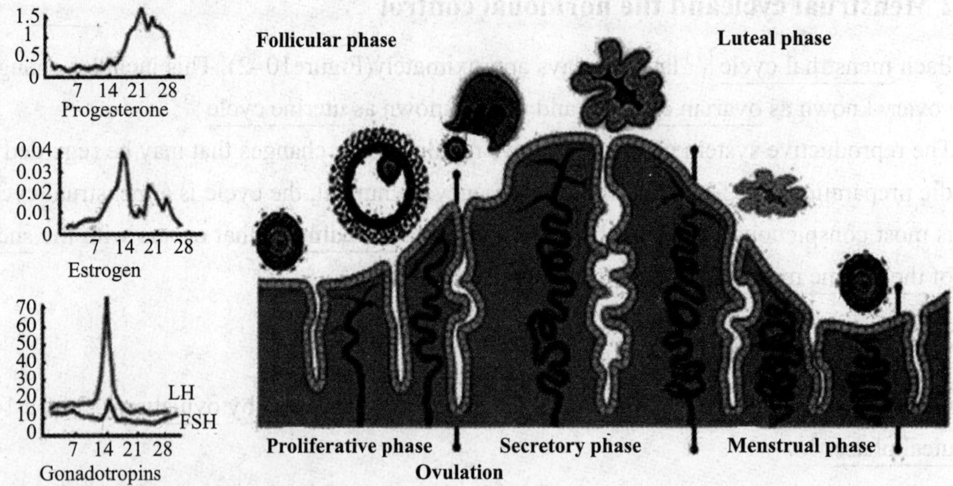

Figure 10-2 Hormonal control of the menstrual cycle

[1] 卵子。

[2] 腔、窦。

[3] 优势卵泡。

[4] 闭锁卵泡。

[5] 黄体。

[6] 白体。

2.2 Uterine cycle

The uterine cycle is divided into three phases: menstrual phase, proliferative phase and secretory phase.

2.2.1 Menstrual phase[1]

When hormonal supporting for the endometrium is withdrawn, theendometrium[2] degenerates. At this phase, spasm and then necrosis of the walls of the arteries lead to spotty hemorrhages[3] that become confluent and produce the menstrual flow. Menstrual flow lasts for about 3 ~ 5 days. The average amount of blood lost is 30 ml. At the end of this phase, the endometrium is very thin.

2.2.2 Proliferative phase

At the end of menstruation, all but the deep layers of the endometrium have sloughed[4]. Under the influence of estrogens from the developing follicle, the endometrium increases rapidly in thickness from the fifth to the fourteenth days of the menstrual cycle. As the thickness increases, the uterine glands are drawn out, but they do not secrete. These endometrial changes are called proliferation, and this part of the menstrual cycle is called proliferative phase[5].

2.2.3 Secretory phase

After ovulation, the endometrium becomes more highly vascularized and slightly edematous under the influence of estrogen and progesterone from the corpus luteum. The glands become coiled and tortuous, and they begin to secrete a clear fluid. The changes are essential for implantation[6] and nourishment for the developing embryo[7]. This phase of the cycle is called the secretory phase[8]. When fertilization fails to occur during the secretory phase, the endometrium is shed and a new cycle starts.

2.3 Hormonal control

Hypothalamic control is exerted by GnRH secreted into the portal hypophysial vessels. GnRH causes the release of gonadotropin (FSH and LH) from the pituitary. FSH is responsible

---

[1] 月经期。

[2] 子宫内膜。

[3] 点状出血。

[4] 脱落。

[5] 增殖期。

[6] 着床：胚泡植入子宫内膜。

[7] 胚胎。

[8] 分泌期。

for the early maturation of the ovarian follicles, and FSH and LH together are responsible for their final maturation. A burst of LH secretion is responsible for trigging ovulation and stimulates follicular remnants to form corpus luteum. LH stimulates the secretion of estrogen and progesterone from the corpus luteum.

During the early part of the follicular phase, FSH is modestly elevated, fostering follicular growth. LH secretion is held in check by the negative feedback effect of the rising plasma estrogen level. At 36 ~ 48 hours before ovulation, the estrogen feedback effect becomes positive, and this initiates the burst of LH secretion (LH surge[1]) that produces ovulation. Ovulation occurs about 9 hours after the LH peak. During the luteal phase, the secretion of LH and FSH is low because of the elevated levels of estrogen, progesterone(Figure 10–3).

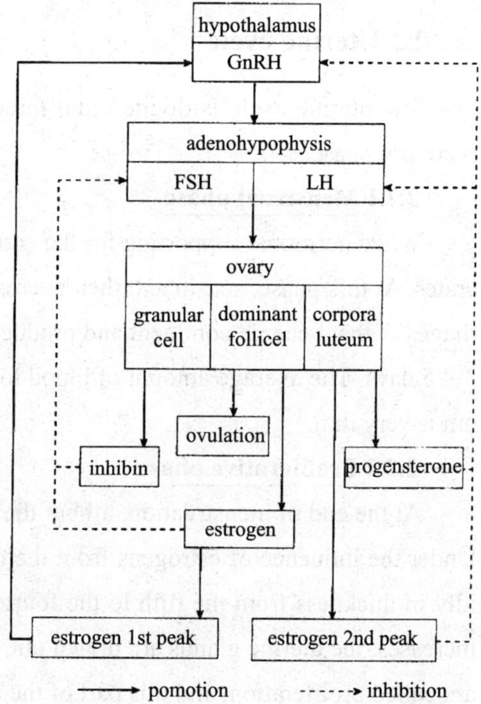

Figure 10–3 Hormonal control of ovarian function

Section 3 Pregnancy and parturition

1 Pregnancy

Pregnancy[2] lasts from fertilization[3] to the birth of the baby.

1.1 Fertilization

Fertilization is the fusion of a sperm and ovum. The two sets of chromosomes—23 from the sperm and 23 from the ovum form the fertilized ovum, termed a zygote. During this process, the ovum is swept into the fallopian tube, and the sperm transports to the fallopian tube. Sperm must exposure to the female reproductive tract several hours to obtain the fertilizing ability. That process is called capacitation[4]. The sperm and ovum binding begin with acro-

[1] LH 峰。

[2] 妊娠：母体承受子代新个体在其体内发育成长的过程。

[3] 受精：精子进入卵子，并与卵子融合成为合子的过程。

[4] 获能：精子表面的糖蛋白被女性生殖道内的酶降解，从而获得受精能力的现象。

some reaction[1]. The sperm head releasesacrosomal enzymes to digest zonapellucida.

1.2 Implantation

The conceptus[2] undergoes a number of mitotic cell divisions at fallopian tube and is transported to the uterus. After reaching the uterus, the developing blastocyst[3] usually remains in the uterine cavity an additional 1 to 3 days; thus, implantation ordinarily occurs on about the fifth to seventh day after ovulation. The trophoblast cells[4] secrete proteolytic enzymes to digest and liquefy the adjacent cells of the uterine endometrium. Once implantation has taken place, the trophoblast cells and other adjacent cells proliferate rapidly, forming the placenta[5].

1.3 Placental hormones

1.3.1 Human chorionic gonadotropin

Human chorionic gonadotropin[6] (hCG) is a glycoprotein produced by the syncytiotrophoblast[7]. Like LH, hCG acts on corpus luteum to prevent the decrease in the progesterone and estrogen, leading to high levels of sex hormones. It can be detected in the urine as early as 14th days after conception and is used for early pregnancy testing. hCG level peaks at about sixtieth days after pregnancy and then decreases gradually, and at about 160th days of pregnancy to a minimum, until the end of pregnancy (Figure 10–4).

1.3.2 Human chorionic somatomammotropin

Human chorionic somatomammotropin[8] (hCS) is secreted by the syncytiotrophoblast. The structure of hCS is similar to that of human growth hormone. hCS promotes fetus growth by decreasing utilization of glucose in the mother.

1.3.3 Progesterone and estrogen

The placenta begins to secrete estrogen and progesterone at the sixth week of gestation, and increases with the duration of pregnancy, reaching the peak before delivery. . The estrogen secreted by the placenta is estriol, and its raw material comes from the fetus. Therefore, the detection of the content of estriol in the maternal blood can be used to determine whether the fetus is alive or not(Figure 10–4).

---

[1] 顶体反应：精子与卵子接触时，精子释放顶体酶溶解卵子的放射冠。

[2] 孕体。

[3] 胚泡。

[4] 滋养层细胞。

[5] 胎盘。

[6] 人绒毛膜促性腺激素。

[7] 合体滋养层。

[8] 人绒毛膜生长素。

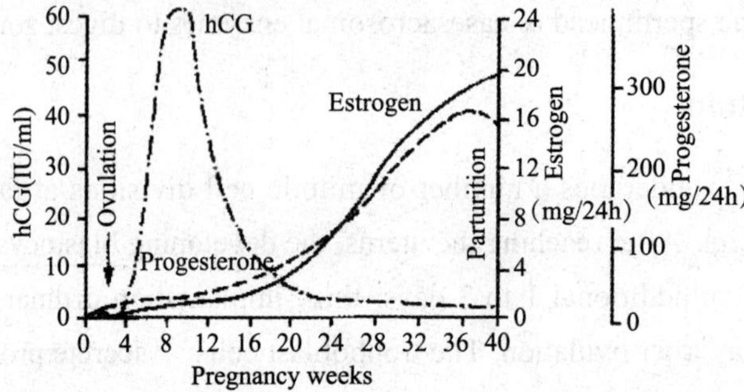

Figure 10–4 Levels of various hormones during pregnancy

2 Parturition

A normal human pregnancy lasts approximately 40 weeks, counting from the first day of the last menstrual cycle. During the last month, the entire uterine contents shift downward. Parturition [1] begins with strong rhythmiccontractions of myometrium. At the onset of labour, the contractions increase in intensity and frequency, the cervix gradually open to approximately 10 cm. At this time, the mother increases abdominal pressure, adding to the effect of uterine contractions, and the baby isdelivered. Finally, the placenta shears off the wall of the uterus and is expelled out of the uterus after child birth.

Section 4 Sex physiology

1 Sex maturation

Sexual development occurs in two main steps: the determination of sex organs during fetal life and onset of full reproduction at puberty. Girls usually begin puberty at 9 ~ 11 years old, about two years earlier than boys. Onset ofpuberty, The two aspect is that: a marked acceleration in height growth and secondary sex characteristics development. These changes are an adult distribution of pubic hair in both sexes, with breast development in females, the penis and testes enlarged in males, the voice breaks and facial and body hair appears. The trigger for the onset of puberty is associated with hormones. GnRH stimulates the release of FSH and LH. These two hormones act upon the gonads, resulting high level androgen or estrogen, leading to spermatogenesis and cyclical follicular development and ovulation in the female.

[1] 分娩：成熟胎儿及其附属物从母体产出的过程。

2 Sexual action

2.1 Sexual action of male

For male, the sex act includes erection[1] and ejaculation[2] stages. Engorgement[3] of the vascular spaces in the erectile tissues of penis results in erection. Sensual stimuli[4] lead to erection and is controlled by activation of parasympathetic nerves and inhibition of sympathetic constrictor nerves. As engorgement processes, the vein draining the penis promote erection. Ejaculation includes two stages: emission[5] and expulsion[6]. Sympathetic nerves stimulate contraction of the smooth muscle in the walls of the epididymis and vas deferens, leading to sperm and secretion mixed together to produce semen. Under the action of somatic motor nerves, skeletal muscle around the base of the penis contracts rhythmically, compresses the urethra, discharging the semen into the vagina, at same time reaching orgasm[7].

2.2 Sexual action of female

For female, stimulated with physical, psychological and hormonal factors, the sex act includes 4 phases: ① Excitation phase can be initiated by multiple internal and external factors, including psychological factors. ② Plateau phase is the culmination of the excitation phase when it reaches its peak. ③ The sexual tension already built up in the whole body released in orgasm phase. ④ the last phase is resolution, in which the sex response goes back to physiological state. All these phases are controlled by Sympathetic and parasympathetic nerves.

---

[1] 勃起。

[2] 射精。

[3] 肿胀。

[4] 性刺激。

[5] 移精：输精管和精囊腺中的精液被运到尿道的过程。

[6] 排射：阴茎根部肌肉收缩，将尿道内精液射出的过程。

[7] 性高潮。

Chapter 11 THE NERVOUS SYSTEM

Section 1 Basic structure and functions of the nervous system

The nervous system is a communication network that allows an organism to interact in appropriate ways with its environment. The nervous system is divided into two parts: ① the central nervous system (CNS)[1], composed of the brain and spinal cord; and ② the peripheral nervous system (PNS)[2], consisting of the ganglions[3] and the nerves that connected between the brain or spinal cord and body's muscles, glands, and sense organs. The peripheral nervous system is divided again into two parts: the somatic nervous system[4] and the visceral nervous system[5].

1 Neuron and nerve fibers

1.1 Neuron

The basic structural and functional unit of the nervous system is the individual nerve cell, called as neuron. It is the basic building blocks of the nervous system, and it has evolved from primitive neuro effector cells that respond to various stimuli by contracting. The human central nervous system (CNS) contains about 10^{11} neurons. The mostly function of neurons operates by generating and transmitting electrical signals. In more complex animals, contraction has become the specialized function of muscle cells, whereas integration and transmission of nerve impulses have become the specialized functions of neurons[6]. Many substances called as neurotransmitter are synthesized[7], and metabolize in the neurons. In most neurons, the electrical

[1] 中枢神经系统。

[2] 周围神经系统。

[3] 神经节。

[4] 躯体神经系统。

[5] 内脏神经系统。

[6] 在更复杂的动物，收缩已成为肌肉细胞的特有功能，而整合和传导神经冲动是神经元的特有功能。

[7] 合成。

signal causes the release of the neurotransmitters, communicating with other cells.

Neurons in the mammalian central nervous system come in many different shapes and sizes. However, most have the same parts as the typical spinal motor neuron[1] with one cell body and processes illustrated in Figure 11–1. They contain three parts: a cell body, dendrites[2] and an axon with terminals. The dendrites highly branched outgrowths and the cell body receive most of the input signals from other neurons.

A typical neuron also has a long fibrous axon that extends from a somewhat thickened area of the cell body, the axon hillock[3]. It carries output to its target cells. The axon hillock is the "trigger zone" where the electrical signals are generated. These signals then propagate away from the cell body along the axon. The main axon may have branches, called collaterals, along its course. Each branch in an axon terminal is responsible for releasing neurotransmitters from the axon. These chemical messengers diffuse across an extracellular gap to the cell opposite the terminal.

The axons of most neurons are covered by myelin[4]. Outside the CNS, the myelin is produced by Schwann cells[5]. The spaces between adjacent sections of myelin where the axon's plasma membrane is exposed to extracellular fluid are the nodes of Ranvier[6]. In the brain and spinal cord these myelin–forming cells are the oligodendrocytes[7] rather than Schwann cells. Not all mammalian neurons are myelinated; some are unmyelinated. They are simply surrounded by Schwann cells without the wrapping of the Schwann cell membrane around the axon that produces myelin. Most neurons in invertebrates[8] are unmyelinated. The myelin sheath speeds up conduction of the electrical signals along the axon and conserves energy. The loss of myelin is associated with delayed or blocked conduction in the demyelinated[9] axons. Nerve fibers are made up of axons. If surrounded with sheath, they are called myelinated fibers; if not, called unmyelinated fibers.

1.2 Classification of nerve fibers

In the general classification, the fibers are divided into types A, B and C, and A is further

[1] 运动神经元。
[2] 树突。
[3] 轴丘。
[4] 髓鞘。
[5] 施旺细胞。
[6] 郎飞结。
[7] 少突胶质细胞。
[8] 无脊椎动物。
[9] 脱髓鞘。

subdivided into α, β, γ and δ fibers. Type C fibers are the very small, unmyelinated nerve fibers that conduct impulses at low velocities. These constitute more than half the sensory fibers in most peripheral nerves and also all of the postganglionic fibers [1]. Over two thirds of all the nerve fibers in peripheral nerves are type C fibers. Their great number contributes to transmit tremendous amounts of information from the surface of the body. The details can be seen in Table 11–1.

Based on the diameter and origin of the nerve fibers, afferent axons can be divided into Ⅰ(Ⅰa and Ⅰb), Ⅱ, Ⅲ, and Ⅳ types.

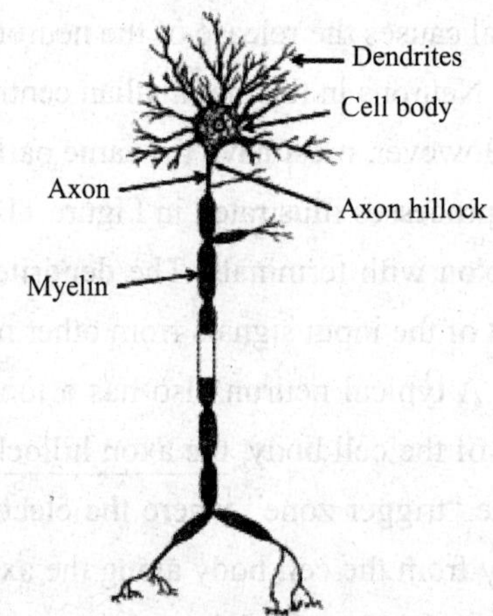

Figure 11–1 The motor neuron

Table 11–1 Electrophysiologic classification in mammalian nerve*

Fiber type		Function	Diameter (μm)	Velocity (m/s)	Spike Duration (ms)	ARP (ms)
A	α(I)	Proprioception; somatic motor	12–20	70–120	0.4–0.5	0.4–1
	β(II)	Touch, pressure	5–12	30–70		
	γ(II)	Motor to muscle spindles	3–6	15–30		
	δ(III)	Pain, cold, touch	2–5	12–30		
B	(III)	Preganglionic autonomic	<3	3–15	1.2	1.2
C(IV)	Dorsal root	Pain, temperature, some mechanoreception[15], reflex responses	0.4–1.2	0.5–2	2	2
	Sympathetic	Postganglionic sympathetics	0.3–1.3	0.7–2.3	2	2

*A and B fibers are myelinated; C fibers are unmyelinated.
ARP: absolute refractory period.

1.3 Characteristics of nerve fibers conducting impulse

There are four features of the nerve fibers, which are, separately, expatiated as blow:

1.3.1 Physiological integrity [2] Normal conduction requires not only the structural integrity of nerve fibers, but also functional integrity of nerve fibers [3]. If the nerve fiber is damaged or cut off, the impulse cannot be conducted. Nerve fibers, with damaged functional

[1] 节后纤维。

[2] 生理完整性。

[3] 正常的神经传导不但要求神经纤维结构完整，而且要求功能完整。

integrity using narcotics, neurotoxicity, or frozen, cannot conduct impulses either.

1.3.2 Insulation[1] The myelin sheath is an excellent electrical insulator that decreases ion flow through the membrane. Thus, the fiber conduction does not interfere with each other. It ensures the accuracy of nerve conduction.

1.3.3 Bidirectional conductivity[2] This means that the effective stimulus is applied to the nerve fiber at any point, the produced excitation can be conducted to the two directions.

1.3.4 Relative indefatigability[3] During the excitation the nerve fiber expends relatively small energy. Therefore, the nerve fibers can work for a very long time without tiredness to insure the impulse conduction.

1.4 Conduction velocity of nerve fibers

Conduction velocity depends on the size of an axon and the thickness of its myelin sheath, if present. Large-diameter axons have less cytoplasmic resistance, thereby permitting a greater flow of ions[4]. This increase in ion flow in the cytoplasm causes greater lengths of the axon to be depolarized, decreasing the time needed for the action potential to travel along the axon. Several factors act to increase significantly the conduction velocity of action potentials in myelinated axons. Glial cells wrap themselves around axons to form myelin, layers of lipid membrane that insulate the axon and prevent the passage of ions through the axonal membrane. Between the myelinated segments of the axon are the nodes of Ranvier, where action potentials are generated. Even though almost no ions can flow through the thick myelin sheaths of myelinated nerves, they can flow with ease through the nodes of Ranvier. Therefore, action potentials are conducted from node to node, this is called saltatory conduction[5]. Conduction velocity is faster for myelinated axons based on size alone. In addition, the myelin acts to increase the effective resistance of the axonal membrane, myelin before they reach the extracellular fluid. This increases the space constant. The layers of myelin also decrease the effective capacitance of the axonal membrane because the distance between the extracellular and intracellular conducting fluid compartments is increased. Because the capacitance is decreased, the time constant is decreased, increasing the conduction velocity. The temperature is one of another factor that affects the nerve conduction velocity. The rise of temperature speeds up the conduction velocity.

---

[1] 绝缘性。

[2] 双向传导性。

[3] 相对不疲劳性。

[4] 直径粗的轴突胞质电阻小，从而允许更多的离子流动。

[5] 跳跃式传导。

1.5 Axon transport of nerve fibers

In order to maintain the structure and function of the cell axon, various organelles and materials must be moved. This movement is termed axon transport. The substances include linking proteins and microtubules in the cell body and axon. The microtubules serve as the "rails" along which the transport occurs. The linking proteins act as the "motors" of axon transport and, as ATPase enzymes, they also transfer energy from ATP to the "motors".

Certain materials, such as growth factors and other chemical messengers, are also transported in the opposite direction, from the axon terminals to the cell body. They can affect the neuron's morphology [1], biochemistry, and connectivity. By the route, certain harmful substances, such as tetanus toxin [2], herpes [3], and other viruses can be taken up by the peripheral axon terminals [4] and enter the central nervous system.

2 Neurogliocytes [5]

In addition to neurons, the nervous system contains neurogliocytes (glial cells). The Schwann cells that invest axons in peripheral nerves are classified as neurogliocytes. The number is estimated to be 10 ~ 50 times of the number of neurons. In the CNS, there are three main types of glia. Microglia are scavenger cells that resemble tissue macrophages [6]. They probably come from the bone marrow and enter the nervous system from the circulating blood vessels. Oligodendrocytes [7] are involved in myelin formation. Astrocytes, which are found throughout the brain, are of two subtypes. Fibrous astrocytes, which contain many intermediate filaments, are found primarily in white matter. Protoplasmic astrocytes [8] are found in gray matter and have granular cytoplasm. Both types send processes to blood vessel, where they induce capillaries to form the tight junctions that form the blood–brain barrier [9]. They also send processes that envelop synapses and the surface of nerve cells. They have a membrane potential that varies with the external K^+ concentration but do not generate propagated potentials [10]. They

[1] 形态，形态学。

[2] 破伤风毒素。

[3] 疱疹病毒。

[4] 轴突末梢。

[5] 胶质细胞。

[6] 小神经胶质细胞是巨噬细胞，类似于组织巨噬细胞。

[7] 少突胶质细胞。

[8] 原浆性星形胶质细胞。

[9] 他们引起毛细血管形成紧密连接从而形成血脑屏障。

[10] 它们有一个随外部 K^+ 浓度而变化的膜电位，但不会产生可传播的电位。

produce substances that are trophic to neurons, and they help maintain the appropriate concentration of ions and neurotransmitters by taking up K^+ and the neurotransmitters glutamate and γ–aminobutyrate (GABA)[1].

Section 2 Synaptic transmission

The site of contact between a neuron and its target cell is called a synapse, which is the anatomically specialized junction[2] between two neurons. All synapses do not operate with one mechanism. Most synapses use chemical transmitter(s), some, however, operate by purely electrical mechanism. In general, synapses can be divided into chemical and electrical synapses[3]. The structural basis of electrical synapses is gap junctions, allowing charged ions to pass information through the channels. The chemical synapse is divided into directional and non directional synapses. The directed synapse is divided into the classical synapses present in the center and the nerve – skeletal muscle junctions existing in the periphery. The non directional synapse is divided into the monoaminergic nerve and the autonomic nerve effector connector existing in the periphery. Here mainly focuses on the directed synapses and electrical synapses.

1 Synaptic structure and classification

Most synapses in the central nervous system are typical synaptic transmissions. A typical synaptic transmissions includes three components: the pre–synaptic membranes, post–synaptic membranes and synaptic cleft[4]. The pre– and post–synaptic neurons are not in continuity. There is a discrete separation, the synaptic cleft, between the presynaptic and postsynaptic elements, having a width usually of 20 to 30 nanometers, and the synaptic knob[5] contains large numbers of vesicles, called synaptic vesicles[6]. Most neurotransmitters are stored in various shaped synaptic vesicles and released upon nerve stimulation by a process of calcium mediated exocytosis; once released, the neurotransmitter binds to and stimulates its receptors briefly before being rapidly removed from the synapse. At most synapses, the signal is transmitted from one neuron to another by neurotransmitters, also including the chemicals by which efferent neurons communicate with effector cells. Almost all the synapses used for signal transmission in the central nervous system of the human being are chemical synapses.

[1] γ–氨基丁酸。

[2] 结构上的特殊连接。

[3] 通常，突触可分为化学性突触和电突触。

[4] 突触前膜、突触后膜和突触间隙。

[5] 突触小体。

[6] 突触小泡。

In the center, the Classification of synapses usually was based on the contacting position of the synaptic, dividing the synapses into three groups: axon–dendritic synapses; axon–somatic synapses; axon–axonic synapses.

2 Directional synaptic transmission [1]

2.1 Presynaptic process

The release of transmitter into the synaptic cleft is triggered when an action potential reaches the axon terminal, and opens voltage–gated calcium channels in the presynaptic membrane, causing calcium influx into the terminal. Calcium influx is necessary for neurotransmitters release [2]. This is followed by movement of vesicles to the presynaptic membrane, fusion of the vesicle membrane with the plasma membrane of the presynaptic terminal, and exocytosis of the vesicle contents into the synaptic cleft.

2.2 Postsynaptic processes

Once released from the presynaptic axon terminal, transmitters diffuse across the synaptic cleft. A fraction of these molecules bind to receptors on the plasma membrane of the postsynaptic cell. The result of the binding of neurotransmitter to receptor is the opening or closing of specific ion channels in the postsynaptic plasma membrane, causing changes of ion flowing across the membrane and by which change the membrane potential of postsynaptic membrane, called postsynaptic potential. There are two kinds of postsynaptic potential:excitatory postsynaptic potentials (EPSPs) and inhibitory postsynaptic potentials (IPSPs) [3].

2.2.1 Excitatory postsynaptic potential

The excitatory transmitter acts on the membrane receptor to open up chemically gated channels. These chemically gated channels allow both Na^+ and K^+ to pass simultaneously. However, because K^+ concentration gradient is not far from equilibrium with the electrical potential, this large opening of the membrane pores mainly allows Na^+ to rush to the inside of the membrane. The large Na^+ concentration gradient and large electrical negativity are inside the neuron. The rapid influx of positively charged Na^+ to the interior neutralizes part of the negativity of the resting membrane potential. This positive increase in voltage above the normal resting neuronal potential. Therefore, the excitatory transmitter causing the depolarization [4] of postsynaptic membrane is called EPSP. At the neuromuscular junction, the EPSP is also called

[1] 定向突触传递。

[2] 钙离子内流对神经递质的释放是必需的。

[3] 兴奋性突触后电位和抑制性突触后电位。

[4] 去极化。

the endplate potential. (Figure 11–2)

2.2.2 Inhibitory postsynaptic potential

The inhibitory transmitter increases the postsynaptic cell's permeability to both K^+ and Cl^-. Consequently K^+ moves out of the cell and Cl^- moves into the cell. Both Cl^- influx and K^+ efflux increase the membrane potential and hyperpolarize the postsynaptic membrane. This inhibits the neuron because the membrane potential is even more negative than the normal intracellular potential. Therefore, the inhibitory transmitter causing the hyperpolarization [1] of postsynaptic membrane is called IPSP.

These membrane depolarizations and hyperpolarizations are integrated and can result in activation or inhibition of the postsynaptic neuron. Because a single action potential in a presynaptic neuron seldom produces an action potential in the postsynaptic cell, and a single action potential usually leads only to EPSP or IPSP in the postsynaptic cells. The process in which postsynaptic membrane potentials are added with time is called temporal summation [2]. This summation of stimulus is rising with increasing frequency.

If the magnitude of the summated depolarizations is above a threshold value, it will generate an action potential [3]. The summation of postsynaptic potentials also occurs with the activation of several synapses located at different sites of contact. This process is called spatial summation [4] (Figure 11–2). This increases with the magnitude of the stimulus.

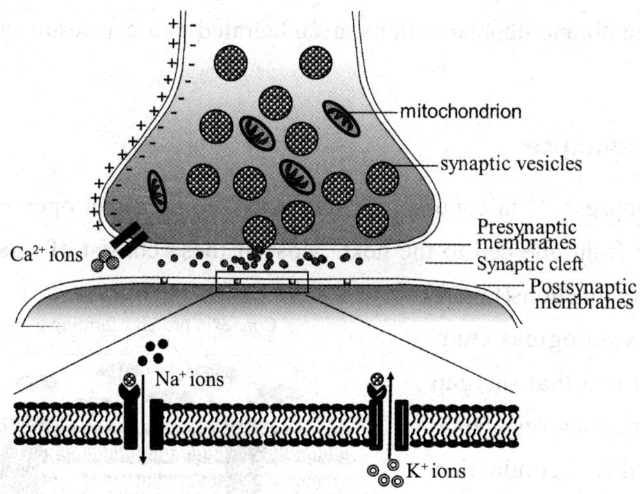

Figure 11–2 The EPSPs and IPSPs

[1] 超极化。

[2] 时间总和。

[3] 如果去极化总和达到阈值时，将产生一个动作电位。

[4] 空间总和。

3 Neuromuscular junction

Synapses in nerve – skeletal muscles are also called neuromuscular junctions. The presynaptic membrane, postsynaptic membrane, and synaptic gap are called the prejunctional membrane, the postjunctional membrane and the junctional cleft respectively. The anterior membrane of the joint is the membrane of the synaptic membrane, and the posterior membrane is the membrane of the skeletal muscle, also called the endplate membrane. The skeletal muscle fibers are innervated by large, myelinated nerve fibers that originate from large motoneurons in the anterior horns of the spinal cord. In the axon terminal are vesicles contain excitatory transmitters–acetylcholine(ACh)[1]. The acetylcholine in turn excites the muscle fiber membrane. ACh is synthesized in the cytoplasm of the terminal, but it is absorbed rapidly into many small synaptic vesicles. In the synaptic space are large quantities of the enzyme acetylcholinesterase[2], which destroys ACh a few milliseconds after it has been released from the synaptic vesicles. When a nerve impulse reaches the neuromuscular junction, vesicles of ACh are released from the terminals into the synaptic space (quantal release). The neurotransmitter ACh binds to a muscle membrane nicotinic cholinergic receptor that increase the membrane's permeability to Na^+. The sudden insurgence of Na^+ into the muscle fiber when the ACh channels open causes the electrical potential inside the fiber at the local area of the end plate to increase in the positive direction as much as 50 to 75 millivolts, creating a local potential called the end plate potential. These membrane depolarizations are integrated and can result in activation of the muscle cell.

4 Electrical synapse

Electrical synapses[3], in contrast, are characterized by direct open fluid channels that conduct electricity from one cell to the next. Most of these consist of small protein tubular structures called gap junctions(Figure 11–3). Electrophysiological studies have demonstrated that the gap junctions represent low–resistance pathways for the direct conduction of electrical activity from one cell to another. Thereby they provide for a more rapid transmission of electrical

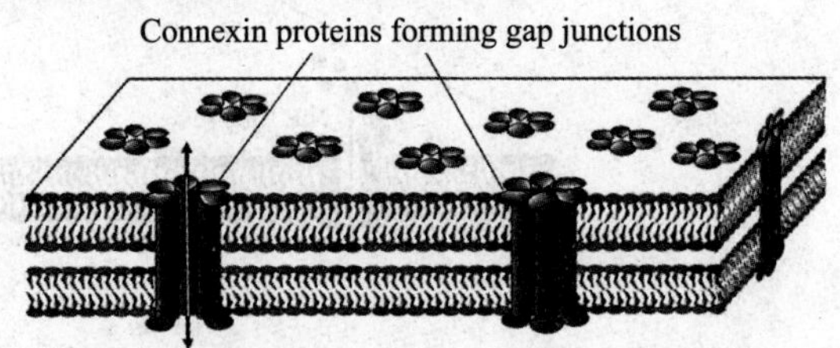

Figure 11–3 Electrical synapses

[1] 乙酰胆碱。

[2] 乙酰胆碱酯酶。

[3] 电突触。

signals between cells than at most chemical synapses. It is therefore interesting to note that gap junctions are present in tissues where the precise synchronization of the activity of many cells is physiologically important. Only a few examples of gap junctions have been found in the central nervous system. They are found not only in the nervous system but also in cardiac muscle, and in smooth muscle cells of the intestine. Their functional role in the central nervous system is not yet to be clarified.

5 Neurotransmitter and receptor

5.1 Neurotransmitter

Central neurotransmitters are substances in CNS that are released by a presynaptic nerve ending on the arrival of an action potential and cross the synaptic cleft to cause either excitation or inhibition in the postsynaptic cell. Strictly speaking, a substance will not be accepted as the neurotransmitters unless the following five criteria are met:

(1) It is synthesized in the neuron.

(2) It is packaged in synaptic vesicles within a neuron and is released from presynaptic membrane by the impulses.

(3) It binds to receptors in the postsynaptic membrane and causes postsynaptic potential.

(4) A specific mechanism exists for removing it from its site of action.

(5) When applied exogenously (as a drug) in reasonable concentration, it would mimic exactly the action of endogenously released neurotransmitter.

The word modulation is used for these complex responses, and the messengers that cause them are called neuromodulators[1]. For simplicity's sake, we use the term neurotransmitter in a general sense, realizing that sometimes the messenger may more appropriately be described as a neuromodulator.

5.2 Receptor[2]

The macromolecular structure to which some chemical substances bind in such a way as to initiate or modify a biological function is called receptor.

The chemical substances which can combine with receptors are called ligand, ligand includes drugs, hormones and neurotransmitter. The classification of ligand is shown below:

(1)Agonists[3] An agonist is a chemical substance that produces the effect when it combines with a receptor.

---

[1] 神经调质。

[2] 受体。

[3] 激动剂。

(2)Antagonist[1] An antagonist is a chemical substance which reduces or abolishes the effect of an agonist.

5.3 Major neurotransmitter and receptor system

5.3.1 Acetylcholine and its receptor

Acetylcholine (ACh) is a major neurotransmitter in the peripheral nervous system at the neuromuscular junction and in the brain. It probably has an excitatory effect either everywhere or almost everywhere that it is released, even though it is known to have inhibitory effects in some portions of the peripheral parasympathetic nervous[2] system, such as inhibition of the heart by the vagus nerves.

ACh is synthesized from choline and acetyl coenzyme A[3] in the cytoplasm of synaptic terminals, and stored in synaptic vesicles. After it is released and activates receptors on the postsynaptic membrane, the concentration of ACh at the postsynaptic membrane decreases due to the action of the enzyme acetylcholinesterase. This enzyme is located on the postsynaptic membranes and rapidly destroys ACh. One chemical weapon, the nerve gas Sarin, inhibits acetylcholinesterase, causing a buildup of ACh in the synaptic cleft. This results in over stimulation of postsynaptic ACh receptors, initially causing uncontrolled muscle contractions, but ultimately leading to receptor desensitization and paralysis.

5.3.1.1 Cholinergic fibers and cholinergic neurons[4]

Neurons that release ACh are called cholinergic neurons. In peripheral nerve system, the preganglionic fibers of the sympathetic and parasympathetic divisions all secrete acetylcholine, and for this reason they are called cholinergic fibers. Cholinergic fibers are: ① most sympathetic and parasympathetic preganglionic fibers; ② most parasympathetic postganglionic fibers; ③ sympathetic postganglionic fibers innervate sweat glands and blood vessels in skeletal muscles (to elicit vasodilatation). In central peripheral nerve system, the neurons which released the acetylcholine as its transmission called the cholinergic neurons.

5.3.1.2 Cholinoceptors[5]

Receptors that bind acetylcholine are cholinoceptors. There are two types of receptors, and they are distinguished by their responsiveness to two different drugs. Some cholinoceptors respond not only to acetylcholine but to the drug nicotine, and have therefore come to be

[1] 拮抗剂。

[2] 副交感神经。

[3] 乙酰辅酶 A。

[4] 胆碱能纤维和胆碱能神经元。

[5] 胆碱能受体。

known as nicotinic receptors[1] (N–receptor, which including N_1 and N_2 subtype). Nicotinic receptors are present at the neuromuscular junction and important in cognitive functions and behavior in the brain. Curare blocks the effect of acetylcholine on the motor end plate of skeletal muscle, whereas synaptic transmission in the autonomic ganglia is blocked by hexamethonium[2].

The other type of cholinergic receptor is stimulated not only by acetylcholine but by the muscarine. The receptors for smooth muscle, cardiac muscle, and glands are called muscarinic cholinoceptors[3] (M–receptor). They are prevalent at cholinergic synapses in the brain and at junctions of neurons that innervate many glands and organs, notably the heart. Atropine is an antagonist of muscarinic receptors with many clinical uses, such as in eye drops that dilate the pupils for an eye exam.

5.3.2 Adrenergic and its receptor

Dopamine[4], norepinephrine (NE)[5], and epinephrine[6] all contain a catechol ring and an amine group; thus they are called catecholamines[7]. The catecholamines are formed from the amino acid tyrosine and share the same two initial steps in their synthetic pathway. Synthesis of catecholamines begins with the uptake of tyrosine by the axon terminals and its conversion to another precursor, L–dihydroxy–phenylalanine (L–dopa) by the rate–limiting enzyme in the pathway, tyrosine hydroxylase. Depending on the enzymes present in the terminals, any one of the three catecholamines may ultimately be released. Autoreceptors[8] on the presynaptic terminals strongly modulate synthesis and release of the catecholamines.

The catecholamine neurotransmitters are also broken down in both the extracellular fluid and the axon terminal by enzymes such as monoamine[9] oxidase (MAO), MAO inhibitors increase the amount of norepinephrine and dopamine in a synapse by slowing their metabolic degradation. They are used in the treatment of mood disorders such as depression.

5.3.2.1 Adrenergic Fibers

In PNS, most of the sympathetic postganglionic fibers secrete adrenaline, so they are called adrenergic fibers. In CNS, the neurons which released the adrenaline as its transmission

[1] 烟碱样胆碱能受体。

[2] 六烃季铵。

[3] 毒蕈碱样胆碱能受体。

[4] 多巴胺。

[5] 去甲肾上腺素。

[6] 肾上腺素。

[7] 儿茶酚胺。

[8] 自身受体。

[9] 单胺氧化酶。

called the adrenergic neurons.

5.3.2.2 Adrenoceptors

Pharmacological evidences indicate that at least two types of adrenoceptors must exist. All catecholamine receptors are metabotropic, that is, they act by initiating metabolic processes that affect cellular function. They are termed alpha and beta adrenoceptors (αR and βR). There are three subclasses of β–receptors, β_1, β_2 and β_3, which function in different ways in different tissues. Alpha–adrenoceptors exist in two subclasses, α_1 and α_2. Noradrenaline (norepinephrine) is most effective at alpha receptors, it is generally excitatory (except in small intestine), resulting in contraction of smooth muscle in blood vessels and other tissues. Adrenaline (epinephrine) has similar actions. The alpha–adrenoceptors respond to a neurotransmitter with an increased permeability to sodium ions, depolarization, and an increased cell discharge frequency. These effects of alpha receptors can be blocked by phentolamine[1]. In contrast, beta–adrenoceptor activation results in relaxation of contracting muscle in blood vessels, bronchioles and intestine but excitation of heart. The beta adrenoceptors are particularly sensitive to a drug, isoproterenol[2] but they are also activated by adrenaline. Beta–adrenoceptor activation results in hyperpolarization and reduced cell firing rates. The effects of beta receptors can be blocked by propranolol[3].

In addition to the cholinergic and adrenergic receptor, there are many other central neurotransmitter receptors, such as dopamine receptor, 5–HT receptor, excitatory amino acid receptors, inhibitory amino acid receptors and opioid receptors. These receptors can be further divided into many subtypes; all have their corresponding receptor blocker.

5.3.3 Biogenic Amines[4]

The biogenic amines are small charged molecules that are synthesized from amino acids and contain an amino group. The most common biogenic amines are dopamine, norepinephrine, serotonin[5], and histamine[6]. Epinephrine, another biogenic amine, is not a common neurotransmitter in the central nervous system but is the major hormone that the adrenal medulla[7] secretes. Norepinephrine is an important neurotransmitter in both the central and peripheral components of the nervous system.

In addition, a type of transmission has been demonstrated in the visceral system in the

[1] 酚妥拉明。

[2] 异丙肾上腺素。

[3] 心得安。

[4] 生物胺。

[5] 羟色胺。

[6] 组胺。

[7] 肾上腺髓质。

gastrointestinal tract. These neurons release polypeptides and are collectively called peptidergic neurons[1]. Beside there are also neurons in the visceral system capable of releasing ATP or adenosine[2] as neurotransmitters.

Section 3 General principles for activities of center

1 Reflex center

Reflection refers to the body's regularity response to the internal and external environmental stimuli. It is the basic way for the nervous system activity. Reflex arc is the basic structure, consisting of five basic aspects of composition, which is receptor, afferent nerve, reflex center, efferent, and effector[3] (Figure 11-4). Reflex center[4] refers to the group of nerve cells in the central nervous system to regulate a particular physiological function.

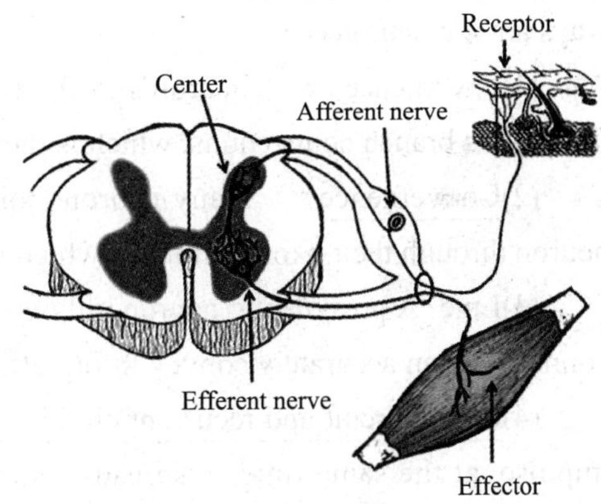

Figure 11-4 Reflex arc

According to the number of synapses in the reflex arc, the reflection is divided into ① Monosynaptic reflex[5]: the simplest form of reflection, only through one synaptic connection, and the shortest reflection mileage. ② Multi-synaptic reflex[6]: more than two synaptic contacts, a longer reflection schedule, more complicated reflection.

According to the formation of the reflection, the reflection is divided into ① Non conditional reflex[7]: the reflection need not to training after birth, which can be divided into defensive reflex, food reflection, sexual reflex and others. This kind of reflection allows the body to adapt to the environment, having important physiological significance for the survival and species breeding. ② Conditioned reflex[8]: refers to the reflection established through training

[1] 肽能神经元。

[2] 腺苷。

[3] 反射弧由五个基本的组成部分组成，即感受器、传入神经、反射中枢、传出神经和效应器。

[4] 反射中枢。

[5] 单突触反射。

[6] 多突触反射。

[7] 非条件反射。

[8] 条件反射。

after birth on the basis of non–conditioned reflex. The establishment of conditioned reflex expands the reaction range of body, and can adapt to the complex environment. Conditioned reflex changes with the change of the living environment. It can create, and can also fade, so the number can be increased.

2 Contact ways of central neurons

According to the different position located in the reflex arc, neuron can be divided into afferent neurons, inter neurons and efferent neurons. [1] There are the following basic contact ways among neurons:

(1)Divergence [2] A neuron's axon terminals make synaptic contact with many neurons through its branch connections, which is more common in the afferent pathway.

(2)Convergence [3] Many neurons jointly establish synaptic connection with the same neuron through their axon terminals, which is more common in the efferent pathway.

(3)Line A presynaptic neuron only contacts with another one postsynaptic neuron. Such connection can accurately convey information.

(4)Chain circuit and recurrent circuit [4] Chain circuit: refers to that inter neuron spreads impulse, at the same time, it spreads impulse directly or indirectly to many other neurons through the collateral.

Recurrent circuit: refers to that a neuron contacts with an interneuron through synapse. In turn, the interneuron then acts directly or indirectly to the neuron. Annular contact is the structural basis of feedback regulation and after discharge.

3 Characteristics of excitatory transmission in reflex center

(1) One–way transmission [5] Excitement can only be spread from presynaptic neurons to postsynaptic neurons, but cannot be spread reversely.

(2) Central delay [6] Excitatory transmission is slower in the central, because it must spend some time in the presynaptic membrane releasing neurotransmitters, dispersion of neurotransmitters and the neurotransmitters contact with postsynaptic membrane.

(3) The summation [7] Temporal summation: Exists mainly in the central nervous system,

[1] 神经元可以分为传入神经元、中间神经元和传出神经元。

[2] 辐散式。

[3] 聚合式。

[4] 链锁式和环状联系。

[5] 单向传播。

[6] 中枢延迟。

[7] 总和现象。

an impulse evoked excitatory postsynaptic potentials is not enough to make the postsynaptic neurons generate action potentials. But if the second impulse or multiple impulse came, before the impulse induced postsynaptic potential disappeared, the new postsynaptic potential can add to the previous phase, the postsynaptic potential increases. Excitatory and inhibitory postsynaptic potential all have temporal summation.

Spatial summation: refers to that a postsynaptic neuron simultaneously or nearly accept different impulse which comes from axon terminals, then postsynaptic potentials generated in each postsynaptic membrane can be summed up. Excitatory and inhibitory postsynaptic potentials all have spatial summation.

(4) Change of excitatory rhythm In the reflex activity, the afferent and efferent nerves have different discharge frequency.

(5) After discharge In a reflex action, when the stimulation is stopped, the efferent nerve can release nerve impulses in a certain period of time.

(6) Sensitivity to variations in the environment and fatigue The synapses can be most easily affected by internal environmental changes. Hypoxia, CO_2, narcotics and other factors all can act on the synapse to change its excitability, and Influence the transfer activities of center. The center is also prone to fatigue, which may be related to the depletion of central peripheral neurotransmitter.

4 Central inhibition

The activity of the central nervous system, in addition to the excited process, There is also inhibitory process. According to the different mechanism, Central inhibition can be divided into presynaptic and postsynaptic inhibition[1].

4.1 Postsynaptic inhibition

It is an inhibition caused by inhibitory interneurons. The inhibitory interneuron is excited, and its peripheral releases inhibitory transmitter, so that the subsequent neuronal postsynaptic membrane produces inhibitory postsynaptic potential and super polarization. It is also called the hyperpolarizing inhibition. According to the different connection ways between neurons, it is divided into afferent collateral inhibition and recurrent inhibition.

4.1.1 Afferent collateral inhibition[2]

Refers to that when a central neuron is excited, the efferent impulses come out along axon, and excites an inhibitory interneuron through the axon collateral branch, and then inhibits another neuron, its activity was inhibited. Because this inhibition often occurs between two

[1] 中枢抑制：可分为突触前和突触后抑制。

[2] 传入侧支性抑制。

centers which is antagonistic in function each other, so it is also called reciprocal inhibition.

4.1.2 Recurrent inhibition [1]

Refers to that when a central neuron is excited, the efferent impulses come out along axon, and excites an inhibitory interneuron through the axon collateral branch, and then inhibits originally launched neuron and another neuron in the same center, its activity was inhibited. This kind of negative feedback is also called the feedback inhibition.

4.2 presynaptic inhibition [2]

Presynaptic inhibition occurs because of the synaptic activity of shaft–axis. The presynaptic excitatory neurotransmitter amount is reduced, and then postsynaptic neuron is inhibited(Figure 11–5).

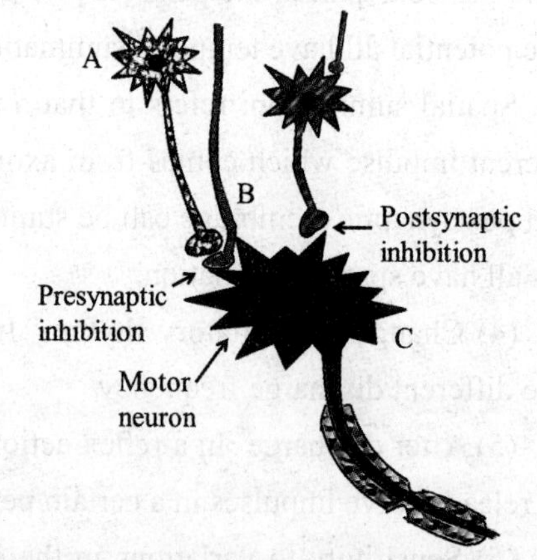

(Neuron A has no direct effect on neuron C, but it exert a presynaptic effect on ability of B to Influence C.

Figure 11–5 Presynaptic inhibition

Section 4 Sensation functions of the nervous system

Sensation from the skin, muscles, bones, tendons, and joints, or somatic sensation, is initiated by a variety of specialized somatic receptors[3]. Some respond to mechanical stimulation on the skin, hairs, and underlying tissues, whereas others respond to temperature or chemical changes. Activation of somatic receptors gives rise to the sensations of touch, pressure, warmth, cold, pain, and awareness of the position of the body parts and their movement. Each sensation is associated with a specific type of receptor. In other words, distinct receptors exist for heat, cold, touch, pressure, limb position or movement, and pain.

1 Neural pathways in sensory systems

Sensory pathways are also called ascending pathways because they go up to the brain. A bundle of parallel, three–neuron chains together form a sensory pathway. The chains in a given

[1] 回返性抑制。

[2] 突触前抑制。

[3] 感受器：是动物体表、体腔或组织内能接受内外环境刺激，并将之转换成神经冲动过程的结构，按感受器在身体上分布的部位和接受刺激的来源可区分为内感受器、外感受器和本体感受器三大类。

pathway run parallel to each other in the central nervous system and, carry information to the part of the cerebral cortex responsible for conscious recognition of the information.

The ascending pathways in the spinal cord and brain that carry information about single types of stimuli are known as the specific ascending pathways. The specific pathways pass to the brainstem[1] and thalamus[2], and the final neurons in the pathways go to specific sensory areas of the cerebral cortex. By and large, the specific pathways cross to the side of the central nervous system that is opposite to the location of their sensory receptors.

1.1 Sensory conduction function of spinal cord

In the sensory conduction process, the spinal cord is an important pathway. Uploaded feeling by spinal cord is somatosensory, whose sensory pathway can be divided into two categories:

1.1.1 Superficial sensory conduction

Conducts pain, temperature sensation and light touch. The afferent fibers enter the spinal cord by lateral root, and then change the neurons in the posterior horn. After changing neurons, the neuron sends fibers which cross to the opposite side before the central tube, respectively upload and arrive in the thalamus by the lateral spinothalamic tract and anterior spinothalamic tract (light touch). This conduction crosses firstly and then uploads.

1.1.2 Deep sensory conduction

Conducts muscle proprioception and deep pressure. The afferent fibers enter the spinal cord by the medial part of the posterior root, and its upstream branches upload in the ipsilateral posterior funiculus, change neurons after arriving to nuclei gracilis and cuneate nuclei in the lower medulla oblongata nuclear. After replacement of neurons, the neurons send fibers, and cross to the contralateral side, arrive at the thalamus by the medial lemniscus. The conduction uploads firstly and then crosses.

1.2 The thalamus and its sensory projection system

Sensory projection system of thalamus: The thalamus plays an important role in the sensory projection system. The thalamus is the transfer station for all kinds of feeling except smelling. That is to say, a variety of sensory pathways will replace neurons in the thalamus, and then project to the cerebral cortex. At the same time, the thalamus can also analysis and synthesis sensory afferent roughly.

According to the different projection ways and functions from thalamic nucleus to cortex,

---

[1] 脑干。

[2] 丘脑：是间脑中最大的卵圆形灰质核团，位于第三脑室的两侧，左右丘脑借灰质团块（称中间块）相连。

sensory projection system of thalamus can be divided into specific projection system[1] and non-specific projection system.[2]

1.2.1 Specific projection system

It refers to the sensory projection system issued from the sensory relay nucleus of thalamic to the specific area of cerebral cortex, which have point to point projection relationship.

Projection of somatosensory can be completed through three levels of neurons: primary neurons locate in the spinal ganglion or related cerebral ganglion; the secondary neurons locate within the dorsal horn of the spinal cord or nerve nucleus of brainstem; the tertiary neurons locate in the sensory relay nucleus of thalamus.

That is to say, in the classical sensory afferent pathway, such as the feelings of surface, the afferent impulses of receptor ascend to thalamic sensory relay nuclei through the spinal cord and brainstem, and then onto a particular sensory area of cerebral cortex, produce specific feeling, and stimulate the cerebral cortex to send efferent impulses.

1.2.2 Nonspecific projection system

It refers to the non – specific sensory projection system which is issued from thalamic intralaminar nuclei group dispersedly arrive to the cerebral cortex wide area.

Therefore, the sensory projection system lost specific sensory conduction function which is the common uplink access of various feeling. Its function is to maintain and change the excited state of cerebral cortex, but does not produce specific sensation.

Some differences between specific and nonspecific sensory projection systems are listed in Table 11–2.

Table 11–2 The differences between specific and nonspecific sensory projection systems

Specific projection systems	Nonspecific projection systems
Respond to a certain stimulus	Respond to various stimuli
Few synapses only	Polysynapses
Point to point to the cortex	Diffuse projection to the cortex
Sensory perception	Maintenance of consciousness

1.3 Sensory function of cerebral cortex

All kinds of afferent impulse finally reach to the cortex and produce sensation through analysis and synthesis. Therefore, the cerebral cortex is the most senior central of feelings. Different regions of the cortex have different effects of function. This is the cerebral cortex function localization. The different feeling has different area in brain cortex.

---

[1] 特异性投射系统。

[2] 非特异性投射系统。

1.3.1 Somatic sensory area

1.3.1.1 somatic sensory area Ⅰ

The projection area of the surface body feeling in the cerebral cortex, mainly locates in the postcentral gyrus, known as the somatic sensory area Ⅰ. The characteristic of the cortical sensory area is the clear position and nature.

The first sensory area has three rules in the sensory projection

(1) Projection fibers cross, namely that one side somatosensory projects to the corresponding region of the other side cortex, but the feelings of head and face project to the bilateral cortical;

(2) Space arrangement of the projection area is inverted, i. e. the lower limb sensory area is at the top of cortex, the upper extremity sensory area is in the middle, head and facial sensory area is at the bottom of cortex, but its internal arrangement is still erect;

(3) The size of the casting zone is related to the sensibility in different body parts. The representing district of the thumb, index finger and lip is large because of their high sensitivity. While back area is small because of its lower sensitivity. Because there are more sensors in the sensitive sites, and there are more neurons associated cortex with these sites, this kind of structure made feeling more precise.

1.3.1.2 Somatic sensory area Ⅱ

In the human and animal brain, there are second sensory area which located between the anterior central gyrus [1] and insula and the area is small. This area can make rough analysis to feeling. Somatosensory projection in this area is bilateral, the spatial arrangement was standing, and the positioning is not accurate. When the second sensory area is removed, the feeling does not have a serious obstacle. It may play an important role in sensory of motor function control.

1.3.2 Proprioception

Proprioception is the motion perception and sense of position in muscle and joint. At present, the precentral gyrus (area 4) is either sport area, or muscle proprioception projection area. The subjects try to launch the subjective feeling of limb movement when the precentral gyrus is stimulated.

1.3.3 Visceral sensation

Projection area of visceral sensation is more dispersed, located on the second somatosensory area of cortex, supplementary motor area and the limbic system.

1.3.4 Special feeling

1.3.4.1 Vision

The main projection area of vision is distributed in the upper and lower margin of calcar-

[1] 中央前回。

ine sulcus[1] in the occipital cortex.

The retina afferent fibers of left temporal and right nasal projects to left occipital lobe cortex; and the retina afferent fibers of right temporal and left nasal projects to right occipital lobe cortex.

In addition, the upper part of the retinal projects to the upper edge of calcarine fissure, the lower part to the lower edge, and the macular region of central retinal projects to the rear part, surrounding area projects onto the front part.

1.3.4.2 Auditory

Auditory projection is bilateral, namely one cortex area receives bilateral impulse from cochlear auditory sensory. Auditory cortical representation is temporal transverse gyrus and superior temporal gyrus in the temporal lobe. So one side area damage will not cause the total deafness.

1.3.4.3 Olfactory and gustatory

The cortical projection area of the sense of smell is located in the anterior basal region of the limbic cortex. The gustatory projection region is located in the central posterior gyrus, the base of the sensory projection area of the head and face. Olfactory and gustatory projection is bilateral.

2 Pain

A stimulus that causes tissue damage usually elicits a sensation of pain. Noxious stimulation can cause tissue injury. The released painful substance by damaged tissue cells, acts on the free nerve endings, and results in nociceptive afferent impulse. The pain is induced by bradykinin, 5– serotonin, histamine, prostaglandins, K^+ and H^+. So the pain receptor is a chemoreceptor. Receptors for such stimuli are known as nociceptor. The primary afferents having nociceptor endings synapse on projection neurons after entering the central nervous system. Glutamate and the neuropeptide, substance P, are among the neurotransmitters[2] released at these synapses.

2.1 Skin pain

2.1.1 Features of cutaneous pain

When the noxious stimulation applies to the skin, two different nature of the pain are produced, firstly is fast pain, then slow pain.

The characteristics of fast pain are: ① happen quickly, disappear quickly, i. e. short incu-

[1] 距状裂。

[2] 神经递质：在突触传递中是担当“信使”的特定化学物质。

bation period, after effect is short; ② it is a sharp, stabbing pain; ③ the clear position; ④ it is often accompanied by reflex flexor contraction.

Chronic pain is characterized by: ① the longer latency and duration; ② there is a strong burning pain; ③ the positioning is not accurate; ④ often with emotional responses and cardiovascular, respiratory changes.

In injury time, the above two kinds of pain appeared. Skin inflammation often produces slow pain.

2.1.2 Afferent pathway of skin pain

There are two kinds of skin pain nerve fibers. The fibers which conduct fast pain are mainly Aδ fiber. This kind of fiber diameter is thick, its transmission speed is fast, and the excitation threshold is low. The fibers which conduct slow pain are mainly C fibers. The fibers have not myelin sheath[1]. Its transmission speed is slow, and the excitation threshold is higher. This may be the reason for the two different pain latency.

The central pathway of pain transmission is very complex. In general, after the dorsal root goes into the spinal cord, pain upload along two ways: One arrives at the sensory relay nuclei in thalamic, and projects to the first body surface feeling area in cerebral cortex, and causes clear positioning pain; Another diffusely goes upward in the spinal cord, through reticular formation in brain stem, arrives at the thalamic kernel group, projects to second somatosensory area in the cerebral cortex and the limbic system after changing the neurons, and causes unclear orientation slow pain, often accompanied by strong emotional reactions.

2.2 Visceral pain and referred pain

2.2.1 Visceral pain

Visceral pain is the pain caused by stimulation to visceral which is a common clinical symptom. The main stimulus of visceral pain is caused by mechanical stretch, spasm, ischemia and inflammation. Myocardial ischemia, cholecystitis, ureteral smooth muscle spasm all can cause severe pain. The stimulation which causes skin pain, such as cutting, burning and pinprick generally does not cause visceral pain. Visceral pain is different from the body pain which is slow, having long duration, unclear position, poor discrimination ability to stimulus, and accompanied by nausea, vomiting, sweating and blood pressure changes.

Visceral pain is also caused by pain substances which effects on free nerve endings and, via the autonomic nerve fibers (mainly afferent nerve fibers in the sympathetic nerve) afferents into spinal cord and projects upward). But the pain afferent nerves in esophagus and trachea

---

[1] 髓鞘：是包裹在神经细胞轴突外面的一层膜，即髓鞘由施旺细胞和髓鞘细胞膜组成。其作用是绝缘，防止神经电冲动从神经元轴突传递至另一神经元轴突。

goes in vagus (parasympathetic fibers), and into the central.

Nociceptive impulses of the trigone the bladder, the prostate, cervix, rectum in pelvic viscera, afferent to sacral along the pelvic nerve.

2.2.2 Referred pain

Visceral disease causes pain at a surface part which is called referred pain [1].

Myocardial ischemia or infarction can produce pain before the heart or at the upper left ulnar. In Gallstones can appear pain at the right shoulder. Kidney stone can appear pain at groin; appendicitis often results to l pain at abdomina or umbilical region.

Referred pain has clear position, and may precede the visceral pain, therefore, in clinical, position of referred pain can assist in early diagnosis of visceral diseases.

The mechanism of referred pain is inconclusive. Most scholars agree 'the central convergence theory', that the skin afferent fibers of referred pain and the sick visceral afferent fiber afferent into the spinal cord at the same spinal dorsal root.

Section 5 Somatic motor function of the nervous system

1 Regulation of spinal cord on somatic motor function

The spinal cord is the lower parts [2] of the central nervous system, with two functions for body motor regulation: ① Transmit the motion command [3]; ② Reflection function: Can do some simple somatic reflex, such as stretch reflex and flexor reflex [4]. Overall, these reflections are regulated by senior center [5], so as to complete many complex physical movements.

1.1 Spinal motor neurons

There are three kinds of spinal motor neurons that innervate skeletal muscles [6], namely alpha beta and gamma neurons whose cell body is located in anterior horn in the spinal cord [7].

---

[1] 牵涉痛。

[2] 低级中枢。

[3] 向下传导运动命令。

[4] 牵张反射和屈肌反射。

[5] 高级中枢。

[6] 支配骨骼肌的脊髓运动神经元。

[7] α，β 和 γ 神经元的细胞体位于脊髓前角。

1.1.1 Alpha motor neurons

Alpha motor neurons have large cell body and large number, whose axon was found out from front root, and have many peripheral branches, direct control extrafusal fibers (i. e. skeletal muscle), and usually every peripheral branche innervates one extrafusal fiber. [1] Therefore, when one alpha motor neuron is excited, the excitation can be spread to many extrafusal fibers which dominate, causing their contraction. A functional unit is composed of one alpha motor neuron and all muscle fibers which dominate. [2]

1.1.2 Gamma motor neurons

Gamma motor neurons are dispersed among alpha motor neurons [3], which have smaller cell body, less number, but have higher excitability, often discharge continuously with high frequency. Gamma motor neuron axon anterior spreads from front root, whose ending branches directly controls intrafusal fibers of skeletal muscle. Therefore, when the gamma motor neurons are excited, intrafusal muscle fibers are excited and contract. [4] But because of the small number, the contractile force is weak, and has little effect on the muscle tension. [5] Gamma motor neurons play an important role on the sensitivity of muscle spindle receptors.

1.1.3 Beta motor neurons

Beta motor neurons send nerve fibers, dominating intrafusal and extrafusal fibers of skeletal muscle. [6]

1.2 Spinal reflex

1.2.1 Muscle stretch reflex [7]

Types of muscle stretch reflex: If the muscle which maintains the normal contact with spinal cord is pulled and stretched, it can reflexively contract. The stretch reflex can be divided into two types, namely, tendon reflex (phasic stretch reflex) and muscle tension (tonic stretch reflex). [8]

---

[1] 其轴突由脊髓前根发出，并有许多末梢分支，直接控制梭外肌纤维（即骨骼肌），通常每一个末梢分支支配一个梭外肌纤维。

[2] 一个运动单位是由 α 运动神经元及其所支配的所有肌纤维组成。

[3] γ 运动神经元分散在 α 运动神经元之间。

[4] 因此，当 γ 运动神经元兴奋时，梭内肌肌纤维是兴奋和收缩的。

[5] 但由于数量小，收缩力较弱，对肌肉张力的影响不大。

[6] β 神经元传出神经纤维，支配梭内肌和梭外肌纤维。

[7]（肌肉）牵张反射。

[8] 腱反射（位相牵张反射）和肌紧张（张力牵张反射）。

1.2.1.1 Type of stretch reflex

(1)Tendon reflex

When tendon is rapidly pulled, the muscle showed a rapid contraction, and cause a shift of the corresponding joint, so it is also called the phasic stretch reflex.[1]

The most typical tendon reflex is the knee jerk reflex[2]: if unit four biceps tendon is rapidly tapped[3], it is pulled, unit four biceps shows a rapid and transient contraction, knee is straightened. Different tendon is tapped; different tendon reflex can be caused.

The tendon reflex is a monosynaptic reflex[4] which only often involves 1 to 2 segments in spinal cord, and the reaction scope is limited to the pulled muscles . In clinical practice, tendon reflex is often used to understand the nervous system function, such as if one tendon reflex disappears, it shows that one segment in the spinal cord central of the reflex arc may be damaged[5]; while if the tendon reflexes shows hyperfunction, the central which control the spinal cord may decreases, suggesting that senior central may have lesions[6].

(2) Muscle tension

Muscle tension is that if the muscle is slowly and continuously pulled, it will weakly and persistently contracts by reflection, thereby preventing the muscle itself lengthen.[7]

Both flexor and extensor muscles have muscle tension, especially the extensor is more obvious. Such as, when the human body is in the vertical, due to the gravity, the joint tends to bend.[8] Joint bending stretches the muscle on the neck, torso back and lower limb, which are all extensor, and makes it tense[9]. Stretch reflex makes muscle tension increases, to resistant joint bending, so the human body can maintain upright posture. Therefore, muscle tension plays an important role in maintaining body posture, which is the foundation of postural reflexes, also the foundation of somatic movement.[10]

---

[1] 肌腱快速牵拉时的伸展反射，肌肉呈快速收缩，并引起相应关节的移位，故也称为位相牵张反射。

[2] 膝跳反射。

[3] 如果快速敲击股四头肌腱。

[4] 单突触反射。

[5] 在临床实践中，肌腱反射经常用于了解神经系统的功能，例如如果一个肌腱反射消失，则表明反射弧的一个部分即脊髓的某个节段有可能被损坏。

[6] 而如果肌腱反射显示亢进，表明控制脊髓的中枢功能可能会下降，这表明高级中枢可能有病变。

[7] 肌紧张是肌肉缓慢而持续被牵拉时，肌肉会持续轻度收缩，从而防止肌肉自身拉长。

[8] 例如，当人体处于站立状态时，由于重力作用，关节倾向于弯曲。

[9] 关节弯曲拉伸颈部肌肉，躯干背部和下肢，它们都是伸肌，使其紧张。

[10] 因此，肌紧张对于维持身体姿势起着重要的作用，这是姿势反射的基础，也是躯体运动的基础。

1.2.1.2 Sensing device and reflex pathway in stretch reflex [1]

Receptors of stretch reflex are muscle spindle [2], which was in the common one piece of muscle with the effectors. The basic central for stretch reflex is in the spinal cord. The afferent and efferent nerve fibers are included in this nerve which controls the muscle. The alpha motor neurons from anterior horn of spinal cord make the muscle contract.

Muscle spindle is a kind of receptor which feels the stretch stimulation, about a few millimeters, and the shape is like spindle. Muscle spindle is wrapped by capsule of connective tissue[3]. The capsule contains 2 ~ 12 specialized muscle fibers, which is divided into nuclear bag fiber and nuclear chain fiber, called intrafusal fibers. [4]

Afferent nerves in muscle spindle have two types: the first type of fiber is Ⅰ a which has coarse diameter, whose nerve endings surround on the nuclear bag fibers and nuclear chain fibers. The other type is class II fiber whose diameter is smaller, and the nerve endings distribute on the nuclear chain fibers.

The muscle spindle attaches to the extrafusal muscle side, and equally arranged with extrafusal fibers. The stripes at two ends of intrafusal fiber can contract, whose middle part is slightly swollen, has no shrinkage function, but the sensory nerve endings are coiled here, so sensing device is located here. Therefore, when the intrafusal muscle contracts, the feeling device is stimulated by stretch, whose sensitivity increases, while, when the extrafusal muscle contracts, stretch stimulation felt by muscle spindle was decreased.

1.2.1.3 Adjust to the stretch reflex by gamma motor neurons

Gamma motor neurons innervate intrafusal muscle [5]. Its excitement can make both ends of intrafusal fibers contract. The excitement of the middle feeling devices can be adjusted through the length and tension change of the intrafusal muscle. Thus gamma motor neurons can regulate muscle spindle sensitivity to stretch [6]. And then through Ⅰ a alpha fiber afferent to change excited state of alpha neuron, and to regulate muscle contraction.

This kind of (gamma neuron→ muscle spindle→ type I fiber→ alpha neuron→ muscle [7]) reflex pathway is called gamma loop. The gamma loop activity is the basis of the regulating the stretch reflex in nervous system [8]. Under normal circumstances, gamma motor neuron

---

[1] 牵张反射中的感受器和反射通路。

[2] 肌梭。

[3] 肌梭由结缔组织囊包绕。

[4] 肌梭囊内含有 2 ~ 12 种分化的肌纤维，称为梭内纤维，分为核袋纤维和核链纤维。

[5] γ 运动神经元支配梭内肌。

[6] 因此，γ 运动神经元可以调节肌梭对牵拉的灵敏度。

[7] γ 神经元→肌梭→Ⅰ型纤维→ α 神经元→肌肉。

[8] γ 环路是调节神经系统中的牵张反射的基础。

activity is mainly regulated by higher central, therefore, senior center can regulate stretch reflex through the gamma loop, to make the posture and body movement adapt to the needs of the body.[1]

1.2.2 Flexion reflex and crossed extensor reflex[2]

When limb skin is damaged, the stimulated limb flexor will contract, and the limb will buckle, which is called the flexion reflex. The flexion reflex can make the limbs to avoid harmful stimuli, which can protect body[3].

When the noxious stimulation increases to a certain intensity, the contralateral limb extensor also begin to activate, and the other side limbs unbend, on the basis of the ipsilateral limb flexion reflex, which is called a crossed extensor reflex. The reflex is a postural reflex, the meaning is that when one side limb buckles which causes the unbalance of body, the other side limb extent to support the body weight, so as to maintain the body balance.

Features: It is a polysynaptic reflex; efferent part of reflex arc can control multiple joint muscle activity, and intensity of reflection is related to the strength of stimulation, the range of reflection can be increased with stimulus intensity.

1.3 Spinal shock

In animal experiments, crosscutting is made at the C3 segment level of the spinal cord, and makes it disarticulate from the senior central[4]. At this time, the animal still keep breathing, but all reflex activities disappear temporarily below section level, this phenomenon is called spinal shock[5].

Main performance: the skeletal muscle tension disappears below the level of spinal cord section; peripheral vasodilatation, blood pressure drops, sweating stops; urine retention[6]. But after a period of time, the lost spinal cord function can be restored gradually, somatic and visceral reflex can be recovered to a certain degree, blood pressure gradually increased to a certain level, but cannot meet the normal needs of the body.

The recovery speed of spinal shock is related to the degree of animal evolution. lower

[1] 正常情况下，γ 运动神经元活动主要由高位中枢调节，因此，高位中枢可以通过 γ 环路调节牵张反射，使姿势和身体运动适应身体的需要。

[2] 屈肌反射和对侧伸肌反射。

[3] 屈肌反射可以使肢体避免有害的刺激，这可以保护身体。

[4] 在动物实验中，在脊髓的 C3 段水平进行横切，使其与高级中枢离断。

[5] 此时，动物仍然保持呼吸，但离断水平以的所有反射活动暂时消失，这种现象称为脊髓休克。

[6] 主要表现：脊髓离断面以的骨骼肌张力消失，外周血管扩张，血压下降，出汗停止，尿潴留。

animal, such as the spinal reflex of frog recovers quickly, just a few seconds to a few minutes are needed. That of cats and dogs needs several hours to several days, of monkey needs several days to several weeks, of human will take several weeks to months to gradually restore[1]. Simple and primitive reflection, such as flexion reflex and tendon reflex recover rapidly, while the complicated reflection recovers slowly. Visceral reflex such as urination, defecation, also has the different degree of recovery, blood pressure also gradually is close to normal level. Some recovery of spinal reflex are increased than normal, some are less than normal. The somatosensory and voluntary movement under the cross-section is lost forever, which is clinically known as paraplegia[2].

It is now believed that the cause of spinal shock is due to the sudden loss of facilitation on the severed spinal cord from higher central nervous system.

2 Regulation of brain stem on muscle tension[3]

Regulation of advanced central on muscle movement have two types, one is that advanced central directly controls muscle movement through exciting or inhibition α-neurons in spinal, the other is to regulate the muscle tension by gamma loop changing muscle spindle sensitivity. [4] The brain stem reticular formation regulates muscle tonus and posture through the facilitation or inhibition of gamma loop[5].

2.1 The facilitation and inhibition zone in brain stem reticular[6]

2.1.1 Facilitation area and its effects

Reticular formation of brain stem can strengthen the muscle tension and muscle movement, which is called the facilitatory area[7]. Stimulation of this area can make the muscle tension strengthen, can also enhance muscle movement induced by cerebral cortex[8].

[1] 脊髓休克的恢复速度与动物进化程度有关。较低的动物，如青蛙的脊髓反射快速恢复，只需几秒到几分钟；猫和狗需要几个小时到几天，猴子需要几天到几个星期，人需要几周到几个月才能逐渐恢复。

[2] 横断面以下的躯体感觉和随意运动的永久丧失，临床上称为截瘫。

[3] 脑干对肌紧张的调节。

[4] 肌肉运动调节的高级中枢有两种类型，一种是中枢直接控制肌肉运动，通过刺激或抑制脊髓中的 α 神经元，另一类是通过 γ 环路调节肌梭敏感度来调节肌张力。

[5] 脑干网状结构通过促进或抑制 γ 环路调节肌紧张和姿势。

[6] 脑干网状结构的易化区和抑制区

[7] 脑干网状结构易化区是指能够加强肌紧张和肌运动的脑干区域。

[8] 刺激这一区域可以使肌肉紧张加强，也可以增强大脑皮质引起的肌肉运动。

Facilitated areas are widely distributed, mainly in the central area of brainstem, including the medullary reticular formation, lateral dorsal pontine tegmentum, midbrain central gray and tegmentum, also extends to the midline nuclear group of thalamus and hypothalamusal cortex, striatum, anterior lobe of cerebellum vermis (intermediate) department.

2.1.2 Inhibition area and its effects

Reticular formation of brain stem can weaken the muscle tension and muscle movement, which is called the inhibitory area. Stimulation of this small area can make the muscle tension weaken, can also decrease muscle movement induced by cerebral cortex.

The inhibition area is located in the medial ventral medullary reticular structure parts, including motor area of cerebral cortex; striatum; anterior lobe of cerebellum vermis (intermediate) department. The effect of inhibition area is to inhibit γ motor neurons in anterior horn of spinal cord through the reticulospinal tract downward, weaken γ loop activity.

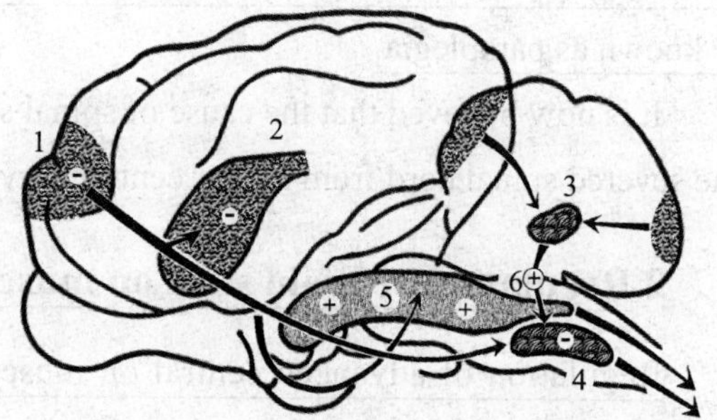

1.Motor cortex; 2.Basal ganglia; 3.Cerebellum; 4.Facilitatory region; 5.Suppressor region; 6.Vestibular nuclei

Figure 11-6 Areas in the cat brain where stimulation produces facilitation (plus signs) or inhibition (minus signs) of stretch reflexes

2.2 Decerebrate rigidity [1]

When the brain stem of an animal is sectioned below the midlevel of the mesencephalon, but the pontine and medullary reticular systems as well as the vestibular system are left intact, the animal develops a condition called decerebrate rigidity. This rigidity does not occur in all muscles of the body but does occur in the antigravity muscles–the muscles of the neck and trunk and the extensors of the legs [2].

The cause of decerebrate rigidity is blockage of normally strong input to the medullary reticular nuclei from the cerebral cortex, the red nuclei, and the basal ganglia. Lacking this input, the medullary reticular inhibitor system becomes nonfunctional; full overactivity of the pontine excitatory system occurs, and rigidity develops. We shall see later that other causes of rigidity occur in other neuromotor diseases, especially lesions of the basal ganglia.

[1] 去大脑僵直。

[2] 这种僵直不会发生在身体的所有肌肉中，但确实发生在抗重力肌：颈部和躯干的肌肉及下肢的伸肌。

3 Regulation of cerebellum on somatic motor function

The cerebellum plays an important role in maintaining posture, muscle tone regulation, voluntary movement coordination.

According to the cerebellar afferent, efferent connections, cerebellum is divided into three parts: the vestibulo cerebellum, spinal cerebellum and cortical cerebellum[1]. They are mainly receive afferent vestibular system, spinal cord and cerebral cortex, whose efferent fibres also go to the vestibular nucleus, spinal cord and cerebral cortex respectively, so three closed neuronal circuits are formed.

3.1 The vestibulo cerebellum – Balance[2]

Vestibulo cerebellar mainly refers to the flocculonodular lobe, and its main function is to regulate the body's balance[3]. Because the flocculonodular lobe and the vestibular nuclei are closely linked. So the balance function is closely related to the activities of vestibular organ and vestibular nuclear[4].

Through vestibular organ→vestibular nucleus→flocculonodular→vestibular nucleus→spinal motor neurons→skeletal device reflex pathways, cerebellum can regulate all muscle tension of body, so as to keep the balance of body.

3.2 Spinocerebellum – regulating muscle tonus and coordination of voluntary movement[5]

Spinocerebellum is composed of anterior and posterior lobe intermediate belt of cerebellum.[6] Regulation of muscle tension is mainly the function of spinocerebellar, especially anterior lobe of cerebellum.[7]

It receives afferent impulses from muscle, joint proprioceptors. Efferent impulses adjust the gamma motor neurons in the spinal cord respectively through the medullary reticular formation (facilitatory area, zone of inhibition) and vestibular nucleus, so as to achieve the effect

[1] 根据小脑传入、传出连接情况，将小脑分为前庭小脑、脊髓小脑和皮质小脑三部分。

[2] 前庭小脑－平衡。

[3] 前庭小脑主要指绒球小结叶，其主要功能是调节身体的平衡。

[4] 因为绒球小结叶和前庭核密切联系。所以平衡功能与前庭器官和前庭核的活动密切相关。

[5] 脊髓小脑调节肌紧张和协调随意运动。

[6] 脊髓小脑由小脑前叶和后叶中间带组成。

[7] 肌张力调节主要是脊髓小脑的功能，特别是小脑前叶。

of regulating muscle tension.

Inhibition of muscle tension is main the function of lobe vermis, whose controlling muscle tension role has certain spatial distribution of location, generally being inverted relationship[1]. Strengthen the muscle tension is mainly the function of both sides, whose spatial arrangement also being inverted.

3.3 Cerebellar cortex – involved in the design of voluntary movement[2]

Cerebellar cortex mainly refers to the outer part of the cerebellar hemisphere. It only accepts incoming information of projection fibers from the contact area of the cerebral cortex which exchanges neurons through pontine nuclei, rather than accepting the spinal cord.

4 Regulation of basal ganglia on somatic motor function[3]

4.1 The composition of the basal ganglia and nerve contacts[4]

Basal ganglia is a group of nerve nucleus deep in brain hemispheres for extrapyramidal main structure. Basal ganglia is mainly composed of caudate nucleus, putamen, globus pallidus, subthalamic nucleus, substantia nigra, and red nucleus.[5]

Its main function is to control muscle tension, adjust and stabilize free movement.[6]

The main pathway of its regulation are two: one is from the cerebral cortex →new striatum globus pallidus→thalamus→cortex (area 4)→the formation of cortical→ inhibition of cortical basal ganglia loops. The loop inhibits on the motor neuron, may be feedback links controlling the basal ganglia activity itself. Another new globus pallidus→ striatum substantia →nigra, red nucleus→ reticular→ anterior horn, thereby regulating the activities of spinal motor neurons[7].

---

[1] 肌紧张的调控主要是蚓叶的功能，其控制肌张力作用具有一定的位置空间分布，一般为倒置关系。

[2] 小脑皮层——参与随意动作的设计。

[3] 基底神经节对运动的调控。

[4] 基底神经节和其神经环路的组成。

[5] 基底神经节是脑半球深部的锥体外主体结构的神经核，基底神经节主要由尾状核、壳核、苍白球、丘脑底核、黑质和红核组成。

[6] 它们的主要作用是控制肌肉神经纤维、调节和稳定随意运动。

[7] 另一条为新苍白球→纹状体质→黑质和红核→网状→前角，从而调节脊髓运动神经元的活动。

4.2 Function of basal ganglia

Basal ganglia deal with the stability of voluntary movement, muscle tension controlling, proprioceptive afferent impulses. There will be two types of motor dysfunction when basal ganglia is damaged[1].

One is too strong muscle tension with movement, muscle rigidity, accompanied by Italian sports reduced, expression dull, often accompanied by resting tremor syndrome symptoms, such as Parkinson's disease, the lesions mainly in the substantial nigra. Meanwhile dopamine (DA) levels also decreased.

The other is excessive involuntary movement with reduced muscle tension syndrome, such as chorea and athetosis psychosis, the lesions mainly in the striatum. The main symptoms of chorea in patients are involuntary arm and head dance-like movements, accompanied by decreased muscle tone[2].

5 Regulation of the cerebral cortex on somatic motor function

5.1 Cortical motor area

5.1.1 The main sports area

The main sports area is located in the medial frontal gyrus and premotor areas, including district 4 and district 6. The basic features of the main sports area are similar to the first somatosensory area.

(1) Cross-dominated (head and facial muscles dominance is mostly bilateral)[3].

(2) Precise positioning capabilities, and its spatial distribution is inverted (head and face arrangements are the upright)[4].

(3) The size of motor areas is related to the fine and complexity of movement, the more sophisticated and complex, the greater cortical corresponding movement area[5].

[1] 基底神经节调节随意运动的稳定性、控制肌紧张和本体感受传入冲动。当基底神经节受损时，症状是运动功能障碍。

[2] 舞蹈病患者的主要症状是不自主的手臂和头部不自主的运动，伴随肌紧张下降。

[3] 交叉支配（头部和面部肌肉大多是双侧支配的）。

[4] 精确的定位能力，其空间分布是倒置的（头部和脸部的排列是直立的）。

[5] 支配区域大小与运动的精细和复杂性相关，运动越精细越复杂，皮质相应运动面积区就越大。

5.1.2 Supplementary motor area [1]

In the side of the area, namely the two hemispheres longitudinal sidewalls, the sport in general were bilateral.

5.1.3 The second movement zone

This area is distributed between central gyrus and insula, i. e. located in Ⅱ somatosensory area. When it is stimulated by a strong electric, can cause bilateral motor response, consistent with the distribution of somatosensory area Ⅱ.

5.2 The motor pathway

Extrapyramidal and pyramidal system are two outgoing functional systems in cerebral cortex, which coordinately activate to achieve a common regulation of body movement [2].

5.2.1 Pyramidal system and its functions

Pyramidal system generally refers to the downstream system which is issued from the motor cortex and control body movement [3], including corticospinal tract issued from cortical and passes through medullary cone and corticobulbar tract issued from cortex and reaches the brain motor nuclei [4].

The function of pyramidal system is coordinately completed by the motor cortex, pyramidal tract and spinal motor neurons. Pyramidal tract can control the activity of α and γ neuron in spinal cord, the former is mainly concerned with muscle movement, while the latter is to adjust the sensitivity of muscle spindles to match the muscle movement [5].

5.2.2 Extrapyramidal system and its functions

Extrapyramidal system [6] refers to the downstream pathways which issued from motor cortex outside of the pyramidal system without passing medullary pyramid. Extrapyramidal originated in a wide area of the cerebral cortex, including almost all of the cerebral cortex, mainly the frontal lobe, parietal lobe, supplementary motor area and the second movement area.

Extrapyramidal downstream pathway is very complex, which includes the basal ganglia, red nucleus, substantia nigra, brainstem reticular formation and cerebellum [7]. During this pathway

---

[1] 辅助运动区域。

[2] 锥体系和锥体外系是大脑皮质中的两个下行功能系统，其功能是实现身体运动的协调运动。

[3] 锥体系通常指发自运动皮质的下行系统，用于控制躯体运动。

[4] 锥体系包括从皮质发出的脊髓束，并通过脊髓圆锥，即皮质脊髓束和从皮质发出的皮质脑干束，并到达脑运动核。

[5] 锥体系的功能由运动皮层、锥体束和脊髓运动神经元协调完成。锥体束可以控制脊髓中 α 和 γ 神经元的活性，前者主要是肌肉运动，而后者则是调整肌梭的敏感度以配给肌肉运动。

[6] 锥体外系。

[7] 锥体外系下行通路非常复杂，包括基底神经节、红核、黑质、脑干网状结构和小脑。

extrapyramidal downstream repeatedly exchange neurons, and finally arrive to the spinal anterior horn, control α and γ neuronal activity. The main function of extrapyramidal system is to regulate muscle tension, to maintain body posture and coordinate muscle activities [1].

Section 6 Visceral activity regulation by nervous system

Generally visceral activity is not controlled by the will, so the neural structure regulating visceral activities is called autonomic nervous system [2]. The central parts of the autonomic nervous system include parts from the spinal cord to the brain. [3] The peripheral parts include the afferent and efferent fibers [4], but traditionally the autonomic nervous system only refers to the efferent fibers. According to the different structure and function, the autonomic nervous system is divided into the sympathetic nervous system and parasympathetic nervous system [5].

1 Characteristics of autonomic nervous system

The main function of the autonomic nervous system is to regulate the body's circulation, respiration, digestion, metabolism, excretion, endocrine and reproduction [6] and other aspects of the function through controlling the activities of myocardium [7], smooth muscle and glands, in order to maintain the internal environment relatively stable, and to support the physical behavior activity. The autonomic nervous system is shown in.

(1) The double controlling: most organs are controlled by both sympathetic and parasympathetic nerve, and the effects of the two kinds of nerve on the dominated organs are often antagonistic [8]. Such as cardiac sympathetic nerve system excites the heart, which shows positive chronotropic, inotropic and dromotropic [9]; while the cardiac vagus nerve depresses the heart, which showing negative chronotropic, inotropic and dromotropic.

Because of the mutual antagonism about sympathetic and parasympathetic nerve, the function of internal organs can balance, and can adapt to the needs of the body. But this antag-

---

[1] 锥体外系的主要功能是调节肌紧张、维持身体姿势和协调肌肉活动。

[2] 内脏活动通常不由意志控制，所以调节内脏活动的神经结构称为自主神经系统。

[3] 脊髓到大脑。

[4] 周围部分包括传入和传出纤维。

[5] 交感神经系统和副交感神经系统。

[6] 循环、呼吸、消化、代谢、排泄、内分泌和生殖。

[7] 心肌。

[8] 双重控制：大多数器官受交感神经和副交感神经共同支配，两种神经对支配器官的作用往往是对立的。

[9] 正性的变时、变力、变传导。

onistic effect is not absolute. In some organs, the functions of sympathetic and parasympathetic nerve show no antagonistic, but synergistic effect[1]. The main function of autonomic nerve is shown in table 11-3.

Table 11-3 The main function of autonomic nerve

Organ	Sympathetic nerve	Parasympathetic nerve
Heart		
Muscle	Increase rate and force	Slowed rate
Coronary arterioles	Dilated	Dilated
Blood vessels	Constricted	None
Abdominal and Skin	Constricted(α receptors)	None
Muscle	Dilated(β receptors)	None
Lungs	Bronchioles dilated	Bronchioles constricted
Glands		
Salivary	Vasoconstriction, slight secretion	Vasodilation, copious secretion
Gastric and Pancreas	Inhibition of secretion	Stimulation of secretion
Lacrimal	None	Secretion
Sweat	Secretion	None
Bladder		
Muscle	Relaxed	Contracted
Sphincter	Contracted	Relaxed
GI tract		
Sphincter	Increased tone	Decreased tone
Wall	Decreased tone	Increased motility
Liver	Glucose released	None
Gallbladder	Relaxed	Contracted
Eye		
Ciliary	Relaxed	Contracted
Pupil	Dilated	Constricted
Sex organs	Ejaculation	Erection
Metabolism	Increased	None

(2) Tonic effects: during resting condition, autonomic nerve often issues low-frequency impulse to affect organ, to make the organs to be in a slight persistent activity, which is called the nervous tonic effects[2]. For example, if the cardiac vagus nerve[3] or sympathetic nerve is cut off, the heart rate will be increased or decreased. It proves that the cardiac sympathetic nerve and vagus nerve have tension effect.

[1] 协同效应。

[2] 紧张性作用：在静息状态下，自主神经常产生低频脉冲作用于器官，使器官处于轻微的持续性活动，叫作神经紧张作用。

[3] 心脏迷走神经。

(3) The influence of effectors function: role of sympathetic and parasympathetic nerve to certain organs is not fixed, but changes with different functional state of organs. For example, sympathetic excitement effect on gastrointestinal smooth muscle [1] is generally diastolic, and on gastrointestinal smooth muscle when being in relaxation state is contraction; effect of sympathetic nerve stimulation on the non–pregnant uterus is inhibiting, while on pregnant uterus is shrinking [2].

(4) The significance of adjustment on overall physiology [3]

The activity range of the sympathetic nervous system is wide. When the body's internal and external environment change quickly, such as strenuous exercise, cold, major blood loss, mental tension, fear and other conditions, the activity of the sympathetic nervous system is strengthened, the adrenal medullary [4] secretion is also increased, so as to promoting the function of circulation, respiration, metabolism and other aspects. At this time, Because sympathetic nerves are related to adrenal medullary function and play the same role, we call them the sympathetic adrenal medullary system. The parasympathetic nervous system excitement causes the activity range is smaller than the sympathetic nervous system. But the system has positive significance on body physiology. When the body is in a relatively quiet state, parasympathetic activity dominates. The vagus nerve can cause enhanced digestive tube motion and increased secretion of digestive juice, accompanied by the increased insulin secretion. Therefore, we call it vago insulin function system [5].

In this way, the parasympathetic nervous system can promote digestion and absorption, energy reserving, restoration and protection of the body.

2 Central function of autonomic nervous system

2.1 Visceral activity regulation by spinal cord

Spinal cord is the primary center for regulation of visceral activities [6]. The spinal cord can complete the vascular tension reflection, sweating reflex, micturition reflx and erection reflex [7]. This indicates that spinal cord has a certain ability to adjust visceral activities. But spinal cord regulation is primary, cannot adapt to the need of the body.

---

[1] 胃肠道平滑肌。

[2] 交感神经刺激对非妊娠子宫是抑制作用，而对妊娠子宫是使其收缩。

[3] 整体生理调节的意义。

[4] 肾上腺髓质。

[5] 迷走 – 胰岛素功能系统。

[6] 脊髓是调节内脏活动的初级中枢。

[7] 血管张力反射、出汗反射、排尿反射和勃起反射。

2.2 Visceral activity regulation by lower brain stem

Autonomic nerve from brain stem dominates all glands of head, heart, throat, esophagus, stomach, bronchial, pancreatic, liver and small intestine[1].

In the brainstem reticular formation, there are many important autonomic nervous centers, such as cardiovascular[2] center, respiratory and digestive center.

2.3 Visceral activity regulation by hypothalamus

There are close connections among hypothalamus, cerebral cortex, subcortical center, thalamus and brainstem reticular formation[3]. In addition, the hypothalamus controls pituitary secretion through hypophyseal portal system and the hypothalamic – pituitary beam[4]. So hypothalamus plays an important role in connecting the autonomic nervous system, endocrine[5] activity and physical activity to regulate food intake, water balance, body temperature, endocrine and emotional reactions which is called integration function[6]. Therefore, the hypothalamus is a more advanced integration center.

2.3.1 Regulation of visceral activity

Stimulation or damaging a part of hypothalamus often causes changes a variety of visceral activity. Therefore hypothalamus is called the autonomic senior center. Stimulation of different parts can cause different organ activities. Compared with the spinal cord and brainstem, the regulating function of hypothalamus is relatively complex, and the regulating function of spinal cord and brainstem is relatively single(Table 11–4).

Table 11–4 Regulation of hypothalamus on visceral activity

Stimulation	Induced effect
The anterior hypothalamus	Detrusor contraction
Lateral hypothalamus or other reaction	Increased blood pressure, mydriasis[7], piloerection Muscle
Dorsal in the middle	vasodilatation
The anterior hypothalamus	Gastric acid secretion
Mammillary body and Gray tubercle	Gastric acid secretion[8] increased

[1] 脑干的自主神经支配头部、心、咽、食道、胃、支气管、胰腺、肝脏和小肠的全部腺体。

[2] 心血管。

[3] 下丘脑、大脑皮层、皮质下中枢、丘脑和脑干网状结构之间有密切联系。

[4] 下丘脑通过垂体门静脉系统和下丘脑－垂体束控制垂体分泌。

[5] 内分泌。

[6] 集成功能。

[7] 瞳孔扩大。

[8] 胃酸分泌。

2.3.2 The regulation of feeding behavior

Food intake is a complex behavior which adapt to the demand of energy. Through the regulation of hypothalamic, the body regulates the feeding activity according to the energy consumption.

Hence, there are two centers associated with feeding activity in hypothalamus: one is the feeding center, located in the lateral hypothalamic area, another is the satiety center, located in the ventromedial nucleus of the hypothalamus[1].

2.3.3 The regulation of water balance

For normal body, water intake and discharge keep dynamic equilibrium[2]. A large number of experimental and clinical practices have proved that the hypothalamus plays an important role in the regulation of the intake and discharge of water.

There is drinking center in lateral hypothalamic area. If this area is destroyed, the animal will refuse feeding and drinking. On the contrary, stimulating this area will increase water in-taking quantity. The function of the hypothalamus to regulate discharge of water is achieved by ADH, which has been described in the eighth chapter. In addition, the hypothalamus has osmotic receptor that regulates intake and discharge of water.

2.3.4 Involved in emotional response regulation[3]

Emotion is a kind of psychological activities, such as joy, anger, sadness, sorrow, fear and so on. In addition to the subjective experience, often accompanied by a series of physiological changes, including changes in autonomic function and body movement, known as the emotional reaction.

In humans, diseases of the hypothalamus are often accompanied by emotional responses. It was also found that mild stimulation of one area of the hypothalamus caused "false anger". In normal circumstances, because the inhibition of the cerebral cortex, the emotional reaction of hypothalamus[4] is not necessarily or fully manifested in emotional reaction, suggesting that the brain plays a more important role.

2.3.5 Control of biological rhythms

All kinds of activities in the body change according to the order of time which is called the biological rhythm[5].

The daily cycle is the most important biological rhythm. For example, the body tempera-

[1] 位于下丘脑的腹内侧核。

[2] 对于正常身体，进水和排水保持动态平衡。

[3] 参与调节情绪。

[4] 抑制大脑皮层，下丘脑的情绪反应。

[5] 生物节律。

ture, the excitability of sympathetic and parasympathetic nerve[1], the blood cell counts in circulating pool, secretion of adrenocorticotropic hormone are all circadian rhythm[2]. The suprachiasmatic nucleus of the hypothalamus[3] may be the control center for daily circadian rhythm.

2.4 Visceral activity regulation by cortical

2.4.1 Neocortex[4]

Experiments show that the neocortex is closely associated with visceral activity, and has characteristics of regional distribution. So the neocortex is the senior center and advanced integration site for autonomic function.

2.4.2 The limbic system[5]

Because the edge leaf structure is closely linked with insula temporal pole, frame in the frontal cortex and amygdala, septum, hypothalamus and thalamus nucleus in subcortical structure. So the edge leaf structure and these structures are all called the limbic system.

The limbic system has a wide range of effects on visceral activities, including regulation of visceral organs, endocrine activity, mood and behavior, so it is also called "visceral brain".

Section 7 Advanced features in brain and electrical activity[6]

The cerebral cortex is the most senior regulating center for various physiological functions of the human body[7]. In addition to its feeling and regulatory function for somatic and visceral motor, the cerebral cortex has more complex integrating functions, such as sleeping and awakening, learning and memory, language and thinking[8]. The cortical activity is accompanied with the changes of biological electricity, which is one of the important indexes of cortical function[9].

[1] 交感神经和副交感神经的兴奋性。

[2] 分泌促肾上腺皮质激素。

[3] 下丘脑视交叉核。

[4] 新皮层。

[5] 边缘系统。

[6] 脑的高级功能和脑电活动。

[7] 大脑皮层是人体各种生理功能中最高级的调节中枢。

[8] 除了感觉和躯体与内脏运动调节功能外，大脑皮层具有更复杂的整合功能，如睡眠和觉醒、学习记忆、语言和思维。

[9] 皮层活动常伴有皮层生物电的变化，这是皮质功能活动的重要指标之一。

1 Bioelectrical activities of cortex

The electrical activity of cerebral cortex has two forms: one is, at rest, the continuous and rhythmic electrical activity which is produced without any obvious external stimulation to the cerebral cortex[1]. It is called the spontaneous electrical activity of the brain[2]. The other one is electrical activity in certain parts of the cerebral cortex induced by artificial stimulation to sensory or afferent nerve, known as evoked brain electrical activity[3].

Electroencephalogram (EEG) refers to the changes of spontaneous potential changes induced and recorded from the scalp with the aid of the instrument. Spontaneous potential changes guided from the cortical surface are called electrocorticogram (ECOG)[4]. In general, the amplitude of ECOG is 10 times bigger than that of EEG, but the rhythm, wave shape and phase are basically the same[5].

1.1 Normal EEG waveform

Normal EEG waveform is similar to sine wave, which can be divided into alpha, beta, delta, theta, according to the different frequency and amplitude[6].

(1) α wave Frequency is 8 ~ 13Hz, the amplitude can be 20 ~ 100μV. The alpha wave occurs in awake state, eyes closed, quiet, and is significant in the occipital lobe[7]. The alpha wave has periodic changes which increase gradually and decrease gradually, and form spindle wave. When participant opens his eyes or accepts other stimuli, alpha waves immediately disappear, and beta waves appear[8]. This phenomenon is called alpha blockade[9]. When he relaxes with eyes closed, alpha waves appear again, so alpha wave is mainly cortical electrical

[1] 大脑皮层电活动有两种形式：一种是在安静状态下，没有明显外部刺激时，大脑皮层产生的连续有节奏的电活动。

[2] 自发脑电活动。

[3] 另一种是通过人工刺激感觉或传入神经诱发的大脑皮层某些部位的电活动，称为诱发脑电活动。

[4] 脑电图（EEG）是用仪器在头皮表面记录到的自发电位变化。由皮质记录的电位称为皮质脑电图（ECOG）。

[5] 总的来说，ECOG 的波幅比脑电图大 10 倍，但节律、波形和相位基本相同。

[6] 正常脑电图波形与正弦波相似，根据频率和振幅的不同，分为 α、β、δ、θ 波。

[7] α 波频率为 8 ～ 13Hz，幅度可以为 20 ～ 100μV。α 波发生在清醒，闭眼安静时，并且在枕叶皮质中最为显著。

[8] α 波具有周期性的变化，振幅逐渐增加后再逐渐减少，形成梭形大波。当受试者睁眼或接受其他刺激时，α 波立即消失，β 波出现。

[9] α 阻断。

activity in the resting state[1].

(2) β wave Frequency is 14 ~ 30Hz, the amplitude can be 5 ~ 20 μV. When a person open his eyes or is in cortical activities, the beta waves appear in the frontal lobe[2]. Generally β wave is believed to be the main wave when cerebral cortex (neocortex) is excited or is in a state of tension.

(3) θ wave Frequency is 4 ~ 7Hz, the amplitude can be 20 ~ 150 μV. It appears in adult sleepy state. So , the appearance of theta wave mainly indicates inhibitory state of the central nervous system[3]. EEG frequency of childhood is slower than that of adult, mainly being theta wave. The alpha wave begins to appear when a people is 10 years old[4].

(4) δ wave Frequency is 0.5 ~ 3Hz, the amplitude can be 20 ~ 200μV. Delta wave almost does not appear when an adult is awake, emerging only during sleep. In addition, when a person is in the depth of anesthesia[5], hypoxia[6], the delta wave can also appear.

Table 11–5 Characteristics and significance of EEG waves

Wave	Frequency (Hz)	Amplitude (μV)	Features
α	8 ~ 13	20 ~ 100	Sober⑦; Quiet; Close eyes
β	14 ~ 30	5 ~ 20	Open eyes; Thinking
θ	4 ~ 7	20 ~ 150	Drowsy⑧; Sleep
δ	0.5 ~ 3	20 ~ 200	Deep sleep

1.2 The formation mechanism of brain waves[9]

Brain wave is mainly formed by the postsynaptic potential sum[10]. Single potential cannot lead to potential changes of cortical surface. Only a large number of neurons produce postsynaptic potential (EPSP and IPSP) at the same time, and a strong electric field is synthesized,

[1] 受试者松弛闭眼时，α 波又出现，所以说 α 波是皮层安静状态下的主要波形。

[2] 当受试者睁开眼睛或皮质活动时，额叶可以记录到 β 波。

[3] 因此，θ 波的出现主要表示中枢神经系统的抑制状态。

[4] 儿童的脑电频率较成人慢，主要为 θ 波。10 岁开始出现 α 波。

[5] 麻醉。

[6] 低氧。

[7] 清醒。

[8] 困倦。

[9] 脑电波的形成机制。

[10] 突触后电位总和。

potential changes can appear in the cortical surface.[1]

1.3 Cortical evoked potential[2]

Potential changes which can be induced in the corresponding region of brain cortex are called cortical evoked potential, when afferent system is stimulated.[3] Evoked potential, which is an important electrophysiological indexes of central nervous system activity, has been widely used in the sensory pathway and localization of cortical function and so on. Especially the cortical evoked potential can be recorded without damage which can be obtained by the computer superposition and average treatment. At present, cortical evoked potential has become an important means for various human sensory function, consciousness, behavior, intelligence and other specific brain activity detection, and used for clinical diagnosis of some diseases of nervous system[4].

2 Wakefulness and sleep

Wakefulness and sleep are two necessary processes presenting the circadian rhythm. An adult needs sleep for 7 ~ 9 h, while a child needs longer, and an elder needs shorter.

2.1 Maintenance of wakefulness

The awakened state depends mainly on the ascending reticular activating system[5] activities. The awakened state includes EEG arousal and behavioral arousal[6]. Behavioral arousal refers to various behavioral performances when one is arousal. Two kinds of awakening state maintenance mechanism is different which is mediated by the different neurotransmitter.

2.2 Sleep

According to the different characteristics of sleep brain waves and physiological activities, sleep is divided into slow wave sleep and fast wave sleep(rapid eye movement sleep or REM sleep)(Figure 11–7).

---

[1] 单细胞电位不能导致皮层表面电位变化。只有大量的神经元在同一时间产生突触后电位（EPSP 和 IPSP），形成强大的电场，皮质表面才有电变化。

[2] 皮层诱发电位。

[3] 当传入系统受到刺激时，大脑皮层相应区域记录到的电位变化，称为皮层诱发电位。

[4] 目前，皮层诱发电位已成为研究人类各种感官功能、意识、行为、智力和特定脑活动检测的重要手段，也应用于神经系统某些疾病的临床诊断。

[5] 网状结构上行激活系统。

[6] 觉醒状态包括脑电觉醒和行为觉醒。

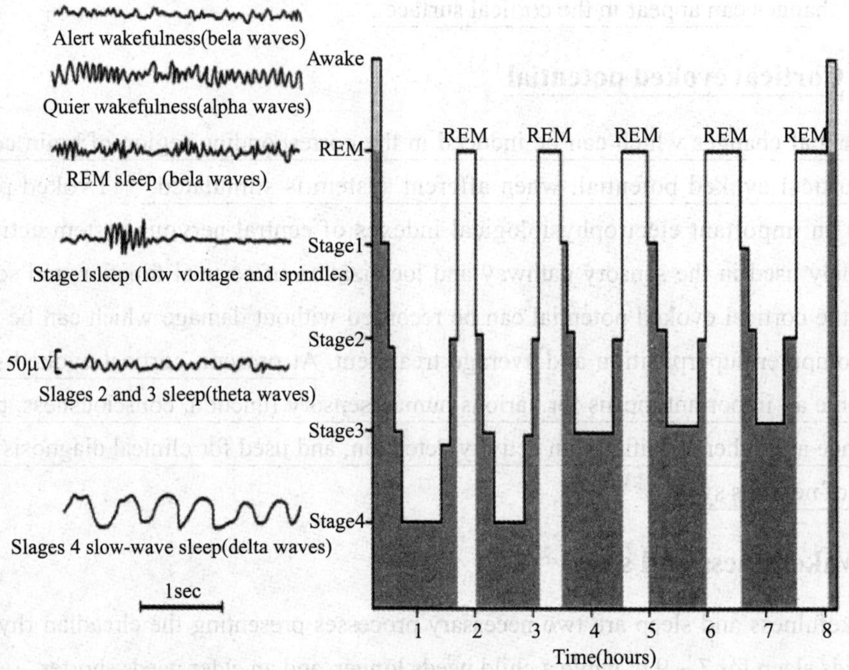

Figure 11–7 Progressive change in the characteristics of the brain waves during alert wakefulness, rapid eye movement(REM)sleep, and stages one through four of sleep

2.2.1 Slow wave sleep

Slow wave sleep is divided into four stages. A person falling asleep first enters stage 1, which is characterized by low–amplitude, high–frequency EEG activity. Stage 2 is marked by the appearance of sleep spindles. These are bursts of alpha–like, 10 ~ 14 Hz, 50μV waves. In stage 3, the pattern is one of lower frequency and increased amplitude of the EEG waves. Maximum slowing with large waves is seen in stage 4. Thus, the characteristic of this stage is a pattern of rhythmic slow waves, indicating marked synchronization.

In this period, the sense function will reduce, muscle tension decreases, voluntary movement disappears, sympathetic nervous system activity decreases, while the parasympathetic nervous system activity enhances[1]. Heart rate and breathing slow down, blood pressure drops, metabolic rate decreases, body temperature, drops, urine volume decreased. But the secretion of digestive juice and the release of growth hormone significantly increase.

So, during slow wave sleep, the body energy consumption reduces, at the same time, growth hormone promotes the body metabolism, which is conducive to the elimination of fatigue, restoring physical strength and promoting the growth[2].

[1] 在慢波睡眠期，感觉功能会下降，肌张力降低，随意运动消失，交感神经系统活动减少，而副交感神经系统活动增强。

[2] 所以在慢波睡眠期，身体的能量消耗降低，同时，生长激素促进身体的新陈代谢，这有利于消除疲劳，恢复体力和促进生长。

2.2.2 Fast wave sleep(REM sleep)

In fast wave sleep period, sleep becomes deeper, the body's sensory function declines further, muscle movement and muscle tension is also weakened further, muscle often twitches irregularly and eyes move rapidly[1]. So, this period is also called REM sleep.

Autonomic nervous function fluctuates irregularly, such as heart rate and blood pressure increase and the dream occurs also in this period[2]. At this phase, the brain protein synthesis rate is the highest, and possibly is important for children's nervous system development, maturation and for adults to establish synaptic contacts and enhance memory[3]. Another phenomenon appears in REM sleep is dream.

In REM sleep, the high-amplitude slow waves seen in the EEG during sleep are sometimes replaced by rapid, low-voltage EEG activity, which exhibits desynchronization trend[4]. So, it can also be called desynchronized sleep. However, the sleep is not interrupted; indeed, the threshold for arousal by sensory stimuli and by stimulation of the reticular formation is sometimes elevated, and most body functions further decrease[5]. This condition is sometimes called paradoxical sleep, since the EEG activity is rapid.

In the entire process of sleep, slow wave sleep and REM sleep phase continuously transform. In adult sleep, slow wave sleep appears first of all, lasting for 90 ~ 120 min, then transferred to fast wave sleep, lasting for 20 ~ 30 min, then transferred to the slow wave sleep again. In a night of sleep, this kind of transformation will repeat 3 to 4 times[6].

3 Learning and memory

Learning and memory are two interrelated process of neural activity. Learning refers to process of obtaining new behavior and experience through the nervous system activity, so as to adapt to the changing environment. Memory is the process of keeping and storing the behavior

[1] 在快波睡眠时间，睡眠变深，身体的感觉功能进一步下降，肌肉活动和肌张力进一步下降，肌肉经常不规则收缩，眼睛快速移动。

[2] 自主神经功能不规则波动，如心率和血压升高，梦也在此期出现。

[3] 在这个阶段，大脑蛋白质合成率最高，这可能对儿童神经系统的发育、成熟起重要作用；此期成人可以建立突触联系，并提高记忆。

[4] 在快波睡眠中，脑电图中的高振幅慢波有时被快速、低振幅的脑电活动所替代，呈现去同步化趋势。

[5] 然而，睡眠是不中断的，事实上，感官刺激和网状结构的觉醒阈值有时升高，大多数身体功能进一步下降。

[6] 在成人睡眠中，慢波睡眠首先出现，持续 90 ~ 120 分钟，然后转移到快波睡眠，持续 20 ~ 30 分钟，然后转入慢波睡眠，这种转换整晚将重复 3 ~ 4 次。

and experience obtaining by learning, which is built on the foundation of learning [1].

3.1 Learning form

Non-associative learning and associative learning [2]. The associative learning is more common, such as the establishment and extinction of conditioned reflexes, including classical conditioning and operant conditioning.

3.2 The basic law of conditioned reflex activity [3]

3.2.1 The establishment of conditioned reflex

It refers to the reflection which is caused by a conditioning stimulus. [4] The establishment of conditioned reflex is formed by irrelevant stimuli and non-conditional stimulation being combined which is based on the non-conditional reflex. [5]

3.2.2 Generalization, differentiation and extinction of conditioned reflex [6]

Generalization: when a reflex is established, if being given similar stimulation to the conditioned stimulus, the conditioned stimulus effect can also be gotten, this phenomenon is called generalization of conditioned reflex [7].

Differentiation: if this approximate stimulation cannot be strengthened, the approximate stimulus will no longer cause reflex, this phenomenon is known as the differentiation of conditional reflex [8].

Extinction: if only use the conditioned stimulus, but not to strengthen the unconditioned stimulus, the effect will be gradually weakened, until finally dissipated [9].

3.3 The two-signal systems

The human brain cortex is highly developed which can form various conditional reflex us-

---

[1] 学习是指通过神经系统活动获得新的行为和经验，以适应不断变化的环境的过程。记忆是储存通过学习获得的行为和经验的过程。

[2] 非联合型学习和联合型学习。

[3] 条件反射活动。

[4] 条件反射指的是由条件刺激引起的反射。

[5] 条件反射的建立是在非条件反射的基础上，由无关刺激和非条件刺激相结合而形成的。

[6] 条件反射的泛化、分化与消退。

[7] 当建立反射时，如果对条件刺激给予类似的刺激，也可以获得条件刺激效应，这种现象称为条件反射的泛化。

[8] 如果这种近似刺激不能增强，近似刺激将不再引起反射，这种现象被称为条件反射的分化。

[9] 如果只使用条件刺激，而不强化非条件刺激，效果会逐渐减弱，直到最后消失。

ing the real concrete signal, more important can establish conditional reflex by abstract word[1]. The specific signal is called the first signal, the corresponding word is called the second signal.

3.3.1 The first signal system

Refers to the use of specific signal, such as light, sound, smell, taste, touch and other physical and chemical properties of objects as a conditioned reflex stimulation which directly stimulate the eye, ear, nose, tongue, body sensor, and so on. It is common to man and animal[2].

3.3.2 The second signal system

People have language and words in social labor and communication which are abstraction of specific signal. Conditioned reflex built by these abstract signal stimulation is called the second signal system which is based on the first signal system, with its high generalization, and is unique to human activity[3].

3.4 The process of memory

The amount of environment information which comes into the brain through the sense organs is great, but only about 1% of the information can be stored for a long time[4]. The long–term storage information is generally significant to Organism.

Memory can be classified as two types as short term memory and long term memory.

3.4.1 Short term memory

It includes sensory memory and the first level memory:

Sensory memory: refers to that the information is stored in cortical sensory area, the memory time is generally not more than one second[5].

The first level memory: if the sensory information is analyzed and processed in one second, discontinuous information will be integrated into continuous new impression, you can enter the first level memory[6]. The information storage can be extended to a few seconds or to a few minutes.

3.4.2 Long term memory

It includes second level and third level memory:

---

[1] 人脑皮层高度发达，可以用真实具体的信号形成各种条件反射，更重要的是可以通过抽象词汇建立条件反射。

[2] 第一信号系统指使用特定的信号，如光、声、嗅、味、触等物理、化学性质的对象作为条件反射的刺激，直接刺激眼、耳朵、鼻子、舌头、身体感应器等。这在人和动物身上很常见。

[3] 由抽象信号刺激引起的条件反射称为第二信号系统是基于第一信号系统，它高度泛化，并且是人类特有的。

[4] 通过感觉器官进入大脑的环境信息量很大，但只有约 1% 的信息可以长期储存。

[5] 感觉性记忆：指信息存储在皮层感觉区，记忆时间一般不超过 1 秒。

[6] 第一级记忆：如果感觉信息在一秒钟内被分析处理，不连续的信息将被整合到连续的新印象中，进入第一级记忆。

The second memory: if the information is repeatedly used, it can be transferred to the second memory, which has a large amount of information, and can be more stored persistently for from a few minutes to several years [1].

Third memory: refers to as one's name or technology operation daily. Because of frequently using, it can become a lifelong unforgettable memory, which is called the third level memory [2].

Long term memory formation process is a highly selective information storage process [3]. Only those meaningful information which repeatedly works on individual can be stored for a long time [4]. While the vast majority of information which comes into the brain cannot be stored and forgotten.

3.5 Loss of memory

Amnesia [5] can be classified as anterograde amnesia and retrograde amnesia [6]. Patients who are unable to establish new long-term memories are called anterograde amnesia [7]. The inability to recall memories from the past is called retrograde amnesia [8].

4 The language center of the cerebral cortex and lateral dominance [9]

4.1 Correlation of the cortical function

There are many combining fibers between both sides of the cerebral cortex, which can transfer the cortical activity from one side to the other side, and associate the function of one side with the other. In mammals. The largest combining fiber is corpus callosum [10].

---

[1] 第二个记忆：如果信息被重复使用，它可以被传送到第二个存储器，它有大量的信息，并且可以存储更持久，几分钟到几年。

[2] 第三记忆：指如姓名或每天的技术操作。因为经常使用，它可以成为终身难忘的记忆，这被称为第三级记忆。

[3] 长期记忆形成的过程是一个高度选择性的信息存储过程。

[4] 只有那些反复使用的有意义的信息才能长期储存。

[5] 健忘症。

[6] 顺行性遗忘症和逆行性遗忘症。

[7] 不能建立新的长期记忆的患者称为顺行性遗忘症。

[8] 无法回忆过去的记忆叫做逆行性遗忘。

[9] 大脑皮层的语言中枢和一侧优势。

[10] 两侧大脑皮层间有许多联合纤维，可将一侧的皮质活动传送至另一侧，从而使两侧大脑皮层功能上能够同步。对于哺乳动物来说，最大的联合纤维是胼胝体。

4.2 The language center of the cerebral cortex

The clinical finds that if one human cortex area is damaged, can cause a variety of special language dysfunction such as motor aphasia, sensory aphasia, alexia, agraphia. This indicates that there is cortical language center in human cortex. ① Motor aphasia: if the Broca area (area 44, speaking central) is damaged, the patient can read text and understand others talking, but she cannot speak, cannot express his thoughts in words; and the muscle associated pronunciation is not paralysis[1]. ② Sensory aphasia: if the back of gyri temporalis superior is (obedient central) damaged, he can speak, write, read text, also can hear the pronunciation, but can't understand the meaning of words, often give an irrelevant answer[2]. ③ Alexia: when the angular gyrus (reading central) is damaged, the patient's visual is normal, other language functions are perfect, but cannot understand the meaning of the text[3]. ④ Agraphia: if the back of gyrus frontalis medius is damaged (Writing Center), the patient can understand others speaking, read text, and can speak himself, but cannot write; the hand's other movement is not affected[4].

4.3 One side advantage of cerebral cortex function

In the right–handed adults, the various language dysfunctions usually are due to the left cerebral cortex being damaged, while the right brain cortex injury does not produce obvious language dysfunction. The phenomenon that the left cerebral cortex dominants in language function, reflects that the human's function of two sides cerebral hemisphere is not equal, and this one side advantage phenomenon is only appeared in humans[5].

Left dominant of language function is associated with certain genetic factors, but mainly is acquired through practice of life, which mainly has a close relationship with human right–handed labor[6].

---

[1] 运动性失语：如果运动语言区 Broca（44 区，口语中心）受损，病人可以阅读文本，理解别人的谈话，但她不能说话，不能用语言表达他的想法；与发音相关的肌肉并无瘫痪。

[2] 感觉性失语：如果颞上回后部（听中枢）受损，则可以说话、写字、读课文，也能听到发音，但不能理解词汇的意思，往往给出一个无关的答案。

[3] 失读症：当角回（阅读中枢）受损，患者的视力是正常的，其他语言的功能是健全的，但不能理解文字的意义。

[4] 失写症：额中回后部受损（写作中心），病人能听懂别人的讲话，可以读文本，可以自己说，但不能写，但手的运动功能并无缺陷。

[5] 左大脑皮层语言功能优势的现象，反映了两侧大脑半球的功能是不平等的，而这一侧优势现象只出现在人类。

[6] 语言功能的左侧优势与一定的遗传因素有关，但主要是通过生活实践获得的，这主要与人的右手劳动有着密切的关系。

Chapter 12 SENSATION

The survival of any organism[1], human included, depends on having adequate information about the external environment[2], where food is to be found and where hazards abound. In addition to that, Not only external ambience but also the internal environment needs to be properly adapted with changes of the input informations for maintaining the homeostasis. Such information is communicated to the central nervous system[3] (CNS) from the skin, muscles, and viscera[4] as well as from the special senses including the visual, auditory[5], vestibular[6], and chemical sensory systems. Events in our external and internal worlds must first be translated into signals that our nervous systems can process. Despite the wide range of types of information to be sensed and acted on, a small set of common principles underlie[7] all sensory sensation processes.

Section 1 Introduction

1 Receptors and sensory organs[8]

Receptors are sensory (afferent) nerve endings that terminate in periphery as bare unmyelinated endings or in the form of specialized capsulated structures. Receptors give response to the stimulus. When stimulated, receptors produce a series of impulses, which are transmitted through the afferent nerves.

Sensory organs include receptors and accessory structure.

[1] 生物体，有机体。

[2] 外界环境。

[3] 中枢神经系统。

[4] 内脏。

[5] 听觉的。

[6] 前庭的。

[7] 成为……的基础。

[8] 感受器和感觉器官。

2 General physiological characteristics of the receptor

2.1 Adequate Stimulus

Most sensory receptors respond preferentially[1] to a single kind of environmental stimulus. Each type of sensory receptors responds much more readily to one form of energy than to others. The type of energy to which a particular receptor responds in normal functioning is known as its adequate stimulus[2]. In addition, within the general energy type that serves as a receptor's adequate stimulus, a particular receptor responds best (i. e. , at lowest threshold) to only a very narrow range of stimulus energies[3]. For example, different individual receptors in the eye respond best to light (the adequate stimulus) in different wavelengths. The minimum stimulus intensity needed to cause a sensation is called the sensory threshold[4].

2.2 Transduction

The process by which a stimulus is transformed into an electrical response is known as sensory transduction. The transduction process in all sensory receptors involves the opening or closing of ion channels that receive information about the internal and external world[5]. The ion channels are present in a specialized receptor membrane located at the distal tip of the cell's single axon or on the receptive membrane of specialized sensory cells[6]. The gating of these ion channels allows a change in the ion fluxes across the receptor membrane, which in turn produces a change in the membrane potential[7]. This change is a graded potential called a receptor potential or a generator potential[8]. Within a certain range, the magnitude of the potential is proportional to the intensity of the stimulus and can be combined. Finally, the corresponding afferent nerve fibers are triggered to produce action potentials.

---

[1] 优先。

[2] 特定感受器在正常运转中响应的能量类型称为适宜刺激。

[3] 在感受器被刺激的一般能量类型中，特定的感受器仅仅是在一个非常窄的刺激能量范围（即在最低阈值）响应最好。

[4] 引起感觉所需的最小刺激强度称为感觉阈值。

[5] 所有感受器的转导过程都涉及通过离子通道的打开或关闭接收内外环境的信息。

[6] 离子通道存在于特殊的感受器的膜上，其位于细胞单个轴突末梢或特殊感觉细胞的接受膜上。

[7] 这些离子通道的门控使感受器膜的离子通量发生变化，从而导致膜电位的变化。

[8] 这种变化是称为感受器电位或发生器电位的分级电位。

2.3 Sensory coding

Coding begins at the receptive neurons in the peripheral nervous system[1]. After the acquisition of sensory stimuli, the process of perception involves the subsequent encoding and transmission of the sensory signal to the central nervous system. Converting stimulus energy into a signal that conveys the relevant sensory information to the central nervous system is termed coding[2]. Important characteristics of a stimulus include the type of energy it represents, its intensity, and the location of the body it affects. These stimulus features can reflected by the different receptors stimulated, frequency of action potential, the number of nerve fibers participated in the information transmission and the specific parts of the cerebral cortex which the afferent impulses reach to.

2.4 Stimulus adaptation

When the same intensity stimulus acts on the same receptor, the action potential frequency produced by the sensory nerve fiber will gradually decrease as the stimulation time increases. This phenomenon is called the adaptation of receptors. Some receptors respond very rapidly at the stimulus onset[3], such as, skin tactile receptor. These are the rapidly adapting receptors. Slowly adapting receptors maintain their response at or near the initial level of firing regardless of the stimulus duration. These receptors signal slow changes or prolonged[4] events, such as those that occur in the joint and muscle receptors. In an adapting receptor, the generator potential[5] and, consequently, the action potential frequency will decline even though the stimulus is maintained. Thus, the sensory input to the CNS is reduced, and the sensation is perceived as less intense. The phenomenon of adaptation is important in preventing "sensory overload," and it allows less important or unchanging environmental stimuli to be partially ignored.

Section 2 Vision

The visual analyzer is the most important sense organ which supplies the brain with90% of the information passing from all receptors. The eyes are composed of an optical portion[6], which focuses the visual image on the receptor cells; and a neural component, which trans-

[1] 周围神经系统。

[2] 编码。

[3] 开始。

[4] 延长。

[5] 发生器电位。

[6] 光学部分。

forms the visual image into a pattern and action potentials.

The adequate stimulus for human visual receptors is light, which may be defined as electromagnetic radiation [1] between the wavelengths [2] of 770nm (red) and 380 nm (violet). The familiar colors of the spectrum [3] all lay between these limits. Out of all other special senses, the vision and olfaction use the common G–proteins as their transducer.

1 Refractive function of eye

1.1 Refractive imaging of the eye

The eye is optically [4] equivalent [5] to the usual photographic camera. It has a lens system [6], composed of four parts of the cornea, the aqueous humor, the lens and the vitreous body. The lens and cornea [7] of the eye are the optical structures that focus impinging [8] light rays into an image upon the retina.

The image is focused on a specialized area known as the fovea centralis[9], the area of the retina that gives rise to the greatest visual clarity. The image that falls on the retina is real and inverted, as in a camera.

When it is fully relaxed, the lens is at its flattest and the eye is focused at infinity (actually, at anything more than 6 meters away). When the ciliary muscle [10] is fully contracted, the lens is at its most curved and the eye is focused at its nearest point of distinct vision. This adjustment of the eye for close vision is called accommodation. The near point[11] of vision for the eye of a young adult is about 10 cm. With age, the lens loses its elasticity [12] and the near point of vision moves farther away, becoming approximately 80 cm at age 60. This condition is called presbyopia [13].

---

[1] 电磁辐射。

[2] 波长。

[3] 光谱。

[4] 光学的。

[5] 等同于。

[6] 透镜系统。

[7] 角膜。

[8] 冲击。

[9] 中央凹。

[10] 睫状肌。

[11] 近点。

[12] 弹性。

[13] 远视眼。

1.2 Reduced eye

If all the refractive surfaces of the eye are algebraically added together and then considered to be one single lens, the optics of the normal eye may be simplified and represented schematically as a "reduced eye[1]. " This is useful in simple calculations. In the reduced eye, a single refractive surface is considered to exist, with its central point 15 millimeters in front of the retina and a total refractive power of 59 diopters when the lens is accommodated for distant vision.

Using reduced eye, the image size on the retina of different distant objects can be calculated conveniently. If AB is a object, ab is a image, Bn = object distance, and nb = image distance, then

$$\frac{AB}{Bn}=\frac{ab}{nb}$$

These relations can be seen in Figure12-1 and nb= 15 mm. The smallest retinal image visible to the human eye, approximately equal to the average diameter of a cone cell in the fovea of the retina.

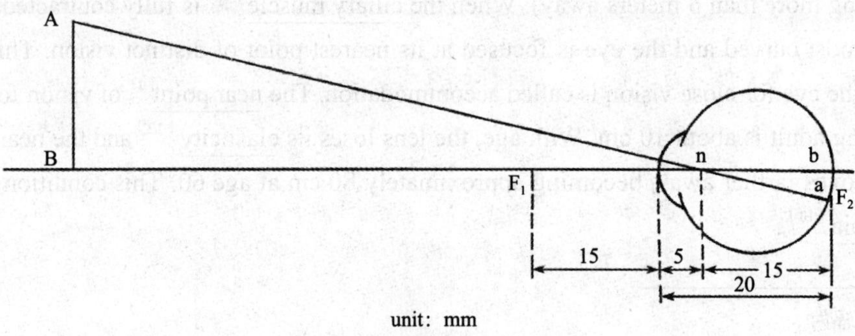

unit: mm

Figure12-1

1.3 Regulation of ocular refractive function

In quiet, the normal eye can make an object more than 6cm far away imaged on the retina. This distance is called far point[2]. If an object is within 6cm, he refractive ability of refractive system must be increased to make image on the retina. This process is completed through reflection, called the eye near reflex[3]. The midbrain is the center of near reflex. There are three

[1] 简化眼。

[2] 远点。

[3] 视近反射。

ways of regulation.

1.3.1 Regulation of lens

In order to see objects within 6cm, the lens must change its shape to increase its refractive power. When focusing on near objects, the ciliary muscle contracts, and the natural elasticity of the lens makes itself to become more spherical. To focus on distant objects, the ciliary muscle relaxes and pulls the lens into a flattened, oval shape. The shape of the lens determines to what degree the light rays are bent and how they project onto the retina. The action of the ciliary muscle exerts the greatest effect on the process of accommodation, though other influences such as constriction of the pupil also contribute(Figure 12–2).

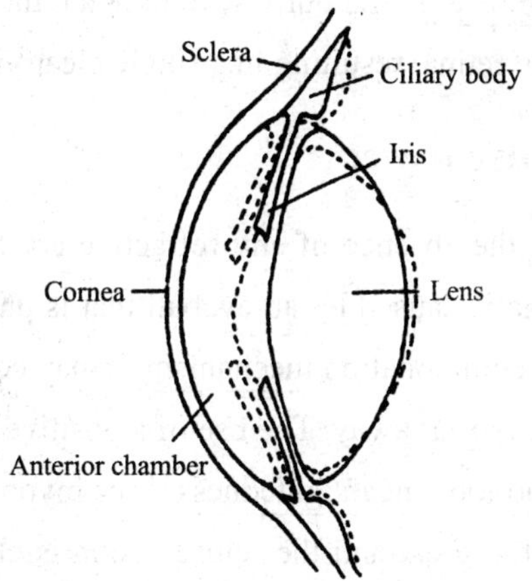

Figure 12–2 Mechanism of accommodation

1.3.2 Pupillary accommodation

The major function of the iris is to increase the amount of light that enters the eye during darkness and to decrease the amount of light that enters the eye in daylight. The amount of light that enters the eye through the pupil is proportional to the area of the pupil or to the square of the diameter of the pupil. The pupil of the human eye can become as small as about 1.5 millimeters and as large as 8 millimeters in diameter. The size of the pupil changes with the intensity of the radiation light. This is called pupillary light reflex [1]. The receptor for light reflex in the pupil is the retina. The reflex center is in the midbrain. The effect is bilateral. That is, when the light shines on one side of the eye, both sides of the pupil shrink at the same time. Clinically, this reflex is used to assist in the diagnosis of neuropathy, to determine the depth of anesthesia, and to assess the severity of the disease. Another kind of pupillary reflex is called the pupillary accommodation reflex [2]. It refers to the fact that when viewed near

[1] 瞳孔的对光反射。

[2] 瞳孔调节反射。

objects, the pupil is narrowed. Its physiological significance makes the imaging of the retina clearer by reducing the amount of light entering the eye and reducing the spherical aberration and chromatic aberration of the near light system. The opening and narrowing of the pupils are accomplished by the constriction of pupil dilatator muscles and the pupillary sphincters [1] respectively, and which are innervated by sympathetic nerves and parasympathetic nerves in the oculomotor nerve [2] respectively.

1.3.3 Convergence

When both eyes are near the object, they turn inward to fix on near objects. This is called eye convergence [3]. It is caused by the reflexophil contraction of two medial rectus muscle, so it is also called convergence reflex [4]. Its purpose is to make the nearby object can fall on the mutual symmetry points of the retina, resulting in a single clear vision and avoid diplopia.

1.4 Abnormal refractive power

Normal vision [5] (i. e. , the absence of any refractive errors) is termed emmetropia [6]. Farsightedness [7] or hyperopia is caused by an eyeball that is physically too short to focus on distant objects. The natural accommodation mechanism [8] may compensate for distance vision, but the near point will still be too far away. The use of a positive (converging) lens can correct this defect. If the eyeball is too long, nearsightedness [9] or myopia is resulted. The converging power of this kind of eye is too great and the close vision is clear, but the eye cannot focus on distant objects. A negative (diverging) lens can correct this defect. If the curvature of the cornea is not symmetric, astigmatism [10] results, objects with different orientations in the field of view will have different focal positions. Vertical lines may appear sharp, while horizontal structures are blurred. This condition can be corrected with the use of a cylindrical lens, which has different radii [11] of curvature at the proper orientations along its surfaces.

---

[1] 瞳孔开大肌和瞳孔括约肌。
[2] 动眼神经。
[3] 眼球会聚。
[4] 辐辏反射。
[5] 正常视觉。
[6] 正视。
[7] 远视。
[8] 结构。
[9] 近视。
[10] 散光。
[11] 半径。

2 Retinal photoreceptor[1] function

2.1 Structure of retina and photoreceptor cells

The retina is only 0.1 ~ 0.5 mm thick but composed of four layers of cells, including a pigment cell layer, a layer of photoreceptors, and a layer of bipolar cells, and a layer of ganglion cells. The pigment cell acts as a protective and trophic agent for photoreceptor cells. Photoreceptor cells are divided into cones and rod cells. The two photoreceptor cells are associated with bipolar cells, and bipolar cells have synaptic connections with ganglion cells. The macular fovea[2] is a minute area in the center of the retina, being composed almost entirely of cones. Slightly off to the nasal side of the retina is the optic disc, where the optic nerve leaves the retina. There are no photoreceptor cells here, resulting in a blind spot in the field of vision (Figure 12–3).

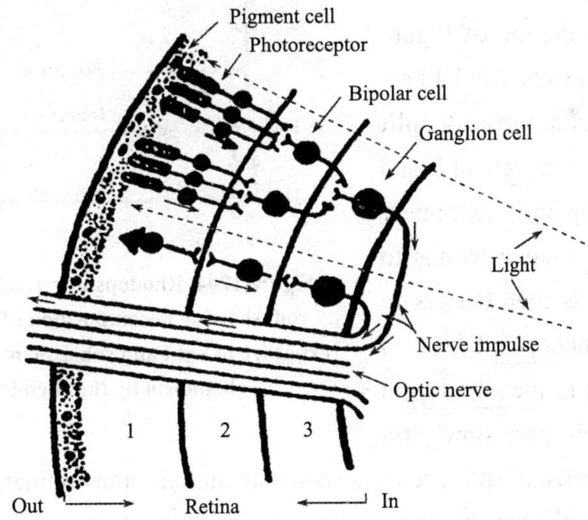

Figure 12–3 Structure of retina

2.2 Photochemistry and photo transduction of vision

The photoreceptors contain molecules called photopigments[3], which absorb light. In the

[1] 感光器。

[2] 黄斑中央凹。

[3] 光色素。

case of the rods, this is rhodopsin[1]; in the cones, it is one of three "color" photopigments, usually called simply color pigments, that function almost exactly the same as rhodopsin except for differences in spectral sensitivity.

2.2.1 The photoreceptor transducing action of rod cells

The outer segment of the rod that projects into the pigment layer of the retina has a concentration of about 40% of the light-sensitive pigment called rhodopsin, or visual purple. This substance is a combination of the protein scotopsin[2] and the carotenoid pigment retinal (also called retinene[3]). Furthermore, the retinal is a particular type called 11-cis retinal[4]. This cis form of retinal is important because only this form can bind with scotopsin to synthesize rhodopsin.

When light energy is absorbed by rhodopsin, the rhodopsin begins to decompose within a very small fraction of a second, as shown at the top of Figure 12-4. The immediate product is bathorhodopsin[5], which is a partially split combination of the all-trans retinal[6] and scotopsin. Bathorhodopsin is extremely unstable and decays in nanoseconds to lumirhodopsin[7]. This then decays in microseconds to metarhodopsin I[8], then in about a millisecond to metarhodopsin II[9], and finally, much more slowly (in seconds), into the completely split products scotopsin and all-trans retinal. It is the metarhodopsin II, also called activated rhodopsin, that excites electrical changes in the rods, and the

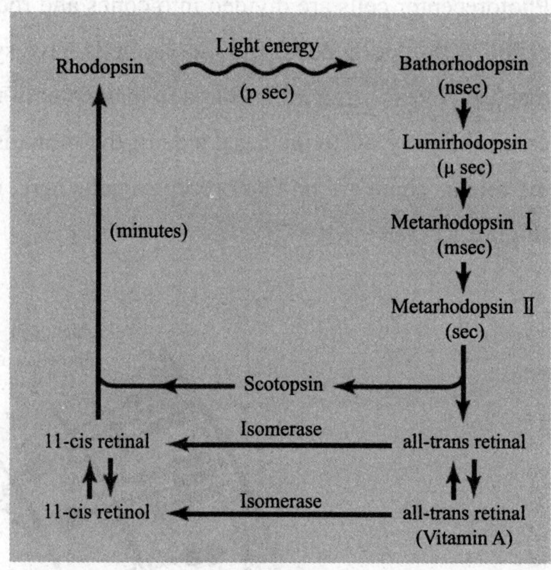

Figure 12-4 Rhodopsin-retinal visual cycle in the rod, showing decomposition of rhodopsin during exposure to light and subsequent slow reformation of rhodopsin by the chemical processes

[1] 视紫红质。

[2] 视暗蛋白。

[3] 视黄醛。

[4] 11-顺视黄醛。

[5] 深紫红质。

[6] 全反视黄醛。

[7] 光视紫红质。

[8] 间视紫红质Ⅰ。

[9] 间视紫红质Ⅱ。

rods then transmit the visual image into the central nervous system in the form of optic nerve action potential, as we discuss later.

Note in Figure 12–4 that there is a second chemical route by which all–trans retinal can be converted into 11–cis retinal. This is by conversion of the all–trans retinal first into all–trans retinol [1], which is one form of vitamin A. Then the all–trans retinol is converted into 11–cis retinol under the influence of the enzyme isomerase [2]. Finally, the 11–cis retinol is converted into 11–cis retinal, which combines with scotopsin to form new rhodopsin. When the body lacks vitamin A, rhodopsin synthesis will disorder, and affect the dark vision ability, cause nyctalopia [3].

2.2.2 The photoreceptor transducing action of cone cells

Only one of three types of color pigments is present in each of the different cones, thus making the cones selectively sensitive to different colors: blue, green, or red. These color pigments are called, respectively, blue–sensitive pigment, green–sensitive pigment, and red–sensitive pigment. The absorption characteristics of the pigments in the three types of cones show peak absorbencies [4] at light wavelengths of 445,535, and 570 nanometers, respectively. These are also the wavelengths [5] for peak light sensitivity for each type of cone, which begins to explain how the retina differentiates the colors.

2.2.3 The photosensitive transducing effect of photoreceptor cells

The outer segment of the photoreceptor cell is the key part for photo electric conversion.

In the absence of light, sodium channels [6] on the outer segment membrane are maintained in an open configuration by the presence cGMP. The resulting influx of sodium ions elevates the membrane potential, causes a steady release of neurotransmitter [7] (glutamate [8]).

When light stimulates the outer segment, the retinal in the disc membrane assumes a new conformation induced by the absorption of energy from photons. This activates a G protein called transducin[9]. In turn, transducin activates an enzyme that inactivates cGMP. The sodium channels close, the membrane potential becomes hyperpolarized, and neurotransmitter release is inhibited.

---

[1] 全反视黄醇。

[2] 异构酶。

[3] 夜盲症。

[4] 吸收能力。

[5] 波长。

[6] 钠离子通道。

[7] 神经递质。

[8] 谷氨酸盐。

[9] 转导蛋白。

Photoreceptor cells themselves do not produce action potentials. The hyperpolarizing potential caused by light stimulation can release the neurotransmitter and cause the changes of slow potential in bipolar cells. This slow potential causes the ganglion cell to be depolarized through summation to reach the threshold potential to produce action potential, thus becoming the visual signal transmitted by the retina to the visual center.

3 Some visual phenomena

3.1 Dark adaptation and light adaptation

If a person moves from a place of bright sunlight into a darkened room, no object could be seen clearly at first. After a period of time, the vision gradually recovered. The process was called dark adaptation[1]. In the dark, vision can only be supplied by the rods, which have greater sensitivity than the cones. During the exposure to bright light[2], however, the rods' rhodopsin has been completely decomposed, making the rods insensitive to light. Dark adaptation occurs, in part, as enzymes regenerate the initial form of rhodopsin, which can respond to light.

In contrast to dark adaptation, light adaptation refers that when one steps from a dark place into a bright one initially, the eye is extremely sensitive to light and the visual image[3] has poor contrast. Only a moment later, the vision will be restored. Rhodopsin is decomposed rapidly, vision is taken over by the cones. Cones are less sensitive to light than are rods, so the visual image becomes less bright.

3.2 Binocular vision and stereopsis

The visual fields of the two eyes overlap[4] in the central part to provide binocular vision[5]. The images falling on the two retinas are not identical but neural mechanisms allow them to be interpreted as[6] single images. Advantages of binocular vision: ① enlarging the visual field of monocular vision; ② making up for blind spot defects in monocular vision; ③ enhancing the accuracy of judging object size and distance; ④ forming stereoscopic vision.

The visual capability of localizing object by two eyes is called stereopsis[7]. Stereoscopic vision allows us to see the height, width, and thickness of objects. It depends on fusion in the

---

[1] 暗适应。

[2] 曝光。

[3] 视觉影像。

[4] 重叠。

[5] 双眼视觉。

[6] 把……理解为。

[7] 立体视觉。

brain of two slightly different view of the same object.

3.3 Visual acuity

Visual acuity[1] is a measurement of the ability of the eye to form a sharply focused image on the retina. It is measured by determining the minimum distance by which two points must be separated in order to appear as two discrete entities. Eyesight is examine using an eye chart. It is represented by the reciprocal of the minimum angle formed by two human light spots. The international eye chart is designed according to this principle. The angle refers to that formed by the lights from two spots in the eyes node. When the human eye can see the gap direction of "E" word 5 m far away on the tenth lines of visual chart. It is normal visual acuity, showed as 1 and the angle of view is 1 cent (Figure 12–5). At this moment, the two points distance of light formed in the retina is 4 ~ 5 cm, just the equivalent of a cone's diameter. In this way, two light rays stimulate two cones, and spaced apart by at least one cone.

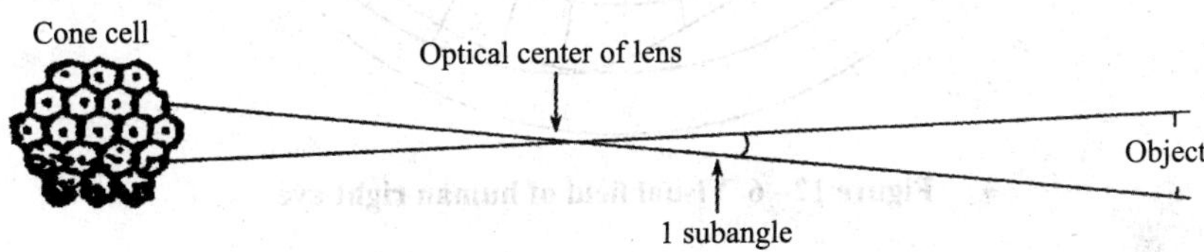

Figure 12–5 Illustrative diagram of visual acuity

3.4 Fields of vision (or Visual field)

The field of vision is the visual area seen by one eye at a given instant. The area on the nasal side[2] is called the nasal field of vision which imaged on the temporal side, and the area on the lateral side is called the temporal field of vision which imaged on the nasal side. Under the same condition, the field of vision of different colors are different in size: white > blue > red > green. In practice it is customarily mapped in a procedure termed optic perimetry[3]. In normal visual field images, the temporal visual field is greater than that of nasal side; lower visual field is greater than the that of upper side. Pathological[4] restrictions of the visual field will occur

[1] 视敏度。

[2] 鼻侧。

[3] 光学视野。

[4] 病理学的。

when the retina, the optic pathway, or the visual cortex [1] are damaged (Figure 12–6) .

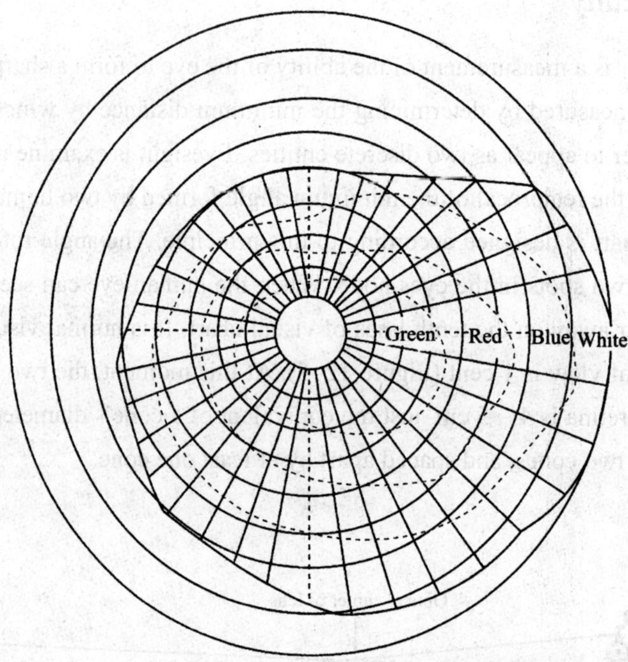

Figure 12– 6 Visual field of human right eye

Section 3 Hearing

The human ear is the special sensory receptor [2] for the sound stimulus. As the stimulus passes from the external medium, the actual receptor are bristle cells in the acoustic labyrinth. The sense of hearing involves the physics of sound, the physiological functions of the external, middle, and inner ear, the nerves to the brain, and the brain processing of acoustic [3] information.

1 The human ear threshold

The normal human ear is sensitive to sound frequency [4] that ranges from about 20 to 20000 Hz, to the sound intensity ranges from 0.0002 ~ 1000 dyn/cm^2. The minimum sound intensity can cause hearing, is called threshold, varying with its frequency. Sound that exceed

[1] 视皮质。

[2] 感受器。

[3] 听觉的。

[4] 频率。

120 dB can cause pain.

2 External and middle ear

2.1 External ear

The external ear includes the pinna and the auditory canal. The pinna may help direct sound into the auditory canal. The auditory canal transmits sound waves to the tympanic membrane[1]. The shapes of the the pinna and the external auditory canal help to amplify and direct the sound.

2.2 Middle ear

The middle ear consists of the tympanic membrane, the ossicles, the eardrum, and the eustachian tube. The main function of the middle ear is to transmit the energy of sound waves in the air efficiently to the inner ear lymph, in which the tympanic membrane and ossicular chain play an important role in the transmission of sound.

The middle ear cavity connects to the pharynx[2] through the eustachian tube[3]. Pressure differences between the external and middle ears can be equalized through this passage. Flying and diving can cause pressure difference, which can stretch the tympanic membrane and cause pain.

The auditory ossicles are connected in turn to form a fixed angle. When the sound wave reaches the oval window[4] from the tympanic membrane through the ossicular chain, its vibration pressure increases and the sound transmission effect increases. Because the oval window is much smaller than the tympanic membrane, the pressure is increased 15 to 20 times.

The middle ear also serves other functions. Two muscles are found in the middle ear: the tensor tympani and the stapedius. These muscles attach, respectively, to the malleus and stapes. When they contract, they dampen movements of the ossicular chain and so decrease the sensitivity of the acoustic apparatus[5]. These muscles help to protect the delicate receptor apparatus of the inner ear from continuous intense sound stimuli produced in the environment or from the proximity of one's own voice.

---

[1] 鼓膜。

[2] 咽。

[3] 咽鼓管。

[4] 卵圆窝。

[5] 听觉装置。

3 Inner ear

The inner ear includes the bony and membranous labyrinths[1]. The cochlea and the vestibular apparatus[2] are formed from these structures. The former is hearing organ, the latter is balance sense organ.

3.1 Structure of cochlea

The cochlea is a spiral–shaped organ[3]. In human, the spiral consists of $2\frac{3}{4}$ turns; it starts from a broad base and extends to a narrow apex. The cochlea is almost completely divided lengthwise by a fluid–filled membranous tube, the cochlear duct[4], which follows the cochlear spiral and contains the sensory receptors of the auditory system. On either side of the cochlear duct are fluid– filled compartments: the scala vestibuli[5] which is on the side of the cochlear duct that begins at the oval window; and the scala tympani[6], which is below the cochlear duct and ends in a second membrane–covered opening to the middle ear, the round window. The scala vestibule and scala tympani meet at the end of the cochlear duct at the helicotrema[7].

The side of the cochlear duct nearest to the scala tympani is formed by the basilar membrane[8], upon which sits the organ of Corti, which contains the ear's sensitive receptor cells. The receptor cells of the organ of Corti, the hair cells, are mechanoreceptors[9] that have hair-like stereocilium protruding from one end. The organ of Corti is located within the cochlear duct. It lies on the basilar membrane and consist of several components, including three rows of outer hair cells, a single row of inner hair cells, a gelatinous[10] tectorial membrane, and a number of types of supporting cells.

3.2 Phonosensitivetransduction in cochlea

3.2.1 Vibration of basilar membrane

Pressure differences across the cochlear duct cause vibration of the basilar membrane.

[1] 膜迷路。

[2] 前庭装置。

[3] 螺旋器。

[4] 蜗管。

[5] 前庭阶。

[6] 鼓阶。

[7] 蜗孔。

[8] 基膜。

[9] 机械性感受器。

[10] 胶状的。

The region of maximal displacement of the vibrating basilar membrane varies with the frequency of the sound source. The properties of the membrane nearest the middle ear are such that this region vibrates most easily, that is, undergoes the greatest movement, in response to high–frequency tones. As the frequency of the sound is lowered, vibration waves travel out along the membrane for greater distances. Progressively [1] more distant regions of the basilar membrane vibrate maximally in response to progressively lower tones.

The hair cells transform the pressure waves in the cochlea into receptor potentials. Movements of the basilar membrane stimulate the hair cells because they are attached to the membrane. The stereocilium [2] of the hair cells are in contact with the tectorial membrane, which overlies the organ of Corti. As the basilar membrane is displaced by pressure waves, the hair cells move in relation to the stationary tectorial membrane, and, consequently, the stereocilium are bent(Figure 12–7).

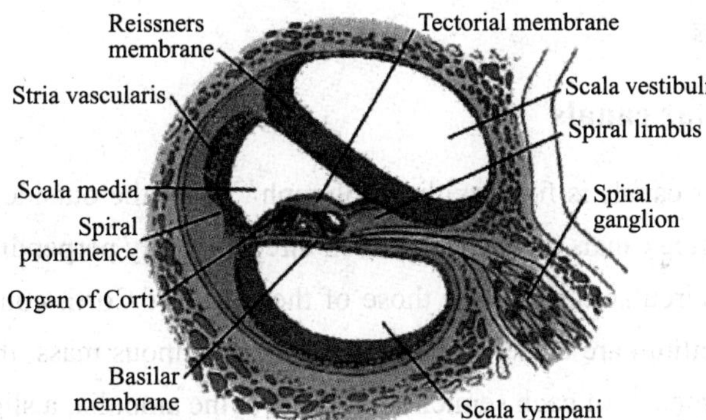

Figure 12–7 Structure of cochlea

3.2.2 Bioelectric phenomena in the cochlea

Whenever the stereocilium bend, cation channels in the plasma membrane of the hair cell open, and the resulting cation influx depolarizes the membrane. This opens voltage–gated calcium channels[3], which triggers neurotransmitter release. In an unusual circumstance, the fluid surrounding the stereocilium has a high concentration of K^+, so the influx of K^+ (rather than Na^+) depolarizes the hair cell.

The neurotransmitter released is glutamate (the same neurotransmitter released by photoreceptor cells), which binds to and activates protein binding sites on the terminals of the 10 or so afferent neurons [4] that synapse upon the hair cell. This causes the generation of action

[1] 日益增多的。

[2] 静纤毛。

[3] 钙离子通道。

[4] 传入神经元。

potentials[1] in the neurons, the axons of which join to form the cochlear nerve (a component of cranial nerve Ⅷ). The greater the energy (loudness) of the sound wave, the greater the frequency of action potentials generated in the afferent nerve fibers.

Section 4 Vestibular sensation

1 Device and appropriate stimulation of the vestibular organs

The ear also has important non-auditory sensory functions. The sensory receptors that allow us to maintain our equilibrium and balance are located in the vestibular apparatus, which consists (on each side of the head) of three semicircular canals[2] and two otolithic organs, the utricle[3] and the saccule[4]. These structures are located in the bony labyrinth of the temporal bone and are sometimes called the membranous labyrinth. As with hearing, the basic sensing elements are hair cells.

1.1 Semicircular canals

The semicircular canals is filled with endolymph[5]; on the outside, they are bathed by perilymph[6]. The three canals on each side lie in three mutually perpendicular planes. Receptor cells of the semicircular canals, like those of the organ of Corti, contain hairlike stereocilium. These stereocilium are closely ensheathed by a gelatinous mass, the cupula[7], which extends across the lumen[8] of each semicircular canal at the ampulla, a slight bulge in the wall of each duct.

Whenever the head is moved, the semicircular canal within its bony enclosure and the attached bodies of the hair cells all move with it. The fluid filling the duct, however, is not attached to the skull[9], and because of inertia[10], tends to retain its original position. Thus, the moving ampulla is pushed against the stationary fluid, which causes bending of the stereo-

[1] 动作电位。
[2] 半规管。
[3] 椭圆囊。
[4] 球囊。
[5] 内淋巴。
[6] 外淋巴。
[7] 壶腹帽。
[8] 内腔。
[9] 颅骨。
[10] 惯性。

cilium and alteration in the rate of release of a chemical transmitter from the hair cells. This transmitter activates the nerve terminals which from synapses [1] with the hair cells. The hair cells are stimulated[2] only during changes in the rate of rotation (that is, during acceleration or deceleration) of the head. The three pair of semicircular canals accept the stimulation of rotational motion consistent with the plane direction in which they are located.

1.2 Saccule and utricle

The proper stimulus the saccule and the utricle, is accelerated motion in a straight line The sensory structures in these organs, called maculae [3], also employ hair cells, similar to those of the ampullar cristae [4]. The macular hair cells are covered with the otolithic membrane, a gelatinous substance in which are embedded numerous small crystals of calcium carbonate called otoliths [5]. Because the otoliths are heavier than the endolymph, tilting of the head results in gravitational movement of the otolithic membrane and a corresponding change in sensory neuron action potential frequency. As in the ampulla, the action potential frequency increases or decreases depending on the direction of displacement. The maculae are adapted to provide a steady signal in response to displacement; in addition, they are located away from the semicircular canals and are not subject to motion–induced currents in the endolymph. This allows them to monitor the position of the head with respect to a steady gravitational field. The maculae also respond proportionally to linear acceleration.

2 Vestibular response and nystagmus [6]

Receptors of semicircular canals give response to rotatory movements or angular acceleration of the head. And receptors of utricle and saccule give response to linear acceleration of head. Thus, the vestibular apparatus is responsible for detecting the position of head during different movements. It also causes reflex adjustments in the position of body postural changes and autonomic nervous responses, such as nausea, vomiting, dizziness, and pale skin. The most specific vestibular response is nystagmus

Nystagmus is the rhythmic oscillatory involuntary movements of eyeball. It is common during rotation. It is due to the natural stimulatory effect of vestibular apparatus during rotational acceleration. Nystagmus occurs both in physiological and pathological conditions.

---

[1] 神经末梢突触。

[2] 受到刺激的。

[3] 斑。

[4] 壶腹嵴。

[5] 耳石。

[6] 前庭反应和眼震颤。

Section 5 Taste and smell

1 Taste

Taste is mainly a function of the taste buds[1] in the mouth. The receptor cells are arranged within the taste buds like the segments of an orange. A long narrow process on the upper surface of each receptor cell extends into a small pore at the surface of the taste bud, where the process is bathed by the fluids of the mouth. Many chemicals can generate the sensation of taste, and these chemicals can come in the air as aromas as well as in food or other objects that are put directly in the mouth[2]. Taste sensations (modalities[3]) are traditionally divided into four basic groups: sweet, sour, salty, and bitter.

Each group of tastes has a distinct signal transduction mechanism[4]. For instance, salt taste begins with sodium[5] entry into the cell through plasma membrane ion channels[6]. This depolarizes[7] the plasma, membrane, causing neurotransmitter[8] release from the receptor cell. This release causes depolarization of another afferent neuron, which carries the signal to the brain. In contrast, organic molecules such as carbohydrates[9] interact with plasma membrane receptors that regulate second messenger cascades.

The pathways for taste in the central nervous system project to the parietal corte[10], near the 'mouth' region of the somatosensory cortex[11].

2 Smell

The receptor organ for smell, or olfaction[12], is the olfactory mucosa, an area of approxi-

[1] 味蕾。

[2] 许多化学物质可以形成味觉，这些化学物质可以来源于散发在空气中的香味，也可以存在于食物中或其他直接放入嘴里的物体。

[3] 模式。

[4] 转导机制。

[5] 钠。

[6] 质膜离子通道。

[7] 去极化。

] 神经递质。

碳水化合物。

皮质。

觉皮质。

mately 5 cm^2 located in the roof of the nasal cavity[1]. The most important functional cell in the olfactory epithelium is the olfactory cell, a bipolar neuron. The cells are specialized afferent neurons that have a single enlarged dendrite[2] that extends to the surface of the epithelium. Several long, nonmotile cilia[3] extend out from the tip of the dendrite and lie along the surface of the olfactory epithelium where they are bathed in mucus[4]. The cilia contain the receptor proteins for olfactory stimuli[5]. The axons[6] of the neurons form the olfactory nerve, which is cranial nerve Ⅰ.

The odor[7] of a substance is directly related to its chemical structure. For an odorous substance to be detected, molecules of the substance must dissolve in the mucus that covers the epithelium and then bind to specific odorant receptors on the cilia. This kind of binding can induce the generate of the second messenger substance(such as cAMP). The Na^+ channels are opened, and Na^+ flow into the cells, resulting receptor potental, and trigger the action potential on the afferent nerves, ultimately exciting smell center.

Although there are many thousands of olfactory receptor cells, each contains one, or at most a few, of the 1000 or so different plasma membrane[8] odorant receptor types, each of which responds only to a specific chemically related group of odorant molecules. Each odorant has characteristic chemical groups that distinguish it from other odorants, and each of these groups activates a different plasma membrane odorant receptor type. Thus, the identity of a particular odorant is determined by the activation of a precise combination of plasma membrane receptors, each of which is contained in a distinct group of olfactory receptor cells.

---

[1] 鼻腔。

[2] 树突。

[3] 无运动纤毛。

[4] 鼻涕。

[5] 刺激物。

[6] 轴突。

[7] 气味。

[8] 质膜。

主要参考书目

1.G McGeown. *Physiology*. Beijing: Peking University Medical Press. 2007.

2. B.R. Mackenna, R. Callander. *Ilustrated Physiology*. Churchil Livingstone Press. 1997.

3. Arthur C. Guyton, John E. Hall. *Medical Physiology*. (13th ed.) Elsevier, Inc. Press.2016.